Practical Neonatology for MRCPCH and Beyond

MRCPCH

DEDICATION

To our respective children – Ben, Matt and Ben, and any yet to come – with love.

To all babies who need the care that we provide. May we continue to learn, and continue to teach, and continue to improve the care that you receive.

Commissioning Editor: Pauline Graham, Ellen Green
Development Editor: Carole McMurray, Hannah Kenner
Project Manager: Frances Affleck
Designer: Erik Bigland

Practical Neonatology for the MRCPCH and Beyond

Catherine Harrison   BMedSci BM BS DTM & H FRCPCH
Consultant in Neonatal Medicine, Leeds General Infirmary, Leeds Teaching Hospitals Trust, Leeds, UK

Alan Gibson   MBBS BSc PhD FRCP FRCPCH
Director of Neonatal Services, Sheffield Teaching Hospitals NHS Trust, Sheffield, UK

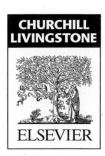

CHURCHILL
LIVINGSTONE

ELSEVIER

Edinburgh   London   New York   Oxford   Philadelphia   St Louis   Sydney   Toronto   2009

CHURCHILL LIVINGSTONE
ELSEVIER

First published 2009

ISBN: 978-0-443-07070-9

British Library Cataloguing in Publication Data
A catalogue record for this book is available from the British Library

Library of Congress Cataloging in Publication Data
A catalog record for this book is available from the Library of Congress

Notice
Knowledge and best practice in this field are constantly changing. As new research and experience broaden our knowledge, changes in practice, treatment and drug therapy may become necessary or appropriate. Readers are advised to check the most current information provided (i) on procedures featured or (ii) by the manufacturer of each product to be administered, to verify the recommended dose or formula, the method and duration of administration, and contraindications. It is the responsibility of the practitioner, relying on their own experience and knowledge of the patient, to make diagnoses, to determine dosages and the best treatment for each individual patient, and to take all appropriate safety precautions. To the fullest extent of the law, neither the Publisher nor the Authors assume any liability for any injury and/or damage to persons or property arising out or related to any use of the material contained in this book.

The Publisher

Printed in China

Contents

Preface   vii
Acknowledgements   ix

1. **Antenatal problems**   1
   Questions   1
   Answers   20

2. **Problems at birth and resuscitation**   69
   Questions   70
   Answers   80

3. **Common postnatal problems**   99
   Questions   99
   Answers   104

4. **Fluid and electrolytes**   117
   Questions   117
   Answers   125

5. **Problems with prematurity**   139
   Questions   139
   Answers   147

6. **Ventilation and blood gases**   163
   Questions   164
   Answers   179

7. **X-rays**   195
   Questions   195
   Answers   223

8. **Scans**   235
   Questions   235
   Answers   248

9. **Feeds and growth**   259
   Questions   260
   Answers   263

10. **Infection**   273
    Questions   273
    Answers   281

Index   297

Preface

Neonatology, to those who have come to practise it recently, appears a well established speciality, yet in truth it is very much in its infancy. It is sobering to think that it is only just over a century ago that obstetricians in France, horrified by high postnatal death rates, proposed that facilities should be established to provide care for the newborn infant. Prior to their intervention nobody did. Midwives briefly reviewed after birth and paediatricians did not take over the care until months or even years had elapsed. The newborn infant was regarded as a disposable and easily replaceable commodity. Attitudes have changed dramatically since then but it was not until 1975 that the American Board of Pediatrics established sub-board certification for neonatology, and local records in the United Kingdom showed little evidence of intensive care activity as we know it today for newborn infants on a widespread basis prior to 1980. Since that time the number of infants being born prematurely has steadily risen as has the proportion successfully resuscitated. As with many other success stories there is another side. Increased survival is associated with an increased proportion of children who develop long-term neurodevelopmental or behavioural problems. The final impact of this is still yet to be fully determined as the longest survival cohorts have only just entered adult life.

The development of neonatal intensive care has always, at least to some extent, been regarded as a temporary measure increasing the quality of care for premature and sick babies in the interim period before advances in obstetric practice reduce the incidence of preterm birth and the need for neonatal services. This hope has yet to be translated into reality and requirements for neonatal intensive care have continued to rise locally, nationally and internationally.

In a world of medicine where super-specialisation is becoming more prevalent and generalisation less, neonatology remains a field where a broad and multi-system knowledge base is essential. It is unlikely that single system or even single organ specialists will become a feature of neonatal units. This need for general neonatal knowledge is reflected in this book. We also hope that the systematic and step-by-step approach that is essential in dealing with neonatal problems is reflected. This is not a textbook – there are truly excellent examples of these already in existence – it is a book of problems for you to work your way through and to consider alternative management decisions. We have deliberately resisted the temptation to include large numbers of photographs and 'what is this typical of' type of questions. Fun as they may be it is rare that 'spot diagnosis' features strongly on a neonatal ward round. What does is the careful assembly of pieces of information to produce a tentative diagnosis and an initial action plan. What frequently then happens is for the plan, and often the diagnosis, to be modified on the basis of the response to that initial action. This we have tried to encapsulate in the format of the questions we have used. We are certain that others will challenge actions we propose and conclusions that we reach. We welcome this and hope that lively debate may be stimulated. We have both had the pleasure of working in many different neonatal units and of being involved in countless discussions with highly knowledgeable and experienced colleagues. We both know that there are different approaches that may be taken in dealing with the problems that we discuss. It is our experience and belief that the best practitioners are those who embrace such differences and work together to achieve best outcome. Those we trust least are those who know that there is 'the right way' and that no other exists.

We hope that you find this book informative and stimulating. We learnt much while writing it and hope that you may by reading it. We hope it will help you to join those of us who are aware that we do not know 'the right way', but are happy to be allowed to continue to explore the alternatives in the hope that individualised care will be the best we can offer at any specific moment in time.

Acknowledgements

Alan would like to thank Cath for being the driving force behind this project and Cath would like to thank Alan for his (occasional and always late) contributions. It is not easy to complete a manuscript of this length and remain good friends. We did and are grateful for it.

We would like to acknowledge the countless colleagues, past and present, who have taught us and inspired us and who we continue to learn from and learn with. Above all we would like to acknowledge the babies and the families we have cared for over many years – we have learned so much from you and been privileged to know you.

Chapter 1

Antenatal problems

A large proportion of the problems that a newborn baby may face do not just happen at the time of birth. Even if they do, there may well have been enough information available to suggest that those problems were possible or probable. They could have been caused by an abnormality that has been present during pregnancy and may well have been detectable by antenatal imaging, or there may have been information in the maternal history that clearly suggested that a problem was possible. Failing to prepare for a problem when there was a well recognised possibility that it could happen is an unacceptable standard of care and is most commonly due to poor communication. In any hospital where obstetric and neonatal services work together, there should be a robust system for notification of problems detected antenatally. Within this system there must be a mechanism for recording a management plan for the newborn infant and a means for ensuring that this information will be readily available at the time of birth, whenever that time may be. Reliance of a letter to be filed with the maternal notes is unlikely to be sufficient. When such a system exists it is interesting to note that possible problems may be reported in up to a third of all pregnancies.

In the cases that you will encounter in this chapter, you have been informed by obstetric or midwifery colleagues that a problem has been identified during a pregnancy. These problems range widely – from medications during pregnancy, through detected physical or anatomical problems, to significant family histories. In each case you are expected to decide what information you are going to give, so that the paediatric staff who will be on call at the time of delivery know what to expect, and the relevance of the problem with a plan of action for the postnatal period. If you think that the obstetricians or midwives could take some action which could help, include this in the plan.

All the cases below have been notified to the paediatricians in one of the hospitals in which the authors have worked.

QUESTIONS

1. A cystic lesion has been seen in the abdomen on the anomaly scan. It is thought that the most likely diagnosis is an ovarian cyst.
   a. What is the significance of this finding?
   b. What is the inheritance?
   c. What postnatal investigations should be performed?

2. This couple's last baby died at 5 days of age from a previously undiagnosed coarctation of the aorta. All antenatal scans, including a detailed cardiac scan, were normal.

a. Is the new baby at an increased risk?

b. Should an echocardiogram be performed?

c. The couple do not want to stay in hospital any longer than necessary due to the memories of their last baby. They would like an early scan and discharge at six hours. Will this be possible?

3. Frequent dropped beats were noted on antenatal scans.

   a. Is this of any significance?

   b. What action would you recommend in the early postnatal period?

4. The baby's mother had episodes of a supraventricular tachycardia that required treatment. She thinks that one of her mother's siblings also had a problem with the heart beating too fast.

   a. What further information would you want to elicit?

   b. Is the newborn baby at an increased risk of having a tachyarrhythmia?

   c. The parents are very anxious and would like their new baby to have an ECG. Is this likely to be helpful?

5. The very experienced ultrasonographer thinks that the fetus has dextrocardia.

   a. What further antenatal investigations would you suggest?

   b. Why?

   c. The parents would like to know the relevance of this finding.

   d. What postnatal investigations would you perform?

6. There is a family history of hypertrophic obstructive cardiomyopathy.

   a. What is the inheritance of this condition?

   b. What antenatal investigations would you recommend?

   c. What postnatal investigations would you recommend?

   d. The family history is of onset of symptoms in early childhood. Is this of any relevance?

7. Antenatal scan at 28 weeks detects a fetal heart rate of about 70 beats/minute that seems to show very little variation.

   a. What diagnosis do you suspect?

   b. What antenatal investigations would you suggest?

   c. What postnatal investigations would you recommend?

   d. The parents would like to know what treatment will be needed if the baby has a very slow heart rate after birth.

8. The fetus at 35 weeks has a very rapid heart rate (about 260 beats/minute) and has developed small pleural effusions and mild oedema.

   a. What is the likely diagnosis?

   b. What antenatal management would you recommend?

   c. What postnatal management would you suggest?

9. A previous child had a complex cardiac malformation that required palliative surgery in the postnatal period. Further palliative surgery has been required. The child is now 4 years old and awaiting a heart–lung transplant.

    a. Is a new baby at increased risk of having a cardiac abnormality?

    b. If the fetal echocardiogram does not show any defect can the parents be reassured?

    c. What postnatal action would you recommend?

10. Mother's brother had a baby with a ventricular septal defect.

    a. Is the new baby at an increased risk of having a heart defect?

    b. What postnatal management would you recommend?

11. The baby was noted to have a moderate increase in nuchal fold thickness. Amniocentesis was performed and karyotyping showed a balanced translocation between chromosomes 4 and 10.

    a. What is the relevance of the nuchal fold thickness?

    b. How is the infant likely to be affected by the balanced translocation?

12. Karyotyping was performed because of maternal age. This has been reported as showing a Turner mosaic.

    a. What significance is this to the infant?

    b. What postnatal management would you recommend?

13. Mother's screening tests have been reported as showing a 'high Down syndrome risk factor'. Antenatal scans have been normal. Karyotyping has been declined.

    a. What is the significance of this observation?

    b. What investigations should be performed? Should this include a postnatal karyotype?

14. Amniocentesis and chromosome analysis has been performed for reasons that are unclear. They have shown that the fetus has a 47 XXYY karyotype.

    a. What is this?

    b. What are the associations?

15. This mother has had a previous baby with trisomy 21.

    a. What is the likelihood of the next baby having the same trisomy?

16. There is a family history of epidermolysis bullosa. Father and a previous child have both been affected.

    a. What are the chances of the baby being affected?

    b. What manifestations may be seen in the early postnatal period?

    c. What investigations should be performed and treatment started in the newborn period?

17. There is a family history of incontinentia pigmenti.

    a. What is the inheritance?

    b. What is the likely outcome for the baby?

    c. What investigations should you perform postnatally?

18. A previous child was noted to have a birth mark on the left leg that steadily increased in size over the first two months after birth. At its largest it extended from the upper thigh to the middle of the lower leg. Over the first year the baby had problems with low platelets and needed platelet transfusions on two occasions. The child is now 2 years old and the mark is still present but fading. The mother is pregnant again and would like to know about possible problems for her new baby.

 a. What is the most likely diagnosis in the previous child?
 b. What is the likelihood of this baby being affected?
 c. What investigations are indicated following delivery of the new baby?
 d. Is there any need to treat this condition should it develop?
 e. Are there any treatments that can be used for the management of this condition?

19. Mother has gestational pemphigoid.
 a. Are there any risks to the fetus?
 b. Are there any risks to the baby once born and is there any treatment?

20. There is a family history of mastocytosis.
 a. What is the inheritance?
 b. Is it likely to present at birth?
 c. What are the usual features of this condition?
 d. How is it diagnosed?

21. Mother is known to be consuming an excessive amount of alcohol during pregnancy. Estimated intake is approximately 10 units each day.
 a. Is the fetus at any risk?
 b. What are the classical features of fetal alcohol syndrome?
 c. Mother has been informed that if her baby shows no dysmorphic features then other effects of fetal alcohol exposure are unlikely. Is this correct?

22. Mother has been on a drug withdrawal programme and has successfully weaned off heroin and has been on methadone, 60 mL daily, for the last 6 weeks.
 a. What further antenatal management would you recommend?
 b. What postnatal management would you recommend?

23. A mother is known to be taking heroin, cocaine, crack cocaine, temazepam, diazepam and methadone. She has not been engaging with the specialist substance abuse midwife or with any other health care professionals. Mother wants a six hour discharge.
 a. Is this safe practice?
 b. What antenatal action would you take?

24. Mother was taking regular heroin (by smoking) and cannabis. She has never used drugs intravenously. She deliberately underwent a detox programme before becoming pregnant and has not taken any illicit substances throughout pregnancy. All urine toxicology screening has been negative.
 a. What postnatal management would you recommend?

25. A mother has been maintained on buprenorphine since before conception and throughout pregnancy. All urine tests for illicit substances have been negative.

    a. Is this drug safe in pregnancy?
    b. Mother wants to breast feed. Is this acceptable?

26. A mother is taking 50 mL of methadone daily. All tests for illicit substances have been negative. Serology for blood-borne viruses is negative. She wishes to breast feed.
    a. Is breast feeding appropriate?
    b. Will breast feeding prevent neonatal abstinence syndrome?

27. A mother has been known to consume alcohol excessively for several years. She has managed to stop drinking during pregnancy and she has been taking acamprosate to help her.
    a. What is acamprosate used for?
    b. Should it be used in pregnancy?
    c. Is it safe to use in a breast feeding woman?

28. A mother is taking amitryptyline for depression. She wishes to breast feed.
    a. Is this safe in pregnancy?
    b. Can she breast feed?

29. A mother is taking atenolol for hypertension. She wishes to know what problems the baby may have.
    a. Are there any risks for the newborn baby?
    b. Is it safe to breast feed?

30. A mother is taking azathioprine for a severe form of inflammatory arthritis. You are informed when the fetus is 10 weeks old. Mother would like to know what problems this might cause the baby and whether she can breast feed.
    a. Are there any risks to the fetus?
    b. Can mother breast feed?

31. Mother is applying betamethasone in relatively large amounts for severe eczema.
    a. Is there any risk to the fetus?
    b. Are any investigations indicated?

32. Mother has fits which are successfully controlled with carbamazepine. It would not be appropriate to stop or reduce this in pregnancy.
    a. Are there any risks to the fetus?
    b. Can mother breast feed?

33. Mother is taking carbimazole which successfully controls her hyperthyroidism. She wishes to breast feed.
    a. Can it have any effects on the fetus?
    b. Can mother breast feed?

34. Mother has been taking chlordiazepoxide during pregnancy.
    a. Is the newborn infant at any risk and if so when are problems likely to develop?
    b. Can mother breast feed?

35. Mother has been working abroad for much of pregnancy and has been taking chloroquine. She will go abroad again with her baby after about a month and intends to continue both chloroquine and breast feeding.

   a. Is this appropriate?

36. Mother has been taking ciclosporin for inflammatory bowel disease. She would like to breast feed.

   a. What is the risk to the fetus?
   b. Is it safe to breast feed?

37. Mother has been taking codeine for chronic back pain.

   a. Is opiate withdrawal possible for the infant?
   b. Are there any other possible side-effects?
   c. Can mother breast feed?

38. Mother has taken diazepam throughout pregnancy, probably in doses larger than prescribed. She wishes to breast feed.

   a. Is there any risk to the developing fetus?
   b. Is there any risk to the baby?
   c. Can the mother breast feed?

39. Mother has been receiving low-dose heparin (enoxaparin) throughout pregnancy because of a past history of deep vein thrombosis.

   a. Is there any risk to the fetus or newborn baby?
   b. If mother has to continue this treatment after delivery would it be safe to breast feed?

40. Mother has been receiving escitalopram during pregnancy. The consultant looking after her is adamant that she must remain on this medication.

   a. What would be your advice to the mother? Should she continue to take this medication during her pregnancy?
   b. Mother does not know whether to breast feed or not. What advice would you give?

41. Mother takes flecainide regularly.

   a. Are there any risks to the fetus and newborn child?
   b. Can she breast feed?

42. Mother takes furosemide regularly for hypertension.

   a. Is it safe to continue this during pregnancy?
   b. Will it be safe to breast feed?

43. Mother has been taking lamotrigine regularly for fits that have been difficult to control with other medications.

   a. Are there any risks to the fetus or newborn baby?

44. Mother received MMR vaccine at approximately seven weeks into the pregnancy. She did not know she was pregnant at the time.

a. Is there any risk to the baby?

b. Are there any investigations you would like to perform?

45. Mother has been taking morphine for regular pain relief. She wishes to breast feed.

    a. Are there any risks to the fetus?

    b. Are there any risks to the newborn infant?

    c. Is it alright to breast feed?

46. Mother has been taking naproxen throughout pregnancy for joint pains. She is now 34 weeks gestation.

    a. Can it have any effect on pregnancy?

    b. Can it have any effect on the fetus?

    c. Is it safe to breast feed?

47. Mother has been taking oxytetracycline for acne for several months. This has just been realised at 22 weeks gestation.

    a. Should it be continued?

48. This lady has been taking paroxetine for depression. It was prescribed six months before she knew she was pregnant and she is now in the second trimester.

    a. Are there any risks to the fetus?

    b. Are there any risks to the newborn child?

    c. Will it be alright to breast feed?

49. On phenytoin for seizures that have been difficult to control. Now 16 weeks pregnant.

    a. Is phenytoin safe in pregnancy?

    b. If not, should it be stopped?

    c. Is it safe to breast feed?

50. A pregnant woman has been taking prednisolone 10 mg daily for the last 3 years for the management of moderately severe rheumatoid arthritis.

    a. Does this represent a risk to the fetus and newborn child?

    b. What investigations would you perform in the newborn child?

51. Mother has Graves' disease and takes propylthiouracil to maintain euthyroid status.

    a. What is the risk to the infant?

    b. What investigations, if any, would you recommend?

52. Taking sodium valproate for control of her epilepsy. Has been stable on this medication for several years.

    a. Is there any risk to the fetus and newborn baby?

    b. Is there any risk of bleeding in the newborn baby?

    c. Can mother breast feed?

53. Mother is a late booker and is taking warfarin. This was started after her last pregnancy when she had a pulmonary embolus and deep vein thrombosis. She is now 22 weeks gestation.

    a. Is there any risk to the fetus?

    b. Can mother breast feed while taking warfarin?

54. Mother has congenital adrenal hyperplasia. She has been stable on medication for many years.
    a. What medication is the mother likely to be on?
    b. Is the fetus likely to be affected?
    c. What are the risks to the fetus and newborn baby? How can this be reduced?
    d. What needs to be done after the baby is born?

55. The last baby was found to have congenital hypothyroidism on the neonatal blood spot test. She is now 3 years old and on maintenance thyroxine.
    a. What is the chance of the next baby being affected?
    b. What tests are required on this baby?

56. The last child, a boy, was found to have neonatal diabetes and has required insulin ever since. He is now 5 years old.
    a. What is the chance of this next baby being affected?
    b. Should this infant be screened?

57. Mother has diabetes and is insulin dependent. Control has been good throughout pregnancy and HbA1c has been within the normal range.
    a. What signs would you examine the baby for?
    b. What symptoms would you monitor for?

58. Antenatal ultrasound has shown a large cystic hygroma. It was seen on the first dating scan and has been present ever since. Now 22 weeks gestation.
    a. What antenatal investigations are required?
    b. What is your management at delivery?
    c. What postnatal investigations are required?
    d. What is the long-term outlook for the baby?

59. A large cleft lip and palate has been detected on the antenatal anomaly scan.
    a. What antenatal interventions are required?
    b. What is your management at delivery?
    c. Who should be involved in the care of the baby?

60. The baby's father and a previous child both had a cleft lip and palate.
    a. Is the next child likely to be affected?
    b. What is your management after birth?

61. Antenatal ultrasound detected an echogenic focus in the bowel at approximately 22 weeks gestation.
    a. What could the antenatal scan findings suggest?
    b. What is your management after delivery?
    c. What investigations are needed?

62. Antenatal scans raise the possibility of duodenal atresia.
    a. How would you manage the newborn baby?

63. Gastroschisis has been detected on antenatal scan.
  a. What is your management after birth?
  b. What is this associated with?

64. There is a family history of Hirschsprung's disease.
  a. What is the likelihood of the next infant being affected?
  b. What is your early postnatal management?

65. The stomach bubble has not been seen on any antenatal scans.
  a. What could the antenatal scan findings suggest?
  b. What is your early postnatal management?

66. A previous child had undescended testes that needed surgical fixation.
  a. What is the likelihood of the next infant being affected?
  b. What is your early postnatal management?
  c. What is the long-term outlook if this child is affected?

67. Bladder exstrophy has been seen on antenatal anomaly scan.
  a. What is your early postnatal management?
  b. What is the long-term outlook for this child?

68. The parents' last child developed acute lymphoblastic leukaemia at 4 years of age. He is currently in remission following chemotherapy.
  a. What is the likelihood of the next infant being affected?
  b. What is your early postnatal management?

69. Mother has anti-Fy^a (Duffy) antibodies.
  a. What problems might the baby have?
  b. What is your early postnatal management?

70. Mother has factor V Leiden deficiency.
  a. What problems might the baby have?
  b. What is your early postnatal management?
  c. What investigations should you carry out and when?

71. This mother is known to be a carrier of factor VIII deficiency. The fetus is thought to be male following a detailed antenatal ultrasound.
  a. What investigations could be carried out?
  b. What advice should be given to the mother about the perinatal period?
  c. What is your early postnatal management?
  d. What follow-up is needed?

72. There is a strong family history of glucose-6-phosphatase dehydrogenase deficiency.
  a. What is your early postnatal management?
  b. What should be avoided?
  c. What follow-up is needed?

73. Mother has Henoch–Schönlein purpura.

   a. What symptoms/signs is the mother likely to have?
   b. Is the infant likely to be affected?
   c. What action is needed after birth?

74. Mother has anti-K (Kell) antibodies.
   a. What may this cause in the infant?
   b. What is your early postnatal management?

75. Mother was found to be polycythaemic on her booking bloods. She has had no problems throughout life. She has been referred for a specialist opinion.
   a. Is the infant likely to be affected?
   b. What is your early postnatal management?

76. There is a family history of protein C deficiency.
   a. Is the infant likely to be affected?
   b. What is your early postnatal management?

77. This lady is 34 weeks pregnant. She is known to have rhesus antibodies and her fetus has been affected. Three in-utero transfusions have been given.
   a. The obstetricians want to deliver now. What information would you need to decide whether this is appropriate?
   b. What problems are likely in the postnatal period?
   c. Outline your early postnatal management.
   d. What follow-up would you arrange?

78. Mother has idiopathic thrombocytopenic purpura. She is currently 32 weeks pregnant and her platelet count is $48 \times 10^6/mm^{30}$.
   a. Is the infant likely to be affected?
   b. What is your early postnatal management?

79. Both parents carry sickle haemoglobin trait.
   a. Is the infant likely to be affected?
   b. What is your early postnatal management?

80. Mother has hereditary spherocytosis.
   a. Is the infant likely to be affected?
   b. What signs and symptoms do you need to watch for?
   c. What is your early postnatal management?
   d. What follow-up is indicated?

81. Mother has von Willebrand disease.
   a. Is the infant likely to be affected?
   b. What is your early postnatal management?

82. Mother had hearing difficulties diagnosed when she was 18 months old. She has bilateral hearing aids. She thinks that her mother also was found to be deaf at an early age.
   a. Is the infant likely to be affected?

b. What is your early postnatal management?

83. Mother has anti-Ro and anti-La antibodies.
    a. What is the mother's diagnosis?
    b. Is the infant likely to be affected?
    c. What other problems might this cause in an affected infant?
    d. What investigations should be carried out?

84. Mother has rheumatoid arthritis for which she is receiving treatment.
    a. What are the risks to the fetus and newborn infant?

85. A previous child was very unsettled in the first three months after birth. A diagnosis of cows' milk protein intolerance was made and he was kept on a soya-based milk until he weaned.
    a. Is the new infant likely to be affected?
    b. What is your management in the early postnatal period?

86. Mother has recently developed chicken pox and is due to deliver in the very near future.
    a. What further information do you need? Is the infant likely to be affected?
    b. What is your management in the early postnatal period?

87. Mother developed chicken pox during the first trimester.
    a. Is the infant likely to be affected?
    b. What is your management in the early postnatal period?
    c. What investigations are needed?

88. Mother has had chlamydia during pregnancy.
    a. What further information do you need to know about the mother?
    b. What investigations are needed?
    c. What follow-up is required?

89. Mother has had hepatitis B in the past.
    a. What further information do you need and how will this affect management?

90. Mother has hepatitis C. Viral titres are low during the mid trimester.
    a. Is the infant likely to be affected?
    b. Can the mother breast feed?
    c. What is the postnatal management of the baby and what investigations are needed?
    d. What follow-up is required?

91. A pregnant woman is known to have HIV.
    a. What is the chance of her infant being infected?
    b. What antenatal action would you take?

c. What action would you take in the immediate postnatal period?
d. What follow-up would you arrange?

92. Mother has had genital herpes in the past.
  a. How should the baby be delivered?
  b. What treatment does the baby need?

93. Mother had mumps at 18 weeks gestation.
  a. Is this likely to have any effect on the infant?

94. Is BCG required for babies born to the following:
  a. Family lives in East London.
  b. Father is Afro-Caribbean.
  c. Parents from the Czech Republic.
  d. Parents from Egypt.
  e. Parents from Lebanon.
  f. Parents from the Philippines.

95. There is a family history of albinism.
  a. Is the baby likely to be affected?
  b. How would it present?

96. Baby's father has alpha-1-antitrypsin deficiency.
  a. Is the infant likely to be affected?
  b. What investigations are needed?

97. Father has hereditary haemorrhagic telangiectasia.
  a. Is the baby likely to be affected?
  b. What clinical signs do you need to look for?
  c. What follow-up is required?

98. Father has Marfan's syndrome. He is known to have mitral valve prolapse.
  a. Is the baby likely to be affected?
  b. What clinical signs do you need to look for?
  c. What follow-up is required?

99. Mother developed renal failure in her teens and a diagnosis of familial juvenile nephronophthisis was made. A kidney transplant was performed in her early 20s but the transplanted organ was rejected. She is currently on haemodialysis three times weekly.
  a. Is the baby likely to be affected?
  b. What is the long-term outlook for an affected child?

100. Mother has neurofibromatosis.
  a. Is the baby likely to be affected?
  b. What clinical signs do you need to look for?
  c. What follow-up is required?

101. A previous child was noted to have an ocular abnormality diagnosed as Peter's anomaly. He was also noted to be small for his gestational age and had some mild dysmorphic features – hypertelorism, round face, long philtrum and mildly malformed ears.
  a. Is the baby likely to be affected?
  b. What is your management in the postnatal period?
  c. What follow-up is required?

102. There is a family history of Waardenburg's syndrome.
  a. How is this inherited?
  b. What are the clinical features?
  c. What are the associations?
  d. What investigations are needed?

103. A previous child has been diagnosed as having Walker–Warburg syndrome.
  a. How is this inherited?
  b. What is your management in the postnatal period?
  c. What investigations and follow-up are needed?

104. A previous child was found to have a Wilms tumour which was subsequently resected and chemotherapy and radiotherapy commenced. Recovery has been uneventful.
  a. Will the next child be affected?
  b. What are the associations?

105. A couple are expecting their first child. Mother's father and her brother both have galactosaemia.
  a. What is the chance of the new baby having galactosaemia?
  b. How may galactosaemia manifest in a newborn infant?
  c. What investigations would you perform in the immediate postnatal period?

106. There is a family history of hereditary hypophosphataemic rickets.
  a. What is the inheritance of this condition?
  b. What antenatal screening is possible?
  c. How does this condition present?
  d. What tests should be performed in the immediate postnatal period?

107. A couple are expecting their second baby. Their first child was found to have medium-chain acyl-CoA dehydrogenase deficiency on the routine neonatal blood spot test.
  a. What antenatal screening would you perform?
  b. What tests should be performed on the new infant in the immediate postnatal period?
  c. What would your management be while waiting for the test results?

108. A couple are expecting their third child. Their first baby had no problems but their second child died shortly after birth. A diagnosis of non-ketotic hyperglycinaemia was established.

a. Can this condition be diagnosed antenatally?

b. What would be your immediate postnatal management?

c. If diagnosed at birth and treated appropriately what is the long-term outlook for this condition?

109. A woman has a twin pregnancy which is found to be mono-chorionic and mono-amniotic. One of the twins dies in utero at 26 weeks gestation.

a. Are there are any risks for the surviving twin?

b. What management would you recommend for the rest of the pregnancy?

c. What investigations would you recommend in the postnatal period?

110. A couple are expecting their second baby. Their first child died at two months. The cause of death according to the death certificate was 'sudden unexpected death of infancy'.

a. What is the chance of the new baby also dying from sudden unexpected death?

b. What investigations would you perform in the immediate postnatal period?

c. What long-term follow-up would you suggest?

111. Antenatal scan suggests that a baby has situs inversus.

a. What further information would you like antenatally?

b. What are the possible associations of situs inversus?

c. Is there an inherited predisposition?

d. What investigations would you perform in the postnatal period?

112. There is a family history of agenesis of the corpus callosum.

a. What is the inheritance of this condition?

b. What postnatal investigations would you perform?

c. What is the long-term outlook for an affected child?

113. A couple are expecting their second baby. Their first child had an uneventful delivery but was later diagnosed as having cerebral palsy. No cause has been identified.

a. What is the likelihood of the new baby being affected?

b. The parents would like you to exclude the diagnosis of cerebral palsy at birth. What will you tell them?

c. What investigations will you perform in the immediate postnatal period?

114. A couple are expecting their first child. Small choroid plexus cysts have been seen on the 20 week anomaly scan. No other abnormalities have been detected and the fetus is growing normally.

a. What are the implications for the newborn child?

b. What investigations would you perform in the antenatal period?

c. What investigations would you perform in the immediate postnatal period?

115. A couple are contemplating having a second child. Their first child had spina bifida and hydrocephalus and is now severely handicapped.

a. What is the chance of another child being affected?

b. What investigations would you perform antenatally?

c. What investigations would you perform following delivery?

116. A couple are expecting their fifth child. The previous children are all healthy. On the 20 week anomaly scan the fetus appears to be microcephalic. The head circumference is well below the 3rd centile but on sequential scans the head does seem to be growing along a line parallel to it.

a. What is the likely outcome for this baby?

b. What further investigations would you consider?

117. A mother has myasthenia gravis.

a. What is the chance of the baby being affected?

b. What investigations will you perform on the newborn baby?

c. How will you manage the infant if affected?

118. There is a family history of myotonic dystrophy. Both mother and a previous sibling are affected.

a. What is the chance of this baby having myotonic dystrophy?

b. What is the genetic basis for this condition and what molecular factors influence the severity of the disease?

c. How may this manifest itself in the newborn period?

d. What investigations would you perform in the immediate postnatal period?

119. There has been a previous child with anencephaly. Mother has just found out that she is pregnant and is worried that this baby may also be anencephalic.

a. What is the chance of another baby being affected?

b. Are there any particular medications that a mother may take that could either decrease or increase the risk?

120. A couple have had a previous child with septo-optic dysplasia. Mother is pregnant again.

a. What are the key features of this condition?

b. What is the chance of the next infant being affected?

c. What investigations would you perform?

121. A couple have had a baby who was affected by West syndrome. They are contemplating a second pregnancy and would like some advice.

a. How might this condition manifest itself in the newborn period?

b. What is the chance of another baby being affected?

c. What antenatal and postnatal investigations would you consider?

122. A 23-year-old woman has aniridia. She is pregnant and would like to know the chances of her child being affected.

a. What is the inheritance of aniridia?

b. What tests would you perform?

c. What associations are there with this condition?

123. A mother and her previous baby were affected by congenital cataracts.
  a. What is the chance of another baby being affected?
  b. At the routine baby check bilateral red reflexes are clearly seen. Are any further investigations warranted?
  c. Are there any associations?

124. A young lady is pregnant for the first time. Her brother has keratoconus. Mother would like more information.
  a. What exactly is keratoconus?
  b. How is it inherited?
  c. What investigations will be performed?

125. A newborn baby is reviewed at two days of age. There is a family history of retinitis pigmentosa – mother and her father were both affected.
  a. What is the chance of this baby being affected?
  b. What are the likely manifestations in the newborn period?
  c. What investigations would you arrange?

126. A couple have had a previous child with a retinoblastoma. They are contemplating another pregnancy.
  a. What is the chance of another child being affected?
  b. What antenatal or postnatal investigation would you perform?

127. A 22-year-old lady had a dislocated hip at birth and needed to be in a harness for six months. No further treatment was needed and she has no significant ongoing problems. She is pregnant with her first baby.
  a. What is the incidence of developmental dysplasia of the hips and what proportion of cases have known risk factors?
  b. What is the chance this lady's baby being affected?
  c. Following delivery the routine baby check is performed and the hips are completely stable. Is it safe to discharge this child without further investigations?

128. A couple have had a child who had ectrodactyly of both hands and who has needed several operations on them. They are considering another pregnancy.
  a. Are there any associations with ectrodactyly?
  b. What is the chance of another infant being affected?
  c. What antenatal or postnatal investigations would you recommend?

129. A couple are expecting their first child. The husband is affected by a form of osteogenesis imperfecta. He had occasional fractures as an infant but there have been none since early childhood.
  a. What is the inheritance of this condition?
  b. What signs would you look for on the routine postnatal examination?
  c. What investigations would you perform?

130. A couple are having their first child and there is a family history of Perthes' disease. Antenatal scans have been normal.

a. What is the likelihood of their baby being affected by Perthes' disease?
b. Are any antenatal tests possible?
c. What investigations would you perform in the postnatal period?

131. A couple have had a previous child with talipes that required surgical correction.
a. What is the likelihood of their next child being affected?
b. Are there any antenatal tests that would be helpful?

132. A couple have had a previous child with congenital nephrotic syndrome (Finnish type). Mother is pregnant again.
a. What is the chance of this infant being affected by congenital nephrotic syndrome?
b. Can the condition be diagnosed antenatally?
c. What investigations would you perform in the postnatal period and what long-term management would you recommend for the baby?

133. A 25-year-old man has recently developed nephrotic syndrome. He is receiving treatment and is improving. His partner is pregnant and the couple are concerned that the unborn child may be affected by this condition.
a. What is the likelihood of the baby developing nephrotic syndrome in the immediate postnatal period?
b. Is there an increased risk of nephrotic syndrome later in life?

134. There is a family history of autosomal dominant polycystic kidney disease.
a. If the fetus is likely to be affected?
b. What is the likely outcome if a fetus is affected by ADPKD?
c. What investigations would you perform in the immediate postnatal period?
d. Is long-term follow-up indicated?

135. A fetus has been found to have a unilateral multicystic dysplastic kidney. This was very large at 20 weeks but was substantially smaller at 32 weeks. The other kidney appears to have shown some compensatory hypertrophy.
a. What would you anticipate to happen over the next weeks?
b. What investigations would you perform in the immediate postnatal period?
c. What investigations would you consider after the immediate postnatal period?
d. Is long-term follow-up indicated?

136. At the 20 week anomaly scan and on subsequent scans there is bilateral dilatation of the renal pelves to approximately 12 mm on the left and 14 mm on the right at 34 weeks. Remainder of the renal tract appears normal.
a. What additional step should be taken prior to delivery?
b. What would be your immediate postnatal management?
c. How would you manage the infant after the immediate postnatal period?

137. The 20 week anomaly scan showed bilateral dilation of the renal pelves. In subsequent scans the dilatation has increased and at 32 weeks there is also ureteric dilation and a thick walled bladder.

    a. Is there any action that should be taken prior to delivery?

    b. What would be your immediate postnatal management?

    c. How would you manage the child after the immediate postnatal period?

138. You are asked to see a couple who had a previous child who died shortly after birth due to pulmonary hypoplasia secondary to renal agenesis. Mother is pregnant again. The 20 week anomaly scan appears normal.

    a. What is the recurrence rate of renal agenesis?

    b. What urgent investigations would you perform in the immediate postnatal period?

139. There is a family history of vesico-ureteric reflux which has affected both the mother and a previous child. Both have had recurrent urinary tract infections and mother had some scarring on her right kidney.

    a. Is there any significant risk to the new baby?

    b. Are any investigations indicated in the postnatal period?

    c. Should the new baby receive prophylactic antibiotics?

    d. Is any follow-up needed?

140. A fetus is thought to have either a single pelvic kidney or a horseshoe kidney. There is no significant family history of renal disease.

    a. What is the incidence of these anomalies?

    b. Are there any associated problems?

    c. What is the inheritance?

    d. How would you manage this infant after birth?

141. On the 20 week anomaly scan a fetus has been seen to have a large cystic lesion which occupies most of the right thorax and seems to be pushing the heart over to the left. It is thought to be a congenital cystic lesion of the lung. The parents have been told that the baby may have severe respiratory distress in the early postnatal period.

    a. The parents would like to know whether termination of pregnancy is possible. What would be your advice?

    b. What may happen to this mass as the pregnancy progresses?

    c. How would you manage this baby in the postnatal period?

142. You are asked to see a couple where there is a family history of cystic fibrosis. Neither parent is affected but they have never been tested. This is their first child.

    a. What is the inheritance of this condition?

    b. What is the likelihood of the new child being affected?

    c. What investigations would you perform in the newborn period?

    d. How accurate is screening?

143. There has been a prenatal case conference. Minutes of the meeting are being circulated.

    a. What important actions must be taken before the delivery of the child?

144. Father has Goldenhaar syndrome.

    a. What are the features of this condition?

    b. What is the inheritance?

    c. What is the chance of the next infant being affected?

145. A couple have had a previous child who could not be resuscitated and died at birth. A diagnosis of Pena–Shokeir syndrome was made. Parents are first cousins.

    a. What are the features of Pena–Shokeir syndrome?

    b. What is the inheritance?

    c. What is the chance of the next infant being affected?

146. You are asked to see a couple who are expecting their first baby because there are members of the family with facial features of Treacher Collins syndrome. Neither parent has obvious facial features but father has had hearing aids since infancy.

    a. What is the inheritance?

    b. What is the chance of their unborn child being affected?

    c. What are the features of the syndrome?

147. You are asked to see a couple in antenatal clinic; they know that the fetus is female. Father has Tourette syndrome and has been told that he can pass it on to his child. No other family members are involved.

    a. What is the inheritance?

    b. What is the possibility of the next child being affected by Tourette syndrome and of needing treatment for it?

    c. Are there any specific investigations?

148. A previous child had biliary atresia and required a liver and small bowel transplant after a failed Kasai procedure. His mother is pregnant again and is worried that her next baby may also be affected.

    a. What is the chance of a second infant being affected by biliary atresia?

    b. What urgent postnatal investigations would you perform?

149. A fetus is thought to have vertebral abnormalities (hemivertebrae) on a detailed anomaly scan. There are also some concerns as to whether a stomach bubble has ever been seen. The heart is thought to be normal.

    a. What other abnormalities would you consider?

    b. What underlying diagnosis are you thinking of?

    c. What investigations would you perform in the immediate postnatal period?

150. A previous baby, a boy, who is currently under the care of his grandmother, was diagnosed as having schizencephaly at 4 years of age following investigation for a mild right-sided weakness. The child's mother is now pregnant again.

a. What are the implications of schizencephaly for a child?
b. What is the possibility of the next infant having the same condition?
c. What antenatal tests for schizencephaly can be performed?

ANSWERS

1. Fetal ovarian cysts.
  a. Almost all ovarian cysts are benign corpus luteal cysts that are derived from germinal or graafian tissues. They enlarge in response to maternal hormone levels and the majority resolve without treatment. Rarely large cysts may cause problems either through haemorrhage or torsion and it is therefore important that they are followed until resolution has occurred.
  b. The vast majority are sporadic. In rare cases they are associated with an inheritable syndrome in which case other anomalies are likely to be present.
  c. A postnatal scan should be arranged – if the cyst is still present follow-up and repeat scanning should be performed. If the cyst is no longer present and the infant remains well they should be discharged without follow-up.[1]

2. Previous baby with coarctation.
  a. Congenital heart disease occurs in about 8/1000 births. Of these approximately 6% are due to coarctation of the aorta giving an approximate incidence of 5/10,000 births.[2] For all left ventricular outflow tract obstructions familial clustering of cardiac defects has been demonstrated as have sibling recurrence rates of 2–9% and higher offspring recurrence rates of 7–13%.[3]
  b. An echocardiogram should be performed and should look for evidence of any defect, not just for the defect that occurred in the sibling.
  c. It would be inappropriate for the infant to be discharged early as an early scan could fail to detect a variety of different defects but would be particularly unlikely to demonstrate a coarctation. An early scan can be performed but should definitely be repeated 2–3 days later. In the region where the authors work the current recommendation from paediatric cardiologists is that in this situation a baby is not discharged until there has been echocardiographic demonstration of ductal closure and the baby remains well at this point in time.

3. Frequent dropped beats.
  a. The impression of a dropped beat is most commonly due to the pause following an extrasystole or an extrasystole that is so early in the cardiac cycle that the stroke volume is too small to be detected. In a study evaluating fetal arrhythmias 88% were due to extrasystoles and the vast majority were atrial in origin.[4] In a much smaller proportion of cases fetal dysrhythmias may reflect a significant abnormality that could have an adverse effect upon the fetus. In the study discussed above the next most common abnormalities were a supraventricular tachycardia occurring in 5% of cases, complete heart block in 2.8% and second-degree atrioventricular block occurring in less than 1%. In all of these, as with

the other potentially serious abnormalities, the presentation is most likely to be with a persisting rhythm abnormality and not with dropped beats.

b. The majority of extrasystoles resolve during pregnancy or in the first few days after birth although some children may have quite frequent, but completely harmless extrasystoles. It would be appropriate to listen to the heart rate of the newborn baby for a period of a few minutes. If no rhythm abnormalities are detected it would be reasonable to take no further action. If any irregularity is detected an ECG could be performed and further action would be decided on the basis of any abnormality that is seen.

4. Mother with a supraventricular tachycardia.

a. It would be helpful if the exact nature of the dysrhythmia could be determined.

b. There is no specific evidence for a familial tendency with SVTs with the exception of Wolff–Parkinson–White syndrome where occasional familial cases have been described.

c. An ECG would seem appropriate if it would help to allay any parental concerns. However, the resting ECG could be normal even if the infant did have Wolff–Parkinson–White syndrome.

5. Fetus thought to have dextrocardia.

a. Further detailed scanning, possibly by a cardiologist with expertise in fetal imaging, would be useful. Karyotyping could be indicated.

b. It is important to make sure that there genuinely is dextrocardia. A heart that is malpositioned on the right side may be due to a left-sided diaphragmatic hernia (dextrocardia is a not uncommon initial diagnosis of CDH). Further scanning should attempt to ascertain whether this is isolated dextrocardia, dextrocardia with situs inversus of the viscera, or dextrocardia with other anomalies. In the latter case dextrocardia could be one component of a syndrome and karyotyping could be indicated.

c. The majority of individuals with dextrocardia lead a normal life and have a normal life span. The presence of other anomalies may affect this and outlook will then be determined by the nature of the other defects rather than by the dextrocardia. Other anomalies are more likely if there is isolated dextrocardia and less likely if there is dextrocardia in association with situs inversus of the viscera.

d. Echocardiography is indicated to confirm the dextrocardia and to look for other cardiac anomalies. Further imaging or investigations may be needed if other problems are suspected.

6. Hypertrophic obstructive cardiomyopathy.

a. Autosomal dominant condition.

b. Fetal echocardiography may be performed as hypertrophic changes occur in utero in a small proportion of affected individuals. Stillbirth has been reported as a direct consequence of this condition.

c. Postnatal echocardiography can be performed but, as with antenatal scans, may be normal in an individual who has the defect. Although the peak occurrence is in the third decade it may present at any age.

d. If symptomatic in infancy the outcome is usually worse than if outcome is at a later age.

7. Fetal bradycardia.

    a. Complete heart block.

    b. Fetal echocardiography is essential. This will confirm the slow heart beat and may also allow detection of other cardiac defects which are commonly associated. Maternal anti-Ro antibodies should be measured as there is a strong association with complete heart block. Studies have reported an association with anti-Ro in up to 75% of cases with a structurally normal heart and complete heart block.[5]

    c. The infant will need careful examination following delivery and an ECG in the postnatal period. The infant should be carefully monitored as symptoms may develop. There is great variation in symptoms from none to very severe.

    d. Drug treatment is rarely effective and pacing is needed if the heart rate is very slow and the infant symptomatic. This is most likely to be indicated if the heart rate is consistently below 55 beats/minute.[5]

8. Fetus with a very fast heart rate, small pleural effusions and oedema.

    a. The infant has a supraventricular tachycardia and is developing hydrops fetalis.

    b. The fetus should be monitored at regular intervals to assess the progression of the effusions and the oedema and whether the tachycardia persists. Echocardiography should look for evidence of any associated cardiac anomalies. As there is evidence that hydrops is developing (effusions and oedema) attempts should be made to convert the rhythm back to sinus. Digoxin has been successfully used for many years but flecainide is now more widely used. No medication is without potential risk to both mother and infant and the risk/benefit ratio should be carefully evaluated. It is generally felt that the presence of hydrops justifies treatment, providing that the parents agree.

    c. The infant should be monitored in the early postnatal period with a formal ECG and echocardiography and other investigations if warranted. If still symptomatic then attempts should be made to treat the tachycardia with a Valsalva manoeuvre or cold applied to the face, with adenosine or with cardioversion if other methods fail. Long-term drug treatment may be needed and this should be initiated in conjunction with paediatric cardiologists.

9. Previous infant with complex cardiac anomaly.

    a. The infant is at an increased risk compared to an infant where there is no sibling history. While the incidence is approximately 0.8% in the general population it increases to 5% with one previously affected infant and 10% if there have been two.

    b. The sensitivity of fetal echocardiography has been reported to be between 60% and 95%. This is influenced by the gestational age at scan, the severity of the defect (more serious defects are more likely to be detected), the index of suspicion and the experience of the person performing the scan.[6]

c. Postnatal echocardiography should be performed, whether or not an anomaly was detected antenatally. If asymptomatic and the index of suspicion is low it is advisable to scan at 48–72 hours so that postnatal haemodynamic changes will have occurred, making detection increasingly possible.

10. Mother's brother had a baby with a VSD.

   a. Although the incidence of cardiac anomalies does appear elevated if there has been an affected sibling (see above) or if the parents have been affected (where the incidence in offspring increases to about 5%) this increased incidence does not apply outside first-degree relatives.

   b. Routine postnatal examination. Some advocate the use of routine pulse oximetry as another tool to detect congenital heart disease. It has been shown to be highly specific with very low false positive rates.[7]

11. Increased nuchal thickening; balanced translocation 5–10.

   a. Increased nuchal translucency has been associated with an increased incidence of both chromosomal and non-chromosomal fetal malformations in numerous publications. In infants with normal chromosomes if the nuchal thickness is greater than the 99th centile but below 4.5 mm at 10–14 weeks there is a 90% chance of a normal healthy baby. If between 4.5 mm and 6.4 mm this falls to around 80% and if above 6.4 mm to 45%.[8]

   b. Approximately 1 in 500 people carry a balanced translocation and no abnormality is present in that person because they still have a full chromosome complement. The likely outcome for a child of that carrier is difficult to predict and is influenced by a number of factors. If a familial translocation has been detected because an individual within that family had an unbalanced translocation, then the recurrence risk of having another child with an unbalanced translocation is 15%. If there has been no member with an unbalanced translocation the recurrence risk is 1–2%. In both cases the spontaneous miscarriage rate is in the order of 25%. A maternal carrier of a balanced translocation is more likely to have a child with an unbalanced translocation than is a paternal carrier.[9] Should an unbalanced translocation result the eventual outcome will be influenced by the amount of genetic material that is missing or in excess.

12. Turner mosaicism.

   a. A 'Turner mosaic' is not a discrete entity. Many different karyotypes fall under the category of 'mosaic'. Some of the most common mosaic karyotypes are 45,X/46,XX and 45,X/46,XY. Generally speaking, individuals with 45,X/46,XX mosaicism have fewer and less severe symptoms of Turner syndrome compared to individuals with 45,X karyotypes. The percentage of 45,X and 46,XX cells in various organs such as the heart, brain or kidneys cannot be determined and it is therefore not possible to predict the severity of Turner syndrome for a mosaic individual. The majority of people who are a mosaic of XY cells and XO cells are externally normal males. Approximately 5% are female with Turner syndrome and approximately 5% are born with ambiguous genitalia. An XY/XO baby may have a streak ovary, a testis, or an ovatestis on either side. The majority of XY/XO babies born with normal male genitals also have normal testes, although they may have reduced fertility. Any XY/XO child may have any of the medical conditions that are more common among girls with Turner syndrome. Whether or not and how a child with a Turner mosaic is affected depends on the distribution of their cell lines during fetal development.[10]

b. The karyotype must be determined if it has not been already. Careful examination of the newborn infant should be performed. Follow-up should be arranged with geneticists and paediatric endocrinologists. For those with a karyotype that includes all or part of a Y chromosome, it is important to investigate the possibility of tumours that can develop in the ovaries.

13. High Down syndrome risk.

a. Different screening methods and times of screening are used in different places and different countries. All use maternal age combined with measurement of specific analytes in the blood that differ with the different screening regimes. Some may combine ultrasound measurements. The classic timing for the screen is the second trimester during which the triple test is performed measuring maternal serum alphafetoprotein, β-HCG and estriol. Some centres are now performing a first trimester screen in which measurements of maternal PAPP-A (pregnancy associated plasma protein A) and free β-HCG are combined with measurement of fetal nuchal thickness. Proponents claim comparable predictive accuracy to the second trimester screen. A screen gives a risk factor (e.g. 1 in 50) which is an approximate estimate of the risk of the baby having trisomy 21. However, all tests have a false positive predictive value and also have a predictive value – the proportion of infants with trisomy 21 that will be detected by an abnormal screen result. For the triple screen in the second trimester this is said to be 60–70%.

b. Although mother has declined an amniocentesis it would be reasonable, with her consent, to perform more detailed ultrasound examination to look for any associated features. When the baby is born it is appropriate to perform a postnatal examination. If there are no suspicions of abnormality no further investigations are indicated.

14. XXYY karyotype.

a. This is often referred to as Klinefelter variant although some feel that it is not appropriate to make this association. It is uncommon, affecting about 1 in 17,000 boys.

b. The following associations have been reported: frequent severe behavioural and psychiatric problems, psychomotor retardation, congenital heart disease, agenesis of the corpus callosum, testicular hypoplasia, undescended testicles, sterility, lower limb ulceration, renal hypouricaemia, acromegaloidism with normal GH, ADD, autistic spectrum, clinodactyly, scoliosis, tall stature, delayed sexual development, flat feet.

15. Mother has had a previous baby with trisomy 21.
    a. An empiric risk of 1–1.5% is quoted for the recurrence of any trisomy. For trisomy 21 this appears to be influenced by the age of the mother. If below 30 when she has the new baby the risk is increased 8-fold above the normal age-related risk, which equates to approximately 1%. If over 30 at the birth of the trisomy 21 infant there is no increase over the age-related risk.[11]

16. Epidermolysis bullosa.
    a. Epidermolysis bullosa is classified into three main groups: epidermolysis bullosa simplex (EBS), junctional epidermolysis bullosa (JEB) and dystrophic epidermolysis bullosa (DEB). Most EBS and DEB are dominantly inherited although recessive forms do exist. There is a recessively inherited form of DEB where metastatic squamous carcinoma is a common manifestation. JEB is normally recessive. As this family has an affected father and an affected child autosomal dominant inheritance is likely and a 50% chance of transmission would be expected. EBS is the most likely form as it accounts for about 92% of all cases.
    b. Epidermolysis bullosa usually presents in infancy and commonly shortly after birth. The skin is usually normal at birth but then shows evidence of blistering at points where the skin is rubbed – nappy contact points at the waist and upper thigh are commonly involved. In a few cases presentation may not be for many months or even years. The family are likely to know the type of EB that they have and how it presented and will have substantial knowledge of the condition.
    c. If no lesions develop there are no investigations to be performed or specific management that should be initiated. If lesions develop the baby should immediately be referred to a specialist in the management of EB.

17. Incontinentia pigmenti.
    a. X-linked dominant.
    b. Females are affected. Most males die in utero but if affected and survive they are likely to be more seriously affected. Most newborns with IP will have skin features at birth or develop discolored skin within the first two weeks after birth. Pigmentation involves the trunk and extremities, is slate-grey, blue or brown, and has an irregular marbled or wavy distribution. The discoloration fades with age. Neurological problems occur in 10–40% and include cerebral atrophy, the formation of small cysts in the central white matter of the brain, and the loss of neurons from the cerebellar cortex. About 20% of children with IP will have slow motor development, unilateral or bilateral muscle weakness, mental retardation, and seizures. Visual problems occur in about one-third of female patients and two-thirds of male patients and these include squint, cataracts and severe visual loss. Dental problems are also common, including missing or peg-shaped teeth.
    c. If the parents are unaffected there is no specific action as the risk is minimal. There are no specific tests that should be performed in the absence of any features. Skin changes are seen at or soon after birth and the diagnosis is normally made clinically.

18. Birth mark and thrombocytopenia.

    a. The combination of an extensive haemangioma/haemangio-endothe-lioma with thrombocytopenia is highly suggestive of Kasabach–Meritt syndrome.

    b. The aetiology of this condition is unknown. There does not appear to be a hereditary element.

    c. No specific investigations are indicated. The lesion may be present at birth (and may even be diagnosed by antenatal ultrasound) and grows rapidly in the first weeks or months after birth. There is no test or investigation that will reveal the potential for this condition in an infant who appears unaffected.

    d. Aggressive treatment of this condition is indicated if an infant becomes seriously symptomatic as there is a reported mortality rate of 10–37%.

    e. A number of different treatment modalities have been used in an attempt to reduce the size of the haemangioma/haemangio-endothelioma. Irradiation has now been discontinued because of a lack of success and the risk of later malignancy. Systemic corticosteroids have been widely used but with little clearly documented efficacy. Interferon has also been used, as have haematological agents such as aminocaproic acid, aspirin, cryoprecipitate, pentoxifylline and dipyridamole, but again with little clear evidence of benefit. Resolution following the administration of vincristine has been described, and there is increasing interest in this treatment.[12]

19. Gestational pemphigoid.

    a. An increased risk of low birth weight and premature delivery has been reported.[13]

    b. A mortality rate in infants born to affected mothers of up to 30% has been reported – but this figure has been disputed.[14] Transient urticarial and vesicular lesions may occur due to transplacental antibody transfer in less than 5% of infants born to affected mothers. Treatment is with systemic steroids.

20. Mastocytosis.

    a. This is a rare condition which may be inherited although the exact pattern of inheritance is uncertain.

    b. It usually presents at 6–9 months although presentation at or soon after birth is recognised.

    c. Presents with macules, papules or orange to yellow nodules which change to wheals on rubbing. Found on any part of the body, most commonly the trunk, and usually become pigmented, and less likely to form a wheal, as the child grows older.

    d. Diagnosis is made clinically and by biopsy.

21. Fetus exposed to alcohol.

    a. Yes. There is no safe lower limit for alcohol exposure. A recent systematic review studied the effect of low–moderate levels of prenatal alcohol exposure and found no convincing evidence of adverse effects. The reviewers however found weaknesses in the evidence and thus could not conclude that drinking at these levels during pregnancy is safe.[15]

b. Classical features include growth retardation, an absent philtrum and a thin upper lip. There is an increased incidence of congenital heart disease, learning difficulties and behavioural problems.

c. No, this is not correct. Although the phrase 'fetal alcohol syndrome' implies the presence of dysmorphic features it is now well recognised that other problems may be present (and serious) in the absence of any dysmorphic features.

22. Mother on drug withdrawal programme, on methadone.

a. Antenatally it would be appropriate to check blood-borne virus status and to screen the urine, with consent, to make sure that she is only taking her prescribed medication.

b. Postnatally the baby should be monitored for signs of neonatal abstinence as well as sedation and respiratory depression. Different hospitals have different policies for doing this, but it is strongly recommended that the baby is kept with mother. The half-life of methadone is long (15–55 hours in an adult and significantly longer in a baby) and withdrawal may occur several days after birth. In the hospitals in which the authors work, the recommended monitoring period is for a minimum of 5 to 7 days. Due to the lifestyle of a substantial proportion of those who use illicit substances there is an increased risk of hepatitis B and TB and immunisation is recommended by many practitioners.

23. Substance misuse and non-engagement.

a. This baby is at high risk. Multiple substance usage, non-engagement with professionals, late booking and an expressed desire to get away from professionals as quickly as possible are all risk factors that should warn of potentially serious child protection issues.

b. A multi-agency child protection meeting must be set up as quickly as possible. A plan must be in place before the delivery and the staff who will be present at birth need to have clear guidance on what to do, particularly if early discharge is attempted.

24. Past substance misuse – successful detoxification.

a. None. A support pathway should be available should this mother need it and she should be made aware that there is easy access to it. No additional care is needed for the mother or baby. Blood-borne virus status should be known and if abnormal then appropriate treatment should be initiated.

25. Buprenorphine.

a. Buprenorphine is typical of many drugs in pregnancy. It is used while the manufacturer's datasheet says it should not be and there is little evidence of any sort. Although there are no human studies suggesting any adverse effects there are none confirming safety.

b. Buprenorphine does cross into breast milk in very low concentrations. It has a short elimination half-life but does bind to the opiate receptor for longer and thus delayed effects are theoretically possible. One study has suggested an association with reduced breast milk output and poor weight gain after extradural buprenorphine following a caesarean section.[16] This has not been duplicated by other studies. A more recent paper found in infants whose mothers had taken buprenorphine, a lower birth weight, 76% incidence of neonatal abstinence syndrome, and worryingly a high number of sudden infant deaths.[17] Prolonged use and breast feeding should probably be avoided but again information is limited.

26. Methadone and breast feeding.
   a. Methadone is transferred into breast milk, but in very low concentrations. In one study the relative infant dose was estimated to be 2.8% of the maternal dose.[18] It is generally accepted that this is not sufficient to present a risk to the breast-fed infant. The American Academy of Pediatrics has classified methadone as 'approved' for breast feeding women.
   b. The amount of methadone transferred into breast milk is not sufficient to prevent neonatal withdrawal, but there is some evidence to suggest that breast feeding may be associated with a reduction in both incidence and severity. In a study reporting the outcome of 190 babies born to mothers taking methadone, 85 of the babies received breast milk and 105 received formula. Treatment for narcotic abstinence syndrome was required in 53% of the breast-fed infants and 79% of those who were formula fed. Breast-fed infants required a shorter duration of treatment when it was needed. It is also of interest to note that those who were breast fed were less likely to be regarded as 'at risk' (31.8% v 68.6%) and less likely to be placed in foster care (9.4% v 29.5%). Although there were other confounding factors (such as that those who fed with formula milk were more likely to be polydrug users) multiple logistic regression analysis clearly showed that being predominantly breast fed was an independent protective factor.[19]

27. Acamprosate.
   a. Used to maintain abstinence from alcohol.
   b. It is contraindicated in pregnancy and breast feeding. Datasheet states: 'Although animal studies have not shown any evidence of fetotoxicity or teratogenicity, the safety of acamprosate has not been established in pregnant women. Acamprosate should not be administered to pregnant women.'
   c. Acamprosate is excreted in the milk of lactating animals. Safe use of acamprosate has not been demonstrated in lactating women. Acamprosate should not be administered to breast feeding women.

28. Amitriptyline.
   a. Amitriptyline is thought to be safe during pregnancy. Mild side effects for the mother include dry mouth, dilated pupils, and sedation. No documented risk for the fetus in utero.
   b. It is thought to be safe in breast feeding. It passes into breast milk in very low concentrations and produces extremely low or undetectable levels in the baby.

29. Atenolol.

   a. β-blockade is possible and the baby may be born with a bradycardia, low blood glucose and low blood pressure. This theoretical risk does not seem to be associated with actual reported adverse events. It would seem sensible to check the pulse rate over the first 48 hours. Some hospitals categorise these infants as having a risk factor for hypoglycaemia and thus have a protocol for monitoring feeding and if necessary blood glucose. There have been reports of intra-uterine growth retardation with atenolol.[20]

   b. One report has given details of a baby who developed hypotension, hypothermia and bradycardia which were attributed to maternal atenolol. This has not been reported in other studies. The American Academy of Pediatrics classifies atenolol as a drug with significant side effects that should be used with caution with breast feeding.

30. Azathioprine.

   a. Azathioprine does not appear to be teratogenic in humans although it is in rabbits. Immunosuppression of the newborn has been documented in isolated case reports as has intra-uterine growth retardation. The latter observation is difficult to interpret as azathioprine is likely to be used when mother has a chronic illness which may well have an effect on the developing fetus.

   b. There is evidence that 6-mercaptopurine (the metabolite of azathioprine) can be measured in breast milk. Concentrations are very low and there have been no documented side effects. There are, however, no recommendations with respect to breast feeding and caution in use is recommended.

31. Topical corticosteroids.

   a. From the manufacturer's datasheet: There is inadequate evidence of safety in human pregnancy. Topical administration of corticosteroids to pregnant animals can cause abnormalities of fetal development including cleft palate and intra-uterine growth retardation. There may therefore be a very small risk of such effects in the human fetus.

   b. It is thought that there may be significant absorption through the skin and there is a possibility of adrenal suppression. There is no consensus as to whether or not this is likely and what appropriate investigations might be. There are practitioners who feel that adrenal function should be assessed by measurement of three random cortisols over 24 hours four to five days after birth. There are others who do not think this is appropriate.

32. Carbamazepine.

   a. There is an increased risk of major and minor malformations including neural tube defects, dysmorphic features, congenital heart disease and many others. Defects appear more likely in combination therapy than with a single antiepileptic drug. The absolute teratogenic risk is uncertain but is definitely significantly raised.

   b. Carbamazepine does cross into breast milk at relatively low concentrations. Sedative effects are possible but concerns have not been reported. Use is regarded as being compatible with breast feeding.

33. Carbimazole.
   a. There is a possible association with aplasia cutis. Mild fetal hypothyroidism may occur and is usually short lived.
   b. Methimazole (the active metabolite of carbimazole) is excreted in breast milk but not in quantities thought to be sufficient to cause the suppression of thyroid function. Although it is unlikely that side effects may occur monitoring of thyroid function in the infant may be indicated.

34. Chlordiazepoxide.
   a. Readily crosses placenta in 1:1 ratio. Neonatal withdrawal consisting of severe tremulousness and irritability has been attributed to maternal chlordiazepoxide. Persisting hypotonia has been reported. Marked depression has been reported in infants within a few hours of delivery and onset of withdrawal on day 26 has also been reported.
   b. There are no reports on breast feeding but chlordiazepoxide is small enough to enter breast milk and have an adverse effect. There is the potential for drug accumulation and toxicity in nursing infants and use is therefore not recommended in breast feeding.

35. Chloroquine.
   a. This is the drug of choice for malaria in pregnancy. A teratogenic effect has not been demonstrated but a small effect cannot be excluded. Small amounts are excreted into breast milk but felt to be compatible with breast feeding.

36. Ciclosporin.
   a. No teratogenic effect has been seen in animals and there has been no evidence of increased risk in pregnancy in humans.
   b. Passes into milk in very low concentrations. No adverse effects have been documented but caution is recommended. Lactation guides give risk as 'moderately safe'.

37. Codeine.
   a. Codeine may be associated with sedation, respiratory depression and narcotic withdrawal. Neonatal apnoea has been reported. The baby should be observed for any signs of an effect.
   b. Codeine is metabolised to its active form morphine. This is dependent upon activity of the cytochrome P-450 oxidase system. There are individuals (approximately 1–2% of the population) who have two copies of the genes coding for this system and they may be ultra-fast metabolisers of codeine. There is a report of a breast feeding baby who died from morphine overdose following maternal consumption of codeine. Mother was an ultra-fast metaboliser.
   c. Low amounts are secreted in breast milk and this is dose-dependent. Sedation has been observed, as have rare cases of severe neonatal apnoea.

38. Diazepam.
   a. There is a possible association with cleft lip and palate and an increased incidence of inguinal hernia has been reported. There is said to be an increased risk of IUGR.

   b. When used close to the time of birth a 'floppy infant' syndrome has been described. Prolonged withdrawal in the form of increased irritability may occur. Both of these effects are dose related.[21]
   c. Diazepam may accumulate in breast milk. The effects are unknown but may be of concern. Parents should be advised to seek advice if there are any worries.

39. Enoxaparin.
   a. There is currently no evidence of fetotoxicity in animal studies and transplacental transfer is said to be minimal. This is not certain in humans.
   b. There is minimal transfer into milk but the manufacturer's data sheet recommends that mothers should be advised against breast feeding. There is no evidence to support this.

40. Escitalopram.
   a. At the time of writing, escitalopram is a relatively new drug and, as is commonly the case with new drugs, there is minimal information about safety in pregnancy or lactation. In this situation advice can be obtained from the datasheet which, in the absence of information, will almost certainly verge on the side of caution. For escitalopram the datasheet states: '…no clinical data are available regarding exposed pregnancies. In rat reproductive toxicity studies performed with escitalopram, embryo-fetotoxic effects, but no increased incidence of malformations, were observed. The risk for humans is unknown. Therefore, escitalopram should not be used during pregnancy unless clearly necessary and only after careful consideration of the risk/benefit.' It is not your role to give advice as to whether medication can be continued (it is used for anxiety disorders and as an antipsychotic). If there are any concerns mother should discuss these with the doctor who prescribed the medication. It may well be that this doctor felt that the risk/benefit ratio justified the use of this medication.
   b. The datasheet states: 'It is expected that escitalopram will be excreted into human milk. Breast feeding women should not be treated with escitalopram or breast feeding should be discontinued.' All that one can do is show this information to the parents and say that you do not have the information to let you give an informed opinion. If mother insists on breast feeding she must accept that this is her decision.

41. Flecainide.
   a. Safety is not proven although there are many case reports of flecainide use for intra-uterine SVT. Flecainide induced arrhythmias and cardiac arrest have been described,[22,23] as has postnatal conjugated hyperbilirubinaemia.[24]
   b. Concentrated in breast milk – breast milk to plasma ratio is about three. Adverse events have not been described and the American Academy of Pediatrics has classified flecainide as compatible with breast feeding.

42. Furosemide.

   a. There are no documented teratogenic effects. Furosemide does cross the placenta and causes fetal diuresis. Administration prior to delivery may lead to diuresis in the newborn infant and elevated urinary sodium and potassium excretion have been reported. Furosemide may alter postnatal plasma volume expansion but no significant impact has been documented.

   b. Furosemide is excreted into breast milk. No adverse effects have been documented. It is classified as compatible with breast feeding.

43. Lamotrigine.

   a. There are insufficient data on use in pregnancy. The datasheet has stated that no teratogenic effects have been documented and that it crosses into breast milk at 40–50% of plasma concentration. No adverse effects have been reported from this either. However, a manufacturer's bulletin in June 2006 stated that 'Emerging data from the North American Antiepileptic Drug Pregnancy Registry suggest an association between lamotrigine and an increased risk of non-syndromic clefts, the incidence being 8.9/1000 births against 0.37/1000 in the general population, relative risk 24; 95% CI 10.0–57.4. Should not be used in pregnancy unless potential benefits outweigh any possible risks.'

44. MMR.

   a. MMR vaccine is a live vaccine and should never be administered during pregnancy, especially early as congenital rubella is possible.

   b. The fetus should be monitored for any sign of anomalies and for normal growth. There should be a normal careful postnatal examination.

45. Morphine.

   a. No fetotoxic effects have been noted.

   b. May cause respiratory depression in the newborn infant – though little evidence that it does. Withdrawal is possible.

   c. No effects have been described from breast feeding. Classified as safe for use while breast feeding.

46. Naproxen.

   a. Naproxen is a prostaglandin synthesis inhibitor and thus has the potential to inhibit labour and prolong pregnancy.

   b. There is no recognised association with congenital defects. There is a potential for fetal toxicity by an effect on the ductus after 34–35 weeks. Use late in third trimester is therefore not recommended.

   c. Very small amounts are secreted into breast milk, but there is a long half-life and the potential for an effect on kidneys, heart, and gastrointestinal system – though problems have not been described. There has been one report of prolonged bleeding and anaemia in a 7-day-old infant.[25]

47. Oxytetracycline.

   a. This should not be taken in pregnancy. There are effects on fetal teeth and bones, maternal liver toxicity, congenital defects, and other miscellaneous effects. It should not be continued.

48. Paroxetine.
   a. No data on effects in human pregnancy – no described fetotoxic effects.
   b. A withdrawal state has been described, and direct toxicity has been proposed.
   c. Lactation appears to be safe in animal studies.

49. Phenytoin.
   a. Known teratogen with clearly defined syndrome associated. This condition has many features including broad nasal bridge, wide fontanelle, low-set hairline, broad alveolar ridge, short neck, ocular hypertelorism, microcephaly, cleft lip and palate, low set ears, epicanthic folds, coloboma, small or absent nails, altered palmar creases and dislocated hips. Features present vary widely between infants.
   b. As discussed earlier, it is not your decision to stop a maternal medication. However, there are safer alternatives and this may be worth discussing with her prescriber.
   c. Phenytoin crosses into breast milk in relatively small amounts and the effects upon the infant are thought to be minimal, providing maternal levels are in the low to normal range. No untoward effect has been observed in infants. The American Academy of Pediatrics considers phenytoin to be compatible with breast feeding.

50. Maternal prednisolone.
   a. Prednisolone and prednisone are widely thought to have little, if any, effect upon the developing fetus. There have been isolated reports of immunosuppression, congenital cataracts and multiple deformities but no firm association has ever been proven. Prednisolone and prednisone are regarded as being compatible with breast feeding.
   b. It is generally felt that in small doses most steroids are relatively safe during pregnancy and are certainly not contraindicated for breast feeding. There are some concerns when higher doses are used although the exact dose being regarded as 'high' is not clear. In one of the authors' practice adrenal suppression has been encountered in a baby whose mother had been receiving relatively low dose prednisolone. As a consequence all babies are screened on day three to four with three cortisols 12 hours apart. Two cortisols less than $100\,\mu mol/L$ are regarded as suggestive of adrenal suppression and babies are referred to the paediatric endocrinologists. Using these criteria a number of babies have been shown to have adrenal insufficiency and following further investigation have needed treatment for several months until intrinsic adrenal function has returned. These data have not been published and the general assumption is that prednisolone is relatively safe during pregnancy.

51. Maternal Graves' disease; taking propylthiouracil.
   a. It is possible that thyroid stimulating antibodies are present and have been transmitted to the fetus. Ideally the presence of such antibody should be established prior to delivery. If thyroid stimulating antibodies are transmitted to the fetus there is a risk of transient neonatal hyperthyroidism. The propylthiouracil will also be transferred across the placenta and can

suppress neonatal hyperthyroidism which will then become apparent after a delay as the PTU levels in the baby fall more rapidly than the thyroid stimulating antibodies. Infants may present with clinically serious hyperthyroidism a few days after birth and goitre may be apparent.

b. With this combination (maternal Graves' disease and taking propylthiouracil) it would be advisable to check formal thyroid function no earlier than day 3–4 and some would advocate screening at least one week after birth to avoid confusion by spurious results in the immediate postnatal period. If there is no thyroid stimulation from the Graves' disease there is a risk of transient hypothyroidism. There is thus a potential for a false positive result on the neonatal heel prick test where TSH is measured.

52. Sodium valproate.

a. Major and minor malformations are possible: IUGR, hyperbilirubinaemia, hepatotoxicity, fetal and/or neonatal distress. Absolute teratogenic risk 1–2%. Distinct dysmorphic syndrome possible.

b. Haemorrhage in the newborn has been shown to be related to the use of anticonvulsant drugs during pregnancy and occurs very early within the first 24 hours after birth, probably due to increased degradation of vitamin K. Their mothers, however, are rarely vitamin K deficient.[26]

c. Compatible with breast feeding.

53. Warfarin.

a. Fetal warfarin syndrome is well recognised – nasal hypoplasia, low birth weight, eye defects, developmental retardation, hearing loss, congenital heart disease, upper airway obstruction and more. The critical period appears to be the 6th to 9th weeks of gestation. Later exposure carries risk of CNS defects. It is also associated with increased rates of spontaneous abortion, stillbirth or neonatal death.

b. Warfarin consumption does not pose a significant risk to normal, full-term, breast-fed infants.

54. Congenital adrenal hyperplasia.

a. The mother is likely to be taking replacement mineralocorticoid in the form of fludrocortisone and replacement glucocorticoids in the form of prednisolone. The glucocorticoids provide a reliable substitute for cortisol, thereby reducing ACTH levels. Reducing ACTH also reduces the stimulus for continued hyperplasia and overproduction of androgens. The mother may also be on other medications to optimise growth, e.g. flutamide (antiandrogen) or testolactone (aromatase blocker) which reduces the conversion of testosterone to oestradiol and thus slows down bone maturation.

b. Congenital adrenal hyperplasia is autosomal recessive and therefore the infant has a one in four chance of being affected and a one in two chance of being a carrier.

c. The risk to the infant is being affected and thus the risk of being virilised. The aim is to detect CAH at the beginning of pregnancy and deliver an effective amount of glucocorticoid to the fetus, without causing maternal harm. Dexamethasone can cross the placenta to suppress fetal adrenal function. Adrenal glands of female fetuses with CAH begin producing excess testosterone by the 9th week of gestation. The most critical stages of virilisation (urogenital closure and phallic urethra) occur between 8 and 12 weeks. The current strategy is for mothers to take dexamethasone as soon as pregnancy is confirmed. Chorionic villus sampling should be done to determine the sex at 9–11 weeks gestation or by amniocentesis at approximately 15 weeks. If the fetus is a girl, further tests are carried out to see if the fetus carries the gene for 21-hydroxylase deficiency; dexamethasone should be carried on until the baby is born. If the fetus is male, the dexamethasone can be stopped. Dexamethasone decreases the virilisation in the fetus but may causes mild cushingoid effects in the mother.

   d. Careful examination after birth. If any doubt on examination discuss with endocrinologists, and take samples for 17-hydroxyprogesterone, electrolytes, cortisol and blood glucose.

55. Congenital hypothyroidism.
   a. If no other significant family history the chance of the next child being affected is very low.
   b. Discuss with mother whether to wait for the Guthrie or perform formal thyroid function, which will need to be done about day 4–5.

56. Neonatal diabetes.
   a. Transient and permanent neonatal diabetes mellitus are rare conditions occurring in 1 in 400,000–500,000 live births. In transient neonatal diabetes, growth-retarded infants develop diabetes in the first few weeks of life and go into remission by a few months. They can have a later relapse as permanent type 2 diabetes, often around the time of adolescence; 46% develop permanent diabetes in the neonatal period, 23% in childhood or adolescence and in 31% it resolves in the neonatal period.[27] In the permanent form, insulin secretory failure occurs in the late fetal or early postnatal period.[28] There is currently interest in the SUR1 gene.[29]
   b. Due to neonatal diabetes being an extremely rare condition, it does not seem appropriate to perform any sort of screening unless the baby is symptomatic.

57. Infant of a diabetic mother.
   a. Careful routine examination looking for macrosomia, hairy ears, sacral abnormalities, cardiac defects, evidence of polycythaemia and respiratory problems.
   b. Hypoglycaemia is the commonest problem to develop and blood glucose should be monitored during the early postnatal period. Although more common if macrosomic, absence of macrosomia does not exclude this. An echocardiogram might be warranted if any signs of cardiac problems.

58. Cystic hygroma.
   a. Imaging and chromosomal analysis with appropriate counselling is required. With the advent of, and more accessibility to, fetal MRI, a scan should be carried out if the cystic hygroma is in the neck. MRI can

delineate the mass and can also identify whether the fetal larynx and trachea are partially or completely compressed. A recent paper found chromosomal abnormalities in approximately 40% cases. The most common abnormality in non-septated cystic hygroma was trisomy 21 (25%) and in septated masses Turner syndrome (21%). Chromosomal abnormalities should therefore be looked for. A detailed antenatal scan should be carried out by a fetal medicine specialist to look for any other abnormalities, e.g. structural heart lesion, associated hydrops.[30]

b. Delivery should be attended by an experienced neonatologist. Approximately 75% occur in the neck, especially on the left, and can distort the anatomy. Large hygromas at birth may cause airway compromise, and thus an experienced team is needed at delivery to secure an airway.

c. The baby must be examined in detail after birth. Hygromas that develop early in pregnancy may well resolve by the time of birth either completely or partially or with some residual redundant skin. After a detailed clinical examination, ultrasound can be helpful to confirm the diagnosis, but MRI scans give more detail of the relationship of the mass to soft tissue, muscle and vascular structures.

d. The long-term outlook for the baby depends very much on the size of the mass and also any other abnormalities present. Surgical excision is the treatment of choice but this is frequently complicated by the size and the location of the mass causing severe respiratory obstruction. There are many complications with surgery including recurrence, infection, damage to vascular structures and nerves, and fistula formation.

59. Cleft lip and palate.

a. In the UK cleft lip and palate services are now regionalised. At the time of first diagnosis on the antenatal scans, the family should be referred to the nearest specialist team so that counselling may be performed and a discussion started about postnatal management, including the approximate schedule for surgical correction.

b. At delivery the infant should be treated as a normal infant. Immediately after delivery contact should be made with the team who will then provide appropriate follow-up. Advice on feeding is often needed with input from speech and language therapists and specialist nurses. There may be some respiratory problems and occasionally specialist respiratory intervention is needed.

c. Where designated teams are not available a local mechanism should exist for referral and support from all relevant specialists – surgeons, speech and language specialist, cleft lip and palate nurses, and appropriate paediatricians.

60. Cleft lip and palate.

a. There is an increased incidence of cleft lip and palate if there is a family history, with the incidence rising the more family members involved and the closer the relationship.

b. Defects are usually, but not always, detectable on anomaly scan. The baby should be examined carefully in the postnatal period with every attempt made to visualise the uvula to exclude a small posterior cleft.

61. Echogenic focus in bowel.
- **a.** Echogenic foci in the bowel can suggest several diagnoses including cystic fibrosis, intra-gut or intra-abdominal bleed, altered composition of meconium in the third trimester, trisomy 21 and other chromosomal abnormalities, intra-uterine growth retardation, fetal infection such as CMV and meconium peritonitis. The most common explanation is a normal variant at term.
- **b.** Examine after delivery. Observe for passage of meconium and watch closely for any evidence of obstruction or abnormal bowel action.
- **c.** If there are any clinical concerns, order abdominal X-ray/ultrasound and discuss with the on-call consultant.

62. Duodenal atresia.
- **a.** The baby should be observed closely in the postnatal period and an abdominal X-ray arranged as soon as possible after birth and before feeding. If the diagnosis is confirmed or the results equivocal, begin an intravenous infusion, leave a large bore nasogastric tube on free drainage in situ and discuss with paediatric surgeons.

63. Gastroschisis.
- **a.** Contact paediatric surgeons as soon as mother is admitted in labour or for induction. Immediately after birth the baby's abdomen should be wrapped with cling film or a similar material (moist sterile wraps or a plastic bowel bag), attempting to maintain bowel position in the midline. Intravenous access should be sought and the baby commenced on intravenous fluids. A large bore nasogastric tube should be passed and left on free drainage. Surgical review should be sought immediately after stabilisation.
- **b.** Gastroschisis is not usually associated with other defects (unlike exomphalos). The aetiology is thought to be vascular and a number of contributory factors have been proposed. These include young maternal age, low socioeconomic status, social instability, the use of aspirin, ibuprofen and pseudoephedrine during the first trimester, as well as alcohol, cigarette and recreational drug use.

64. Hirschsprung's disease.
- **a.** There is polygenic inheritance and variable expression. Males are more commonly affected than females. If there is a previously affected child, there is a 17% risk if the next child is a boy, and 13% if a girl.
- **b.** Keep baby under observation until bowels open regularly without any abdominal distension. If any concerns get an abdominal X-ray and discuss with paediatric surgeons.

65. Absence of a stomach bubble.
- **a.** Absence of a stomach bubble on antenatal scans can be associated with a left-sided diaphragmatic hernia, tracheo-oesophageal atresia or fistula or oesophageal atresia. Occasionally it can be due to neurological abnormalities that prevent swallowing. These conditions present with polyhydramnios. It can however be a normal variant.

b. Careful examination after birth and observe baby in the postnatal period. If any concerns pass a nasogastric tube.

66. Undescended testes.
  a. Undescended testes occur in 3% of term infants and 33% of preterm infants. It is more common for the right to be undescended. There does not appear to be any specific familial predisposition.
  b. Examine the infant carefully after birth.
  c. It is important to review these babies regularly as undescended testes are associated with development of hernias. It has normally resolved by 1 year of age at which point the prevalence is approximately 1%. Orchidopexy is usually carried out between 1 and 2 years to bring the testes down into the scrotum.

67. Bladder exstrophy.
  a. Bladder exstrophy is a rare condition and surgery is complicated. Management of this condition is normally only in a small number of supraregional centres and discussion with the nearest centre should have been started antenatally to make sure that an appropriate management pathway is decided. After birth the baby should be admitted to a neonatal unit and prophylactic antibiotics started. Treatment requires closure of the bladder and pubic ring within the first few days after birth. Following surgery is then in a staged approach to correct the epispadias and reconstruct the bladder neck.
  b. Children who are affected will require long-term follow-up, but after surgery the majority are socially continent.

68. Acute lymphoblastic leukaemia.
  a. There is no hereditary component and no reason to suppose that the next infant is more vulnerable than any other infant.
  b. A blood test at birth or at any other time without a clinical indication is really not indicated although could be considered if parental anxiety is extreme and would be reduced by doing this. The parents must be aware that an early blood test is of no value however and a normal result is of no prognostic value.

69. Duffy antibodies.
  a. The baby is at risk of haemolytic disease.
  b. Cord blood for FBC, SBR, direct Coombs test should be taken. Monitor the baby for jaundice.

70. Factor V Leiden.
  a. Factor V Leiden deficiency does not normally cause problems in early childhood.
  b. No routine investigations should be done at birth. It is an investigation that is carried out as part of a thrombophilia screen in neonatal stroke where there is growing evidence of an association in the pathogenesis of perinatal stroke, and in the risk of recurrence. The largest study to date suggests recurrence rate of 2–5% in infants where factor V Leiden deficiency is known.[31]

c. Current recommendations are to allow the child to make decision re testing in early teenage.

71. Haemophilia – factor VIII deficiency.

  a. Where the mother is known to be a haemophilia carrier, there should be antenatal discussion regarding testing of the baby to see if the fetus is affected. Tests are performed to establish whether the affected gene has been inherited and this may be done by direct mutation analysis, gene tracking techniques or a combination of the two in specialist laboratories. The outcome of this test then leads to further counselling regarding mode of delivery, delivery in specialist centre, and the need for treatment on the day of birth. In prenatally diagnosed infants, there is no evidence to suggest that elective caesarean section eliminates the risk of bleeding. Vaginal deliveries are thought to be safe, but vacuum extraction should be avoided as it is associated with a high rate of subgaleal bleeds.[32]

  b. Give oral (not intramuscular) vitamin K to all male infants born to haemophilia carriers (unless you can be certain that the infant is not affected). Intramuscular injections should be avoided in haemophiliacs. Furthermore, if the infant is a haemophiliac the parents should be informed that all vaccinations will need to be given subcutaneously or intradermally. Newborns with reduced FVIII/IX levels should have a head ultrasound scan on the day of birth and if any haemorrhagic abnormalities are seen, the case should be discussed with a paediatric haematology consultant on-call. All newborns with severe haemophilia will be offered treatment on the day of birth to cover birth trauma.

  c. In every case where a haemophilia carrier is delivering a male fetus, take a cord sample to assess the clotting. The sample should be taken into a tube with citrate anticoagulant, i.e. the one normally used for all the routine coagulation tests. Inform the local laboratory that the sample could be from a haemophiliac and you require a clotting screen and FVIII/IX level urgently. The sample will need to be processed on-call. After performing a local clotting screen, the sample will need to be sent to the appropriate centre for FVIII/IX estimation. The sample will be analysed on-call on arrival.

  d. The cord FVIII/IX should be known before the mother is discharged from hospital. If the FVIII/IX levels on the infant are normal (i.e. the infant is not a haemophiliac) no further action is necessary. If the levels are low (i.e. the infant is a haemophiliac) an appointment should be made with the local Haemophilia Centre who will see the family for advice and counselling.

72. Glucose-6-phosphate dehydrogenase deficiency.

  a. Take cord blood for G6PD levels, full blood count and reticulocytes. Remember G6PD levels may be falsely elevated and thus appear normal if the reticulocyte count is high. Make sure that blood is sent off and the laboratory is aware. The baby can have vitamin K and it can be given as normal. Although it is widely stated that vitamin K may cause problems in this condition there is no evidence-based support of this conclusion and there is evidence that it may be administered safely. In the USA the Council for Responsible Nutrition concludes that 'There is no known reason for concern about the usual supplemental forms of vitamin K for G6PD deficient persons'. The laboratory may need a second sample of blood for testing.[33]

b. Other drugs should be avoided until enzyme status is established, e.g. quinolones – ciprofloxacin, sulphonamides including co-trimoxazole and antimalarials.

c. Monitor the baby closely for jaundice but this may not present until day 3–5 after birth. If G6PD levels are abnormal discuss with paediatric hae-matologists immediately.[34]

73. Henoch–Schönlein purpura.

a. HSP is a systemic vasculitis characterised by prominent tissue deposition of IgA-containing immune complexes, especially in the skin and kidney. The mother is likely to have prominent cutaneous involvement similarly seen in mixed cryoglobulinaemia and hypersensitivity vasculitis; palpable petechiae or purpura is a major finding in these disorders. The pathogenesis is similar to that of IgA nephropathy, with similar histological findings in the kidney.

b. There is no apparent inherited predisposition.

c. No specific action is indicated after birth.

74. Kell antibodies.

a. Haemolytic disease of the newborn is possible. Although anti-Kell antibodies are less common than anti-D, they can cause severe fetal and neonatal anaemias. They cause haemolysis as well as inhibiting erythropoiesis.

b. Cord blood should be taken for haemoglobin, serum bilirubin, group and Coombs' test. The infant should be monitored for jaundice. Mother and baby should not be discharged until FBC and SBR results have been reported.

75. Maternal polycythaemia.

a. The infant is unlikely to be affected. The majority of the causes of poly-cythaemia are either secondary to another process or idiopathic. There are very rare congenital cases where there is an abnormality of the eryth-ropoietin receptor. Unless the family history is of congenital polycythae-mia there does not appear to be any specific intervention or investigation indicated.

b. It would be sensible to try and get more information about the nature of the condition in the family, but no specific tests are needed for the baby and no specialist treatment is indicated.

76. Protein C deficiency.

a. Protein C deficiency is a rare disorder occurring 1 in 160,000–360,000 births.[35] Babies will only be affected if they are homozygous or double heterozygotes for protein C deficiency. A clear family history should be taken to elucidate who is affected and to what extent.

b. Postnatal management should involve close observation for symptoms. Heterozygotes rarely present with symptoms in the neonatal period. Affected babies present within hours or days after birth with rapidly spreading bruising. Thrombosis in dermal vessels leads to life-threatening haemorrhagic necrosis, along with DIC. Thrombosis in renal and cerebral veins can also occur.

77. Rhesus disease.
  a. The presence of rhesus disease is not an indication for early delivery, nor necessarily is the presence of hydrops. If, however, there is evidence of fetal compromise that cannot be improved with fetal transfusion, delivery at this gestation may be appropriate.
  b. Haemolytic disease of the newborn is possible but may not be dramatic if there have been in-utero transfusions and the baby has little of its own red cells. If haemolysis is significant, severe and rapidly progressing jaundice may develop and there may be severe anaemia.
  c. Cord blood should be taken for haemoglobin, serum bilirubin, blood group and Coombs' test. The tests must be requested urgently and the results chased. Serial bilirubin measurements should be performed until a safe plateau or continuing decline has been reached. Prompt and effective phototherapy must be utilised and can avert the need for exchange transfusion. However, if exchange transfusion looks likely, appropriate steps must be taken so that an exchange can be performed as soon as indicated.
  d. Although jaundice will improve, haemolysis can continue and progressive anaemia develops. This can be quite rapid in onset and haemoglobin should be measured within one to two weeks of discharge so that the rate of decline can be assessed. Follow-up for several weeks may well be necessary.

78. Idiopathic thrombocytopenic purpura.
  a. There is no correlation between mum's platelet count and that of the baby. Severe neonatal thrombocytopenia is an infrequent complication of maternal autoimmune thrombocytopenia and is not reliably predicted by maternal characteristics.[36]
  b. Cord blood should be taken for platelet count. Even if normal, counts should be repeated on venous samples on the first two to three days.

79. Sickle cell disease.
  a. Sickle disease and sickle trait are possible.
  b. Haemoglobins will be measured on heel prick blood at time of routine heel prick testing – no specific action needed in early postnatal period.

80. Hereditary spherocytosis.
  a. Hereditary spherocytosis is the commonest red cell membrane disorder and is an autosomal dominant condition. However, 25% of cases are sporadic due to new mutations. The infant therefore has a 50% chance of being affected.
  b. The commonest presentation is an unconjugated hyperbilirubinaemia. Most infants do not become anaemic, but a small proportion will require transfusions.

c. Cord blood should be taken for Hb, FBC, SBR, and blood film to look for spherocytes.

d. These infants require haematological follow-up. They should also be monitored for jaundice and should receive folic acid supplementation for their first year of life.

81. von Willebrand disease.

a. There are several types of von Willebrand disease, which have different genetic inheritance and presentation. There are, however, only two that present in the neonatal period. Type 2b is autosomal dominant and causes thrombocytopenia but no bleeding. The autosomal recessive form, type 3, is the most severe form and presents like haemophilia.

b. The baby should receive oral rather than intramuscular vitamin K. There is no reason for paediatric presence at the delivery. Problems in the postnatal period are extremely uncommon and early postnatal diagnosis difficult. Send cord blood to coagulation for factor VIII assay.

82. Family history of hearing loss.

a. It is difficult to predict whether the infant will be affected as hearing loss can be due to many reasons. A detailed family history might reveal more information.

b. Hearing screen before discharge is needed with audiological follow-up.

83. La and Ro antibodies.

a. The mother is likely to have systemic lupus erythematosus. Pregnancy in these patients can be associated with a high risk of maternal disease exacerbation and adverse fetal outcome if the disease is unstable. Patients should be evaluated before pregnancy for pregestational risk factors and be closely followed during pregnancy.[37]

b. The risk to the baby is said to be about 2%.[38]

c. There is an association with fetal and neonatal heart block of varying degrees. The heart disease is thought to be permanent but there are reports of a transient effect.[39,40] It is also associated with skin lesions (transient) and thrombocytopenia. Examine the infant carefully in immediate postnatal period.

d. If there is any doubt, admit, monitor, perform ECG and echocardiogram. Check platelets.

84. Rheumatoid arthritis.

a. Rheumatoid arthritis does not present a specific risk to the infant. However, the mother may well be taking some medication that can pose a risk. For example, maternal prednisolone may cause adrenal suppression and azathioprine is associated with intra-uterine growth retardation and immunosuppression. Methotrexate is contraindicated.

85. Cows' milk allergy.

a. Milk allergy is the most common food allergy. It affects 2–3% of infants in developed countries, but approximately 85–90% of children lose clinical reactivity to milk once they pass 3 years of age. There is no reported familial predisposition.

b. There is no specific management in the postnatal period. Milk allergy is an immunologically mediated adverse reaction to one or more cows' milk proteins. The principal symptoms are gastrointestinal, dermatological and respiratory, which may manifest as skin rash, urticaria, wheezing, vomiting, diarrhoea, constipation and distress. The clinical spectrum extends to diverse disorders: anaphylactic reactions, atopic dermatitis, wheeze, infantile colic, gastroesophageal reflux (GER), oesophagitis, allergic colitis and constipation. The symptoms may occur within a few minutes after exposure in immediate reactions, or after hours (and in some cases after several days) in delayed reactions.

86. Recent chicken pox and will deliver soon.
  a. You need to know when mother was in contact, specifically the number of days pre-delivery. This will affect whether the infant needs to be treated or not.
  b. If mother developed the rash more than five days before giving birth immunoglobulins will have been transferred and outcome is good. If rash developed less than five days before birth or in the two weeks after delivery risk is markedly increased and zoster immunoglobulin should be given. If the baby is born within 7 days of the maternal presentation aciclovir is also recommended.

87. Mother had chicken pox in the first trimester.
  a. Congenital varicella syndrome can occur if maternal infection occurs in the first and second trimester. From the Green Top Guideline (September 2007) from the Royal College of Obstetricians and Gynaecologists: 'Pooled data from nine cohort studies detected 13 cases of FVS following 1423 cases of maternal chickenpox occurring before 20 weeks of gestation: an incidence of 0.91%. The risk appears to be lower in the first trimester (0.55%).'
  b. Routine postnatal examination is indicated. Congenital varicella is characterised by one or more of the following: skin scarring in a dermatomal distribution, eye defects (micro-ophthalmia, chorioretinitis and cataracts), hypoplasia of the limbs and neurological abnormalities (e.g. microcephaly, cortical atrophy).
  c. No specific investigations are indicated unless any abnormalities are picked up on routine examination.

88. Maternal chlamydia.
  a. You need to know if the mother has been treated. If she has been the baby is at minimal risk.
  b. If conjunctivitis develops send specific swabs for chlamydia and treat topically and systemically.
  c. Notify GP as symptoms often present late.

89. Mother has had hepatitis B in the past.
  a. Further information needed: do we know the e antigen and e antibody status?
    i. If e Ag +ve, the baby will need Hep B immunoglobulin and Hep B immunisation.

ii. If e Ab −ve will only need immunisation. Immunise as soon as possible after birth and at 1, 2 and 12 months. In some centres immunoglobulin may also be given in cases of acute hepatitis or particularly high viral loads and when e antigen and antibody status are negative.

90. Mother has hepatitis C.

    a. It is estimated that 1150 pregnancies annually in the UK involve a woman infected with HCV, leading to approximately 70 infected infants being born each year.[41] Vertical transmission is almost always confined to women who have detectable HCV RNA. Risk of transmission is increased by level of maternal HCV viraemia and maternal HIV co-infection.[42] Therefore this infant is at risk of being infected.

    b. Currently breast feeding appears appropriate providing mother is not HIV +ve.[43]

    c. Blood needs to be taken from baby at about 8 weeks for Hep C serology (Ab + PCR). Cord blood is unreliable due to contamination. Although there is agreement that testing should be delayed to at least 4 weeks of age, some recommend waiting until 3 months. A practical recommendation is to delay testing until at least 8 weeks, which could coincide with routine childhood immunisation.[44] If negative, repeat at 6–12 months. If positive, discuss with supraregional liver team.

    d. Follow-up is required in clinic. Repeat serology may be needed. Long-term outcome is thought to be satisfactory although long-term follow-up data are needed.

91. Maternal HIV.[45,46]

    a. The risk of transmission of HIV infection from an infected mother to her infant is around 25–30% without any medical intervention. This rate is increased further to around 45% if the infant is breast fed. With appropriate management transmission can be reduced to <1%. It is therefore clearly crucial that HIV infected women are identified in pregnancy.

    b. Antiretrovirals should be commenced during pregnancy if not started already. These may have a significant effect upon transmission to the fetus as well as an effect upon the mother. Mother's viral load should be determined throughout pregnancy as this will determine the nature of the treatment she receives as well as the medication that will be given to the newborn child.

    c. Appropriate antiretrovirals should be prescribed for the infant immediately after birth with the first dose being given within two hours. The exact nature of the medication to be prescribed will be determined by the maternal viral load, the medication mother is receiving and any evidence of viral resistance. For a low-risk infant zidovudine alone may be adequate but in a high-risk baby zidovudine, lamivudine and nevirapine may be indicated (or another combination of at least three antiretrovirals). Blood should be sent for HIV DNA PCR. Other investigations may be indicated according to local protocols. The infant should not be breast fed.

    d. Infants should have regular follow-up and regular serology should be performed. Current recommendations are that co-trimoxazole should be started at 6 weeks after birth. All medications are usually discontinued at around 3–4 months if serology remains negative and there are no other factors causing concern.

92. Mother had genital herpes.

a. Current recommendations are that the baby should be born by caesarean section if there is any evidence of active herpetic lesions. This can reduce the risk of herpes infection from around 50% down to 20%. There is no evidence to support routine section for asymptomatic carriers and vaginal delivery should be permitted.

b. The only babies who routinely need treatment are those born vaginally to mothers with overt genital herpes. These babies should receive intravenous aciclovir. Those with no evidence of infection need no screening or treatment.

93. Mother had mumps.

a. In infected experimental animals mumps virus has been shown to induce congenital malformations. No definite evidence for teratogenic potential has been shown in humans. There has been one controlled prospective trial.[47] This concluded that congenital malformation rate was the same in infected mothers as in those who were not affected. Endocardial fibroelastosis has been proposed as a complication[48] – there is no definitive evidence.

94. Tuberculosis and recommendations for BCG.

Current Health Protection Agency recommendations for the UK are that BCG should be given to:

1. All infants in areas within the United Kingdom where the incidence of tuberculosis is greater than 40 per 100,000 population per year.

2. Infants, wherever they live, with one or more parent or grandparent born in a country with a tuberculosis incidence of greater than 40 per 100,000.

3. Previously unvaccinated new immigrants from high incidence countries.

Up-to-date prevalence of TB can be found at http://www.globalhealthfacts.org.

a. Incidence is very high in areas of East London: by PCT – Newham >80; City and Hackney, Tower Hamlets 60–79.9; Redbridge, Waltham Forest, Haringey, Camden, Islington, Lambeth 40–59.9. Other regions currently <40.

b. Afro-Caribbean: rather non-specific – most African countries have a very high incidence; some Caribbean ones do not. Find out which country the person comes from.

c. Czech Republic 10/100,000 – no BCG required.

d. Egypt: 27/100,000 – no BCG required.

e. Lebanon 11/100,000 – no BCG required.

f. Philippines: 463/100,000 – BCG required.

95. Family history of albinism.

a. Most forms of albinism result from the inheritance of recessive alleles from both parents of an individual, though some rare forms are inherited from only one parent. Albinism usually occurs with equal frequency in both sexes. The only exception to this is ocular albinism which has an X-linked inheritance. There are other genetic mutations which are proven to be associated with albinism. About 1 in 17,000 human beings has some type of albinism, although up to 1 in 70 are carriers of albinism genes.

b. Albinism (hypomelanism or hypomelanosis) is a congenital hypopigmentary disorder, characterised by a lack of melanin pigment in the eyes, skin and hair, more rarely the eyes alone, and is known to affect mammals, fish, birds, reptiles and amphibians. There are several different types and subtypes of both oculocutaneous and ocular albinism. Affected individuals are generally as healthy as the rest of the population with growth and development occurring as normal, and albinism by itself does not cause mortality – though the lack of pigment is an elevated risk for skin cancer and other problems.

96. Baby's father has alpha-1-antitrypsin deficiency.
    a. Autosomal recessive condition so 1:4 chance of next child being affected.
    b. Do Pi typing and measure alpha-1-antitrypsin level.

97. Father has hereditary haemorrhagic telangiectasia.
    a. The infant has a 50% chance of being affected as it is an autosomal dominant condition. The most frequent form of hereditary haemorrhagic telangiectasia maps to the long arm of chromosome 9. There is evidence of genetic heterogeneity. Highly penetrant – 97% involvement by 40 years, 67% by 16 years.
    b. It is a vascular dysplasia leading to telangiectases and arteriovenous malformations of skin, mucosa and viscera (lung, liver and brain). Epistaxis and gastrointestinal bleeding are frequent complications of mucosal involvement.
    c. It is unlikely to be present at birth and this should be explained to the parents. Geneticist referral should be made.

98. Father has Marfan's syndrome.
    a. Marfan's is an autosomal dominant condition with very variable expression. The infant has a 50% chance of being affected.
    b. Clinical signs include arachnodactyly (but not always), tendency to tall, thin stature, and decreased upper to lower segment ratio. Features may not be clear at birth.
    c. Open appointment follow-up should be offered to the parents. There are local variations on timing and accessibility of screening echocardiogram.

99. Mother has familial juvenile nephronophthisis.
    a. Familial juvenile nephronophthisis (also called nephronophthisis 1 – NPH1) is inherited as an autosomal recessive trait. There is a 1 in 4 chance the infant may be affected. The gene for the NPH1 disease is on chromosome 2 in region 2q13 and is designated NPHP1. It codes for a protein called nephrocystin. About 70% of cases are caused by large deletions in the 2q13 region in both of the child's number 2 chromosomes. The deletions can be readily detected by PCR. For NPH2 the defect is in the inversin protein coded at 9q22-q31. For NPH3 the defect is at the nephrocystin 3 gene coded at 3q21-q32.

b. It was first described by Guido Fanconi and his colleagues in 1951. It is a childhood genetic kidney disease in which there is progressive symmetrical destruction of the kidneys involving both the tubules and glomeruli, characteristically resulting in anaemia, polyuria, polydipsia, decreased ability to concentrate urine, progressive renal failure and death with uraemia. Hypertension and proteinuria are conspicuous by their absence. The chronic kidney failure affects growth and leads to short stature. The median ages of onset of ESRD are 13 years in NPH1 (juvenile), 1–3 years for NPH2 (infantile), and 19 years for NPH3 (adolescent). End stage renal disease is inevitable. The age at death ranges from around 4 to 15 years without a renal transplant. Disease does not recur in transplanted kidneys.

100. Mother has neurofibromatosis.
  a. Neurofibromatosis is an autosomal dominant condition with very variable expression.
  b. Diagnostic criteria are frequently/usually not present at birth. Café-au-lait spots usually appear over first 1–2 years. Other features (Lisch nodules, freckling) appear over 5–10 years. Neurofibromas seen after 10 years.
  c. Follow-up for the first 1–2 years to detect signs. If affected, long-term multidisciplinary paediatric input is required.

101. Peter's anomaly.
  a. Peter's anomaly is a defect of the anterior chamber of the eye with a thinning of the posterior aspect of the cornea, iridocorneal adhesions and a central corneal opacity. It usually occurs as an isolated anomaly in otherwise normal individual. In association with prenatal onset growth deficiency, craniofacial anomalies (round face, prominent forehead, hypertelorism, long philtrum, cupid bow upper lip, small mildly malformed ears, micrognathia and others), short limbs, fifth finger clinodactyly and other problems (as described in the question), it become Peter's plus which is an autosomal recessive condition.
  b. Careful examination for above features.
  c. Refer for formal ophthalmological opinion.

102. Waardenburg syndrome.
  a. Autosomal recessive.
  b. Clinical features are a white forelock, depigmentation, sensorineural deafness, increased distance between inner canthi, heterochromia of the irides, synophrys and a high nasal bridge.
  c. It is associated with a cleft lip and palate, Hirschsprung's disease and congenital heart disease.
  d. Careful postnatal examination and consider an echocardiogram.

103. Previous child with Walker–Warburg syndrome.
  a. Walker–Warburg syndrome is a lethal autosomal recessive condition, with characteristic brain and eye malformations.
  b. Careful postnatal examination and cerebral USS.

c. OPD follow-up and a postnatal MRI to look for structural abnormalities such as lissencephaly and cerebellar abnormalities. There is a test available for mutations in the POMGn-T1 gene – discuss with genetics.

104. Previous child with Wilms tumour.

a. Approximately 2% of Wilms tumour patients have a family history, and even sporadic Wilms tumour is thought to have a strong genetic component to its aetiology. Familial Wilms tumour cases generally have an earlier age of onset and an increased frequency of bilateral disease, although there is variability among Wilms tumour families, with some families displaying later than average ages at diagnosis. One Wilms tumour gene, WT1 at 11p13, has been cloned, but only a minority of tumours carry detectable mutations at that locus, and it can be excluded as the predisposition gene in most WT families. It is thought that most cases of bilateral disease and 25% of unilateral have a genetic component. Understanding of the molecular genetics is continuing to evolve and there has been recent work to suggest that a significant number of otherwise unexplained cases may have evidence of inactivation of a previously unknown gene on the X-chromosome.[49]

b. When associated with aniridia, genital abnormalities and mental retardation there is a known association with a deletion at 11p13, 11p15. There is also an association with Beckwith–Weidemann syndrome.

105. Family history of galactosaemia.

a. The family history is on one side of the family and there is a possibility that the mother may be a carrier. The population incidence of this condition is approximately 1:60,000–80,000 and therefore the likelihood of the new baby being affected is very small.

b. There are two variants of the gene responsible for galactosaemia. One variant causes so-called classic galactosaemia, in which there is an extreme deficiency in galactose-1-phosphate uridyltransferase (GALT). The gene for GALT has been mapped at 9p13. In individuals with galactosaemia, GALT activity is severely diminished, leading to build up of toxic levels of galactose in the blood, resulting in hepatomegaly, renal failure, cataracts and brain damage. Without treatment, mortality in infants with galactosaemia is about 75%. The variant gene, responsible for Duarte galactosaemia, leads to about half the normal levels of GALT. Individuals with Duarte galactosaemia may experience few or none of the serious symptoms of classic galactosaemia. Presentation in infants with classical galactosaemia is normally towards the end of the first week of life with vomiting, failure to thrive and jaundice. Neurological symptoms are common and 30–40% may have concomitant septicaemia, particularly with *E. coli*. Cataracts may be present.

c. Cord blood should be sent for a galactosaemia screen and a heel prick sample should also be sent on the routine sample card on day 1. The diagnosis is confirmed by the measurement of subnormal levels of erythrocyte GALT.

106. Hereditary hypophosphataemic rickets.
  a. There are autosomal dominant, recessive and X-linked forms of this condition.
  b. No antenatal testing is available.
  c. Autosomal dominant hypophosphataemic rickets is characterised by isolated renal phosphate wasting, hypophosphataemia, and inappropriately normal 1,25-dihydroxyvitamin D3 (calcitriol) levels. Patients frequently present with bone pain, rickets and tooth abscesses. This form shows incomplete penetrance, variable age at onset (childhood to adult), and resolution of the phosphate-wasting defect in rare cases. X-linked hypophosphataemia is an X-linked dominant disorder characterised by growth retardation, rachitic and osteomalacic bone disease, hypophosphataemia, and renal defects in phosphate reabsorption and vitamin D metabolism. Hereditary hypophosphataemic rickets with hypercalciuria (HHRH) is an autosomal recessive form that is characterised by reduced renal phosphate reabsorption, hypophosphataemia and rickets. It can be distinguished from other forms of hypophosphataemia by increased serum levels of 1,25-dihydroxyvitamin D resulting in hypercalciuria.
  d. There may well be no abnormalities detectable in the newborn infant. If there are suspicions that this condition may be present there should be serial measurements of plasma calcium, phosphate and alkaline phosphatase, and urine phosphate excretion should be measured.

107. Medium-chain acyl-CoA dehydrogenase deficiency (MCAD).[50]
  a. This is technically possible by demonstrating a marked reduction in octanoate oxidation in cultured amniotic cells obtained via amniocentesis. Although antenatal screening is practically possible it is not routinely offered. Molecular genetic testing is available if the nature of the mutation is known.
  b. Where screening is available blood samples can be sent at 48–72 hours for tandem mass spectrometry. The sample can be sent on the routine heel prick card. Urine should also be sent off for organic acid analysis.
  c. Problems arise if the infant becomes unwell or is fasted; therefore any baby where this condition is suspected should be treated as if affected, with the implementation of three-hourly feeds and a change to intravenous dextrose if unwell or vomiting. Regular carnitine has been administered although evidence of benefit remains poor.

108. Non-ketotic hyperglycinaemia.[51]
  a. Prenatal testing is possible on CVS using enzymatic analysis of elements of the glycine-cleavage pathway. This is not routinely available and would need to be arranged if there were any concerns because of a pre-existing family history. DNA diagnosis may be performed in families where a specific mutation is known.
  b. If an infant is normal at birth there is debate as to whether investigations are warranted. Infants normally have a relatively short symptom-free period with 66% becoming symptomatic by 48 hours. Feeding normally deteriorates and as it does so the baby becomes lethargic and hypotonic.

Routine laboratory investigations are commonly unremarkable and the diagnosis is usually confirmed by a plasma/CSF glycine ratio of >0.08. A number of different therapeutic strategies have been adopted – as yet none have proved consistently effective. Reduction of glycine intake has no effect. NMDA antagonists such as strychnine, ketamine and dextromethorphan have been used but without evidence of long-term benefit. Sodium benzoate has been used as this may conjugate glycine and permit its excretion in the urine. Once again the long-term benefit is not established.

    c. The prognosis is extremely poor. The majority of infants die in the early postnatal period or within the first year. Those who survive usually have intractable seizures and profound mental retardation. A minority of affected infants develop symptoms either later in infancy (usually after a symptom-free first six months) and present with seizures and a variable degree of mental retardation. There is a very rare late-onset form in which presentation is in childhood with progressive spastic diplegia and optic atrophy. In these children intellectual function is normally preserved and there are no seizures. Five neonatal cases have been described where the infants present in an identical manner to normal neonatal NKH but symptoms resolve within 8 weeks.

109. Mono-chorionic twins – demise of one twin.

    a. Although intra-uterine demise of one twin is not an uncommon event, occurring in 21% of twin pregnancies, it usually has no effect upon the surviving fetus. However, the risk of neurological morbidity is significantly increased in a mono-chorionic twin pregnancy. In a series of 434 twin pregnancies where one twin had died, cerebral palsy was reported in 10.6% of surviving twins and other neurological injuries in 11.4%. In another series multicystic encephalomalacia was reported in 12% of surviving twins.[52,53]

    b. The risk of neurological morbidity is present from the moment of demise and there is thus debate about the optimal management following the death. There is no evidence to suggest that immediate delivery can protect the living twin. Close monitoring of the surviving fetus is recommended and many practitioners deliver the baby at 37 weeks.

    c. If antenatal monitoring revealed no evidence of any problems with the surviving twin the chances of this baby being affected are reduced but by no means eliminated. The infant should have neurodevelopmental follow-up for a significant period of time following delivery. Cranial ultrasound scanning during the postnatal period should be considered and further imaging determined by subsequent clinical progress.

110. Sudden infant death syndrome in previous child.

    a. Eight studies have reported on the incidence of sudden infant death in families where one child has already been affected. A relative risk of between 1.7 and 10.1 has been reported. These data have recently been reviewed and have been challenged.[54] The overall risk in the population is currently in the region of 1 in 3300 and if the most recent estimates of a six-fold increase in risk are used an approximate estimate of 1 in 600 would be obtained.

   b. In the absence of any family history or any known cause of the previous death no specific investigations are warranted.

   c. Advice should be given about any factors which it is thought may influence the incidence of sudden infant death in infancy such as smoking, the possibility of overlying and the correct sleeping position. In some areas specific follow-up is arranged for families where there has been a previous death from SIDS. This may involve more frequent input from health visitors, a general practitioner, a community paediatrician or some other form of support. If available the family would normally be referred for this form of ongoing surveillance.

111. Situs inversus.

   a. Further imaging should be performed to see whether this is situs inversus totalis (i.e. with dextrocardia) or situs inversus incompletus (i.e. with the heart remaining on the left side).

   b. In situs inversus totalis (occurring in 0.01% of the population) all major structures within the thorax and abdomen are affected, with all organs transposed. The heart is located on the right side of the thorax, the stomach and spleen on the right side of the abdomen and the liver and gall bladder on the left side. The left lung has three lobes and the right lung two, and other organs and vessels are also inverted (the aorta running to the right of the vertebral column and the inferior vena cava to the left, for example). Much less commonly (one in 22,000 cases) the heart remains in the normal left side of the thorax – situs inversus with levocardia or situs inversus incompletus. In this condition, as in dextrocardia without situs inversus, congenital defects are more likely than when situs inversus occurs with dextrocardia. There is a 5–10% prevalence of congenital heart disease in individuals with situs inversus totalis, most commonly transposition of the great vessels. The incidence of congenital heart disease is 95% in situs inversus with levocardia.[55]

   c. Situs inversus is generally an autosomal recessive genetic condition, although it can be X-linked.

   d. The infant should be examined in the immediate postnatal examination. An echocardiogram and abdominal ultrasound should be performed and a chest and abdominal X-ray may well be indicated.

112. Agenesis of the corpus callosum.

   a. This is a relatively common condition with an incidence reported at between 0.7% and 3.5% of all births with a higher incidence in males compare to females. The majority of cases are thought to be sporadic but recessive and X-linked forms have been described. It is also found in association with over 40 syndromes including Aicardi, Andemann, Shapiro, Acrocallosal, Menkes and septo-optic dysplasia. It also may be found in association with maternal nutritional deficiencies and infections, metabolic disorders and fetal alcohol syndrome.

b. A cranial ultrasound is indicated in the immediate postnatal period and may help delineate the abnormalities that are present. An MRI scan is the imaging procedure of choice as it permits a more detailed examination and an accurate diagnosis of agenesis of the corpus callosum and any associated anomalies. Associated abnormalities such as neuronal migration anomalies or atypical forms of holoprosencephaly may be subtle and difficult to image reliably on either CT or US.

c. The degree of impairment that may be associated with agenesis of the corpus callosum is directly related to the magnitude of the defect and any associated abnormalities. Agenesis may be partial, total or atypical and a wide range of other brain defects may be associated including schizencephaly, lissencephaly, pachygyria, Dandy–Walker cyst, hydrocephalus, porencephaly and holoprosencephaly. Some children with mild degrees of agenesis and no associated abnormalities are thought to have normal outcome while others with more severe problems may have major degrees of neurodevelopmental impairment.[56]

113. Previous child with cerebral palsy.

a. Inherited factors are thought to contribute about 2% of all cases of cerebral palsy in European populations. It is also thought that some de novo mutations and recessive disorders may be classified as non-genetic in origin. An increased incidence has been noted in consanguineous partnerships in comparison with those where the relationship is not consanguineous. In the absence of any history suggestive of an inherited pattern there is very little reason to suppose that a new child is more likely to be affected than any other baby without such a history.[57]

b. Routine postnatal examination should be performed unless there are any concerns expressed beforehand.

c. No investigations are indicated in this situation.

114. Choroid plexus cysts.

a. Choroid plexus cysts are a common finding occurring in upwards of 15% of normal pregnancies. In the absence of other abnormalities these cysts are almost certainly a normal variant. There is a weak association with trisomy 18 and trisomy 21. This association appears weaker as more studies report on the outcome of infants in whom these cysts are detected.[58]

b. An antenatal anomaly scan should be performed to make sure that the fetus is growing normally and that there are no other abnormalities visible. If there are no abnormal findings, no further investigations are warranted.

c. The routine postnatal examination should be performed. In the absence of other abnormalities no further investigations are warranted.

115. Previous child with spina bifida and hydrocephalus.

a. There is a genetic predisposition towards spina bifida. The incidence varies in different societies and has decreased significantly over recent years. Recent sources have quoted an incidence in the UK and USA in 2006/07 of approximately 1 in 1300 pregnancies. However if a parent or previous child has been affected the incidence increases to somewhere in the region of 1 in 25 to 1 in 40. If an aunt or uncle is affected the incidence is in the region of 1 in 50 and 1 in 200 if a cousin is affected.[59]

   b. Both spina bifida and hydrocephalus are normally relatively easily identified on antenatal ultrasound. An anomaly scan should therefore be performed at which point the defect should be seen. It may well be regarded as prudent to repeat an ultrasound later in pregnancy.

   c. If antenatal ultrasound is normal, specific investigations are not warranted. However, many parents will find a postnatal ultrasound examination reassuring. Spina bifida should be easily visible but making sure that the infant is examined while crying may help to exclude a spina bifida occulta.

116. Microcephaly.

   a. When severe, microcephaly is likely to be associated with significant neurodevelopmental problems. There is, however, overlap between the normal small head and the pathologically small head. A head that is growing along a centile that is below, but parallel, to the bottom centile line may be small but normal. It is often not possible to predict outcome with any certainty in cases such as this. However, if head growth is such that measurements progressively fall further away from the centiles, poor outcome becomes increasingly likely.

   b. On occasion moderate microcephaly may be a family trait and it is therefore advisable to measure the head circumferences of other family members. Other investigations that may be considered include amniocentesis or chorionic villous biopsy for karyotyping, detailed antenatal ultrasound to look for any other anomalies which may imply a syndromic origin and evidence of congenital infection involving particularly cytomegalovirus or rubella.

117. Myasthenia gravis.

   a. Myasthenia gravis is an autoimmune disorder where antibodies block the acetylcholine receptor at the neuromuscular junction. There should therefore be no specific risk of inheritance although more than one case in a family has been documented. The newborn infant may be affected if there has been transplacental transfer of maternal antibodies. This occurs in 10–15% of mothers with myasthenia and does not appear to be related to the severity of the maternal disease. Symptoms usually subside within 6–8 weeks. Rarely there are cases of a congenital myasthenia syndrome. This term is used to describe a heterogeneous group of hereditary disorders which are characterised by abnormalities of acetylcholine transmission at the neuromuscular junction. These conditions are rare and autosomal recessive inheritance has been proposed.[60]

   b. The need for investigations will be determined by the symptoms. If an infant is symptom-free, no investigations are warranted, irrespective of the severity of maternal disease. If symptoms are present an edrophonium test can be performed or neostigmine may be used. It is also possible to measure ACh receptor antibody levels in the baby.

c. Management of this condition will be determined by the severity of symptoms. If there is respiratory weakness that is compromising the ability to breathe, ventilation may be required. Virtually all cases respond to anticholinesterases and neostigmine is normally used for maintenance treatment.

118. Myotonic dystrophy.

a. Myotonic dystrophy has an autosomal dominant inheritance and therefore if one parent is affected there is a 50% chance of the offspring being affected.

b. Type 1 muscular dystrophy is due to a defect in the DMPK (myotonic dystrophy protein kinase) gene on the long arm of chromosome 19. There is a triplet repeat of cytosine–thymine–guanine in this disorder and the number of repeats is associated with the severity of the condition. In unaffected individuals there are between five and 37 repeats where those affected by this condition may have over 50 and as many as 2000 or more. In type 2 muscular dystrophy, which is normally a milder condition, there are defects in the ZNF9 gene on chromosome 21. The repeat expansion is larger in this condition, involving from 75 to over 11,000 repeats.

c. Infants may be completely unaffected by this condition and develop symptoms later. However, in some infants affected by type 1 myotonic dystrophy, there may be a congenital form of the condition characterised by profound hypotonia. The infant may need support with ventilation and there may be difficulty with sucking, swallowing and the clearance of secretions. There will be a paucity of movement and a lack of facial expression. Although respiratory problems usually improve with time it may be several weeks before this is apparent.

d. If the infant is symptom-free there is no specific indication for testing and, as the condition is untreatable, it is acceptable to await the development of symptoms before considering testing. If a child remains symptom-free, they can decide for themselves at a later age as to whether they want the test to be performed. For a baby who is symptomatic at birth, molecular testing for the number of triplet repeats should be performed.

119. Anencephaly.

a. The cause of anencephaly is unknown but in general neural tube defects do not follow direct patterns of heredity. Studies have shown that a woman who has had one child with a neural tube defect such as anencephaly has about a 3% of having another child with a neural tube defect.

b. This risk can be reduced to about 1% if the woman takes high dose (4 mg/day) folic acid before and during pregnancy. It is known that women taking certain medication for epilepsy and women with insulin dependent diabetes have a higher chance of having a child with a neural tube defect.

120. Septo-optic dysplasia.

a. Septo-optic dysplasia is a congenital malformation syndrome manifested by optic nerve hypoplasia, hypopituitarism, and absence of the septum pellucidum. In the most severe cases this may be associated with deficiencies of pituitary hormones, blindness and mental retardation. With less severe forms there may be milder degrees of each of these three problems and in some individuals only one or two are involved. Problems reported on cranial imaging include agenesis of the corpus callosum, schizencephaly, and lobar holoprosencephaly. The optic nerve hypoplasia is generally manifested in nystagmus which typically appears by 1–4 months, and a smaller-than-usual optic disc. The degree of pituitary deficiency ranges from normal function through deficiency of a single hormone, to deficiency of both anterior and posterior hormones. Hypopituitarism in this syndrome is most often manifested by growth hormone deficiency. The impact on brain development is variable and ranges from normal intelligence to severe mental retardation. Seizures sometimes occur. It is often difficult to accurately predict the degree of intellectual impairment.

b. The cause of septo-optic dysplasia is not known. Rare familial recurrence has been reported, suggesting at least one genetic form, but in most cases it is a sporadic birth defect of unknown cause and does not recur again with subsequent pregnancies.

c. Unless there is a significant familial history or there are obvious abnormalities at the time of birth there are no specific investigations warranted.

121. West syndrome.

a. West syndrome consists of the triad of epileptic spasms, hypsarrhythmia and psychomotor regression. Onset is nearly always within the first year of life, most commonly between three and seven months of age.

b. In the majority of cases (85–90%) a cause can be established. In the majority of the remainder no cause can be established but in a very small number of cases some form of inheritance appears. This most commonly affects boys, therefore suggesting X-linked inheritance.

c. In the absence of symptoms or signs no specific investigations are warranted.

122. Aniridia.

a. Most cases of aniridia are inherited as an autosomal dominant trait with almost complete penetrance but variable expression. It is due to a mutation of the PAX6 gene on chromosome 11p – one of a family of genes that codes for transcription factors that regulate expression of other genes during ocular development. It may be familial or sporadic, the latter being associated with a larger deletion.

b. The eye must be carefully examined and the iris clearly visualised. Defects are apparent. Nystagmus is usually present and there may be other defects including abnormalities in the cornea, the lens, the retina and the optic nerve. Should any abnormality be suspected a detailed ophthalmological review is essential.

c. Approximately 20% of individuals with sporadic aniridia developed a Wilms' tumour.

123. Congenital cataracts.[61]

a. The aetiology of cataracts is diverse and can be established in approximately half of those with bilateral cataracts and a smaller proportion with unilateral ones. More than 90% of unilateral, and 40% of bilateral cataracts, are idiopathic in origin. Some are hereditary and autosomal dominant; autosomal recessive and X-linked cases have also been reported. Other causes include metabolic (e.g. galactosaemia), congenital infections and in association with a number of syndromes. With this particular history a hereditary form seems likely.

b. Although an abnormal red reflex is to be anticipated if a cataract is present not all cataracts arc fully formed (or even partially in some cases) and an abnormal red reflex may not be seen. With a significant family history it is essential that a formal ophthalmological review is performed shortly after birth.

c. Other causes include metabolic (as in galactosaemia), congenital infections (rubella and toxoplasmosis) and in association with a number of syndromes including Soto, Hallermann–Strieff, Cockayne, myotonic dystrophy, and others.

124. Keratoconus.

a. Keratoconus is a corneal dystrophy with onset in teenage years. The name, literally translated, means cone shaped cornea. It is normally an isolated condition with no known associations.

b. One large cohort study suggested a familial rate of about 25% but the inheritance was unclear.[62] Genetic heterogeneity and the phenotypic diversity of keratoconus means that genetic analysis continues to be a complex process but some authorities maintain that predisposition to develop the condition is primarily inherited. A more recent paper estimated that keratoconus prevalence in first-degree relatives was approximately 3% which is up to 67 times higher than that in the general population.[63]

c. Keratoconus commonly presents around the time of puberty and the diagnosis is made by late teenage or early adulthood. In rare cases it may occur in later adult years or in childhood. Neonatal presentation has not been documented and no specific investigations or follow-up are warranted.

125. Retinitis pigmentosa.

a. Autosomal dominant, recessive and X-linked (both dominant and recessive) patterns of inheritance have been reported. In addition, retinitis pigmentosa may be a part of many different syndromes. In the latter case therefore inheritance will be determined by the inheritance of the syndrome.

b. Neonatal problems have not been reported. Visual impairment usually develops well into adult life although it has been reported in children.

c. A referral for an ophthalmological opinion is indicated. There are at least 35 different genes or loci known to be involved. Gene testing is available for a small number of these on a regular clinical basis, but not the majority.

126. Retinoblastoma.

a. Approximately 40% of cases are inherited. There is an autosomal dominant pattern with virtually total penetrance, but genetic counselling is made more difficult as in a significant proportion of cases there is evidence of genetic mosaicism of the gametes. Where a positive family history exists, there is a significant risk of inheritance but it is difficult to quantify exactly. If there is no history inheritance is unlikely.

   b. In a large population-based cohort study the mean age at diagnosis in patients with fundus screening was 4.9 months, with a range from one day to 48 months. This was substantially earlier than the mean age of 17.2 months in patients without fundus screening. It is therefore appropriate for children to be followed up with regular eye checks for the first four years but after that screening is no longer necessary. In families where there is a known gene mutation genetic screening may be possible but at present this is only so for a relatively small proportion of cases.[64]

127. Developmental dysplasia of the hip (DDH).

   a. Sonographic DDH incidence is quoted as from 55 to 69.5 per 1000 live births but only a small proportion of these remain abnormal and require treatment, indicating the incidence of true DDH as 5–6/1000.[65,66] A number of large population studies have been performed and have suggested that between 60% and 80% of infants with DDH have no identifiable risk factors.

   b. Family history is a well documented risk factor which has been quantified. Where there is one affected child there is a 6% risk, with one affected parent this rises to 12% and there is a 36% risk with one affected child and one affected parent.[67]

   c. In some reported studies as many as 70% of cases of DDH have not been detected by clinical examination.[68] Although sensitivity of the test is to some extent influenced by the experience of the examiner there are studies which have shown that even very experienced examiners can be unable to detect a dislocation even when they know it to be present. Most orthopaedic specialists agree that clinical examination does not reliably detect ultrasonographically defined developmental dysplasia of the hip in infants being screened for this disease, and in some centres in the UK, universal ultrasound screening is being carried out after birth.[69]

128. Ectrodactyly.

   a. Ectrodactyly is found in isolation or as part of a syndrome. In EEC syndrome, ectrodactyly is linked with ectodermal dysplasia and clefting. The commonest limb abnormality is a cleft of the hand or foot, although syndactyly and oligodactyly have been reported. Ectodermal dysplasia manifests with sparse, fair and dry hair, absent eyebrows and eyelashes, hypohidrosis (lack of sweat glands) and hyperkeratosis. The teeth will be small and may be partially formed. Nails are thin, brittle and ridged. Ectrodactyly has also been associated with tibial aplasia.

   b. If isolated there is no specific risk to this infant. If ectrodactyly is part of a syndrome then there is a possible inheritance. Both the syndromes above are inherited with an autosomal pattern.

   c. Severe ectrodactyly may be visible on antenatal ultrasound scan. In the absence of obvious features no specific investigations are indicated. If ectrodactyly is present, and EEC syndrome is suspected, a renal ultrasound scan should be performed as urogenital anomalies including megaureter, vesicoureteric reflux, hydronephrosis and hypospadias are reported.

129. Osteogenesis imperfecta (OI).
  a. Autosomal dominant and recessive forms have been described and there is therefore a significant chance of an affected child if a parent is affected.
  b. The baby should be examined in the immediate postnatal period looking for evidence of fractures. Blue sclerae are possible, particularly in type III OI.
  c. In the absence of any evidence of fractures, or anything else to suggest OI, there are no specific investigations that are warranted. There are no definitive biochemical tests and marked heterogeneity of the genetic mutations makes assessment difficult. If any bony lesions are suspected appropriate imaging is indicated. If the diagnosis is suspected the infant should be referred to a specialist centre.

130. Ischaemic necrosis of the femoral head.
  a. There is no clear pattern of causation of ischaemic necrosis of the femoral head. The incidence is reported as approximately 1 in 2000 and a 3% recurrence rate in siblings has been quoted. There are occasional reports of occurrence in twins. No clear pattern of inheritance is documented and the risks in this case are probably not much higher than in the general population.
  b. There are no antenatal tests.
  c. There are no postnatal tests.

131. Previous child with talipes.
  a. In a large population-based study of idiopathic congenital talipes equinovarus (CTEV) 194 cases were identified and pedigrees were obtained in 167. In one-quarter of these there was a family history of CTEV. In some families an autosomal dominant inheritance was suggested.[70]
  b. Significant talipes is usually visible on a careful antenatal ultrasound examination. As this is routinely performed it is appropriate to look for talipes but specific investigations are not indicated for a condition which is normally correctable.

132. Congenital nephrotic syndrome.
  a. Congenital nephrotic syndrome is an autosomal recessive condition and there is therefore a one in four chance of another infant being affected.
  b. Enlarged kidneys may be visible on antenatal ultrasound. The placenta is characteristically bulky. Amniotic fluid alpha-fetoprotein may be markedly elevated before 20 weeks gestation. Clinically evident oedema and ascites may be evident before delivery.
  c. The baby should have a detailed postnatal examination. Plasma and urine albumin should be measured. Other investigations will be determined by the level of suspicion. Although most infants show signs by the time of birth this is not always the case and later presentation (within the first three months) has been recorded. An apparently unaffected child does not necessarily warrant follow-up and parents should be aware of the

small chance of later onset symptoms and signs. A child who is thought to be affected should be transferred to a specialist nephrology unit where dialysis and transplantation are possible.

133. Family history of later onset nephrotic syndrome.
  a. Providing that the nephrotic syndrome was not congenital there is no specific risk to infant and no specific investigations are warranted.
  b. There are a few reported cases of familial nephrotic syndrome but these appear to be very rare and the risks to an infant if another family member has had idiopathic nephrotic syndrome appears extremely small.

134. Family history of autosomal dominant polycystic kidney disease.
  a. Although autosomal dominant polycystic kidney disease does not normally present with problems in infancy this is not always the case. There are documented cases of severe neonatal illness which is indistinguishable from autosomal recessive polycystic kidney disease. Asymptomatic renal cysts have been found and hypertension has been reported in infants with normal renal function.
  b. One study has reported outcome of 26 infants over a 25-year period where renal cystic disease was diagnosed prior to delivery or on day one of life. Nineteen of these children were asymptomatic at a mean of 5.5 years, five had hypertension at a mean of 8.5 years, two had proteinuria at a mean age of 9.7 years and two had chronic renal impairment at a mean age of 19 years.[71]
  c. A renal scan can be performed and would be expected to be normal but will detect abnormalities in the rare cases where present. Parents should be aware that a normal scan does not mean that cysts may not develop later.
  d. As the condition is autosomal dominant there is obviously a one in two chance that an infant will be affected if one parent is. It is therefore appropriate to continue to monitor an infant and child with approximately annual assessments for haematuria, hypertension or palpable abdominal masses. There are no specific recommendations as to the point at which to commence such checks.

135. Multicystic dysplastic kidney.
  a. The majority of multicystic dysplastic kidneys are asymptomatic and a large proportion show progressive involution which may commence antenatally in some cases. In a few cases expansion may occur and a large abdominal mass be present following delivery. This is a very rare phenomenon. In one study of 61 patients, associated urological anomalies were noted in 16 (26%). Complete involution occurred in 25 patients (41%) and partial regression in 18 (30%). The size of the multicystic dysplastic kidney increased in 1 patient (1.6%) and was unchanged in 17 (28%) without any pathological manifestations. Median age at complete involution was 2.1 years (range 36 days to 13.7 years).[72]
  b. An ultrasound scan should be performed at some point in the relatively early postnatal period to assess the size of the kidney and any evidence of ureteric or contralateral pelvicalyceal dilatation. In the past it has been

recommended that antibiotics are commenced but this is no longer the case.

   c. No specific investigations are warranted unless additional problems are detected. Some authorities recommend a routine MCUG but others suggest that it is deferred unless abnormal ultrasound features are present in the contralateral kidney or ureter.[73] Although vesico-ureteric reflux is a common association with reported incidence of 28–43%, any reflux affecting the contralateral upper tract is generally low-grade and self-limiting. In the study referred to above,[72] urinary tract infection developed in 6 patients, of whom 1 was ultimately found to have reflux and 1 had uretero-pelvic junction obstruction.

   d. For long-term follow-up, clinical review and infrequent ultrasound should be carried out. The primary care provider should monitor patients for hypertension, abdominal mass and urinary tract infection. Longer-term renal follow-up should continue in children with renal remnants and those with impaired GFR.[73]

136. Antenatally dilated renal pelves.

   a. Ultrasound scan should be repeated at intervals through the remainder of the pregnancy to assess progression of the dilatation.

   b. Most authorities are agreed that a postnatal ultrasound examination should be performed although the recommended interval between birth and the first scan varies widely. The urgency of investigation will be partly determined by the magnitude of the dilatation present in the scan performed closest to delivery.

   c. Although a significant proportion of dilated renal pelves resolve over time, a significant number do not and there is an association with other abnormalities, particularly vesico-ureteric reflux. The possibility of associated problems is related to the magnitude of the dilation. The need for longer-term follow-up will be determined by the appearances on postnatal ultrasound and any possible associations with other abnormalities.

137. Bilateral dilation of the renal pelves, ureteric dilatation and bladder wall thickening.

   a. Although antenatal drainage of unobstructed urinary tract has been performed there is currently no consistent body of evidence to suggest that this is of proven benefit.

   b. An urgent ultrasound should be performed shortly after birth and a MCUG should be considered. The infant should be monitored for urine output and bladder distension. If posterior urethral valves are suspected urgent referral should be made to a urologist for valve ablation.

   c. This will be determined by the abnormality detected. Posterior urethral valves will require surgical intervention and follow-up. If there is pelvicalyceal dilatation to a lesser degree, repeat ultrasound monitoring may be indicated with further investigations based on the degree of dilatation.

138. Renal agenesis in a previous child.

   a. The method of inheritance of renal agenesis is unknown but genetic factors do play a role in some cases. Concordance in twins has been reported, as has familial recurrence.[74] In a series of 199 cases, seven had siblings who were similarly affected.[75]

b. When there is a family history of renal agenesis or dysgenesis, parents and siblings should have a renal ultrasound. In one study of 71 parents and 40 siblings of 41 index patients with bilateral renal agenesis, bilateral severe dysgenesis or agenesis of one kidney and dysgenesis of the other, 10 of 111 (9%) had asymptomatic renal malformations (most often unilateral renal agenesis). This is significantly higher than the background frequency of 0.3% in 682 adults reported in the same paper.[76]

139. Family history of vesico-ureteric reflux.

a. There is a risk to the newborn baby. Vesico-ureteric reflux is usually familial and is inherited as a Mendelian dominant trait with partial expression. The gene frequency is approximately 1 in 600. Studies have suggested an incidence of approximately 35% if a previous child has been affected.

b. Ultrasound examination of the kidney should be performed to look for evidence of pelvicalyceal dilatation. At some point a micturating cystourethrogram should be performed. There is no consensus as to exactly when either investigation should be performed. Some practitioners recommend an ultrasound examination approximately two weeks after birth and a MCUG at three months. Others recommend a longer time interval.

c. There is again difference of opinion over this issue. There are review articles that categorically state that prophylactic antibiotics should be commenced at birth and others have stated antibiotics are only needed as cover during an MCUG.

d. Where there is a family history of vesico-ureteric reflux infants should be followed up until the diagnosis is established or excluded. This may be difficult as VUR can be intermittent and may not be detected by routine screening tests. Parents should be aware of the association with urinary tract infections and given advice as to what to do if there are any concerns.[77]

140. Single or horseshoe kidney.[78]

a. Unilateral renal agenesis is reported to have an incidence of between 3 per 1000 and 1 in 550. Horseshoe kidney has been reported with an incidence of between 1 in 400 and 1 in 1000.

b. Unilateral renal agenesis has a high incidence of renal and other anomalies of the urogenital tract including renal dysplasia, renal ectopia, vesico-ureteric reflux, pelvi-ureteric junction obstruction and other abnormalities of the Müllerian system. Horseshoe kidney is associated with other congenital genitourinary tract abnormalities in approximately 20% of cases and with other system anomalies in approximately 30%.

c. Both conditions are found with a high incidence in a number of syndromes, some of which are of unknown origin and some where there is a definite chromosomal abnormality. There are well documented familial cases but there is no clear inheritance pattern.

d. It would be appropriate to perform a renal ultrasound examination in the postnatal period. This should not be performed too early as reduced urine flow in the early postnatal period may make detection of some urinary tract abnormalities less likely. Further investigations may be indicated depending upon the result of the ultrasound examination.

141. Cystic abnormality within the fetal lung.

   a. It would not be your role to advise termination under any circumstance. It is your role to provide accurate information which will allow the parents to make a decision for themselves. In this case, the information is that it is not possible, at this stage in pregnancy, to say what the likely outcome will be. Termination on the basis of the appearance at 20 weeks may be very ill-advised.

   b. There is good evidence that many infants who appear to have large cystic lesions in their lungs early in pregnancy show considerable resolution before term and in some cases there may be no lesion visible at term. Occasionally some lesions may enlarge, particularly ones with large cysts.

   c. This will be determined by the baby's symptoms. A very small number of infants may require emergency or urgent surgery in the newborn period if the cystic abnormality is sufficiently large to be compressing the normal lung. However, the majority of infants are asymptomatic and no early intervention is required. All infants will need further investigations including computerised assisted tomography. The majority of authorities advise that even totally asymptomatic infants will require removal of the affected lobe at some point in the future for cystic adenomatoid malformations, intra-pulmonary sequestration and bronchogenic cysts. A few authorities suggest expectant management, particularly if the cystic abnormality was thought to be congenital lobar emphysema or extra-pulmonary sequestration.[79]

142. Family history of cystic fibrosis.

   a. Cystic fibrosis has an autosomal recessive inheritance.

   b. If the carrier status of the parents is not known it is not possible to predict the likely outcome for the new infant. It is always wise to elucidate the full family history and to discuss with parents whether they wish their carrier status to be determined in the antenatal period. In some areas it is offered as a routine to one parent and only if that parent is found to be positive for the gene defect will the other parent be tested. If neither are carriers the risk is very low.

   c. Postnatal screening will depend on the degree of suspicion. All infants may be screened by measurement of immunoreactive trypsin on blood taken by heel prick at the same time as other screening tests are performed. This currently remains the most accurate test for population screening but is not available universally, either in different countries or in different regions within one country. An elevated trypsin will warrant further investigation but this test is only valid in the first few weeks after birth as trypsin levels will subsequently fall as pancreatic insufficiency develops. If the index of suspicion is higher it may be deemed appropriate to send blood for gene mutation analysis.

d. Gene screening is not 100% accurate. There are now more than 1400 gene mutations on chromosome 7 that have been identified as being responsible for this condition. The ΔF508 defect is responsible for approximately 65% of the disease worldwide and a small number of other defects account for the majority of the remainder. The majority of commercially available tests look for 32 or less mutations. There is thus always the possibility that one of the rarer mutations may be present but not detected.

143. Prenatal case conference.

a. Prenatal case conferences may be held for a wide variety of different problems. For any conference to be called there must be some concerns that there are likely or possible problems for the child when born or for the mother or some other member of the family. In some cases there may be sufficient concerns to feel that the newborn child will be at significant risk. Unfortunately, although the fact that there has been a case conference has been mentioned it is by no means uncommon for none of the details of the case conference to be recorded anywhere. It is therefore very important that full details are found and recorded and that any antenatally determined actions are completed. Under no circumstances should the baby be discharged unless all parties are certain that it is safe to do so.

144. Goldenhaar (facio–auriculo–vertebral) syndrome.

a. Characteristic features of this syndrome include asymmetric facial hypoplasia, macrostomia, microtia, pre-auricular pits or tags, hearing defect, hemivertebrae or vertebral hypoplasia, and epibulbar dermoid. There are many other less common features.[80]

b. Aetiology is unknown. Goldenhaar syndrome is normally sporadic. Irregular dominant families have been described

c. Estimated recurrence in first-degree relatives is about 2%.

145. Pena–Shokeir syndrome.

a. Pena–Shokeir 'syndrome' is thought to be a common phenotype resulting from a number of separate entities. An affected baby will characteristically have multiple ankyloses, pulmonary hypoplasia, facial anomalies, and polyhydramnios. Some may display congenital myopathy and others have specific neurological abnormalities (anterior horn cell degeneration, abnormalities of the cortex and cerebellum). In a few cases post mortem has revealed evidence of long-standing ischaemic–hypoxic damage of the brain.[80]

b. Some, but not all, cases appear to be autosomal recessive.

c. In the absence of a specific diagnosis a recurrence risk of 10–15% is normally quoted.

146. Treacher Collins syndrome.

a. Inheritance is autosomal dominant and is due to mutations in the TCOF1 gene at 5q31.3–32. The gene encodes for a protein named Treacle – function unknown. More than half of all cases are thought to be new mutations because there is no significant family history of this condition.

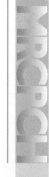

b. There is wide variability in expression but there are usually, at the very minimum, subtle features that are diagnostic. If neither parent is affected then it is extremely unlikely that a new child will be affected. In this specific case, although neither parent has abnormal features, father does have bilateral hearing aids. This could be unrelated but may not be.

c. Antimongoloid slant of the eyes (89%), malar (81%) and mandibular (78%) hypoplasia, lower lid coloboma (69%), partial to total absence of lower eyelashes (53%), malformation of the auricles (77%), external ear canal defect (36%), conductive deafness (40%), visual loss (37%), cleft palate (28%), incompetent soft palate (32%), and projection of scalp hair on to lateral cheek (26%).[81]

147. Tourette syndrome.[82]

a. In the past Tourette syndrome has been regarded as an autosomal dominant condition. This is no longer thought to be the case although the exact pattern of inheritance is not completely understood. The condition is now thought to be polygenic with a number of genes having a substantial effect and possibly many genes contributing a smaller effect. Environmental factors may also play a role in the development.

b. Genetic predisposition may not necessarily result in full-blown Tourette syndrome but may instead be manifest in either a milder tic disorder or an obsessive–compulsive behaviour pattern. It is also possible that an individual carrying the abnormal gene may exhibit no symptoms at all. At-risk males are more likely to have tic disorders and at-risk females are more likely to have obsessive–compulsive disorders. Only around 10% of affected children will ever have symptoms severe enough to need medical treatment.

c. There are no specific investigations.

148. Biliary atresia.

a. Biliary atresia is a rare condition of unclear aetiology. It is almost always an isolated event and there does not appear to be an inherited predisposition.

b. No specific investigations are indicated unless the baby becomes jaundiced. Any investigations should follow the normal pathway for investigation of jaundice. Additional investigations for biliary atresia are not indicated because of the family history.

149. Vertebral anomalies and absent stomach bubble.

a. Cardiac abnormalities, imperforate anus, tracheo-oesophageal fistula, renal abnormalities, limb abnormalities.

b. VATER or VACTERL association.

c. Postnatal investigations will be determined by the degree of suspicion. If it is thought that the baby may have this association, screening to detect abnormalities in all of these systems would be appropriate. A nasogastric tube should be passed and a chest X-ray should be performed. If there are thought to be any limb abnormalities a skeletal survey may be indicated. Ultrasound of the renal tract should be performed and there should be careful examination to make sure the anus is patent. Although in this case the heart was thought to be normal antenatally it would be prudent to perform an echocardiogram as postnatal imaging of the heart does not detect all abnormalities.

150. Schizencephaly.

    a. Schizencephaly is a rare developmental disorder characterised by abnormal slits, or clefts, in the cerebral hemispheres. Individuals with bilateral clefts are often developmentally delayed and have delayed speech and language skills and corticospinal dysfunction. Individuals with smaller, unilateral clefts (clefts in one hemisphere) may have a hemiparesis and may have average or near-average intelligence. Where clefts are bilateral there is an increased likelihood of significant neurodevelopmental impairment. Patients with schizencephaly may have varying degrees of microcephaly, mental retardation, hemiparesis or quadriparesis and may have hypotonia, seizures and hydrocephalus.[83]

    b. There is no universally accepted theory of the causation of schizencephaly. There is thought to be focal destruction of the germinal matrix early in brain development. It is thought that this is probably the end result of a variety of different insults. No specific prenatal events have been identified. It is likely that the aetiologies are multiple and include genetic, toxic, metabolic, vascular or infectious causes. Familial cases have been reported and there have been suggestions that there is involvement of the Emx^2 gene. This is now no longer thought to be the case.[83]

    c. There are reports of successful antenatal diagnosis using both ultrasound and MRI imaging. These techniques have been able to detect even relatively small clefts.[84]

REFERENCES

1. Sanders RC. Structural fetal abnormalities. The total picture. Mosby, New York, 2002
2. Jordan SC, Scott O. Heart disease in paediatrics. Butterworth, Oxford, 1989
3. Lewin MB, McBride KL, Pignatelli R et al. Echocardiographic evaluation of asymptomatic parental and sibling cardiovascular anomalies associated with congenital left ventricular outflow tract lesions. Pediatrics 2004;114:691–96
4. Kleinman CS, Nehgme R, Copel JA. Fetal cardiac arrhythmias. In: Creasy RK, Resnik R (eds) Maternal-fetal medicine. Saunders, Philadelphia, 2004
5. Archer N, Burch M. Pediatric cardiology. Chapman & Hall, London, 1998
6. Meyer-Wittkopf M, Cooper S, Sholler G. Correlation between fetal cardiac diagnosis by obstetric and pediatric cardiologist sonographers and comparison with postnatal findings. Ultrasound Obstet Gynecol 2001;17(5):392–97
7. Thangaratinam S, Daniels J, Ewer AK et al. Accuracy of pulse oximetry in screening for congenital heart disease in asymptomatic newborns: a systematic review. Arch Dis Child Fetal Neonatal Ed 2007;92:F176–F180
8. Souka AP, Snijders RJ, Novakov A et al. Defects and syndromes in chromosomally normal fetuses with increased nuchal translucency thickness at 10–14 weeks of gestation. Ultrasound Obstet Gynecol 1998;11:391–400
9. http://en.wikibooks.org/wiki/Handbook of Genetic Counseling
10. http://www.turner-syndrome-us.org
11. Jenkins TM, Wapner RJ. Prenatal diagnosis of congenital disorders. In: Creasy RK, Resnik R (eds) Maternal-fetal medicine. Saunders, Philadelphia, 2004
12. Krafchik BR, Hendricks LK, Faguet GB, Kuthiala S. Kasabach-Merritt syndrome. e-medicine 2007.www.emedicine.com/med/topic1221.htm

13. Al-Fouzan AW, Galadari I, Oumeish I et al. Herpes gestationis (pemphigoid gestationis). Clin Dermatol 2006;24(2):109–12
14. Shornick JK, Black MM. Fetal risks in herpes gestationis. J Am Acad Dermatol 1992;26(1):63–68
15. Henderson J, Gray R, Brocklehurst P. Systematic review of effects of low-moderate prenatal alcohol exposure on pregnancy outcome. Br J Obstet Gynaecol 2007;114(3):243–52
16. Hirose M, Hosokawa T, Tanaka Y. Extradural buprenorphine suppresses breast feeding after caesarean section. Br J Anaesth 1997;79(1):120–21
17. Kahila H, Saisto T, Kivitie-Kallio S. A prospective study on buprenorphine use during pregnancy: effects on maternal and neonatal outcome. Acta Obstet Gynecol Scand 2007;86(2): 185–90
18. Wojnar-Horton RE, Kristensen JH, Yapp P et al. Methadone distribution and excretion into breast milk of clients in a methadone maintenance programme. Br J Clin Pharmacol 1997;44(6):543–47
19. Abdel-Latif ME, Pinner J, Clews S et al. Effects of breast milk on the severity and outcome of neonatal abstinence syndrome among infants of drug-dependent mothers. Pediatrics 2006;117:e1163–e1169
20. Cissoko H, Jonville-Béra AP, Swortfiguer D et al. Neonatal outcome after exposure to beta adrenergic blockers late in pregnancy. Arch Pediatr 2005;12(5):543–47
21. Swortfiguer D, Cissoko H, Giraudeau B et al. Neonatal consequences of benzodiazepines used during the last month of pregnancy. Arch Pediatr 2005;12(9):1327–31
22. Ackland F, Singh R, Thayyil S. Flecainide induced ventricular fibrillation in a neonate. Heart 2003;89:1261
23. Rasheed A, Simpson J, Rosenthal E. Neonatal ECG changes caused by supratherapeutic flecainide following treatment for fetal supraventricular tachycardia. Heart 2003;89:470
24. Vanderhal AL, Cocjin J, Santulli TV et al. Conjugated hyperbilirubinemia in a newborn infant after maternal (transplacental) treatment with flecainide acetate for fetal tachycardia and fetal hydrops. J Pediatr 1995;126(6):988–90
25. Fidalgo I, Correa R, Gómez Carrasco JA et al. Acute anemia, rectorrhagia and hematuria caused by ingestion of naproxen. An Esp Pediatr 1989;30(4):317–19
26. Cornelissen M, Steegers-Theunissen R, Kollée L et al. Increased incidence of neonatal vitamin K deficiency resulting from maternal anticonvulsant therapy. Am J Obstet Gynecol 1993;168(3):923–28
27. Shield JP. Neonatal diabetes: new insights into aetiology and implication. Hormone Res 2000;53(Suppl 1):7–11
28. Polak M, Shield J. Neonatal and very early onset diabetes mellitus. Semin Neonatol 2004;9(1):59–65
29. Ellard S, Flanagan SE, Girard CA et al. Permanent neonatal diabetes caused by dominant, recessive, or compound heterozygous SUR1 mutations with opposite functional effects. Am J Hum Genet 2007;81(2):375–82
30. Gedikbasi A, Gul A, Sargin A et al. Cystic hygroma and lymphangioma: associated findings, perinatal outcome and prognostic factors in live-born infants. Arch Gynecol Obstet 2007;276(5):491–98
31. Grabowski EF, Buonanno FS, Krishnamoorthy K. Prothrombotic risk factors in the evaluation and management of perinatal stroke. Semin Perinatol 2007;31(4):243–49
32. Kulkarni R, Ponder KP, James. AH et al. Unresolved issues in diagnosis and management of inherited bleeding disorders in the perinatal period: A White Paper of the Perinatal Task Force of the Medical and Scientific Advisory Council of the National Hemophilia Foundation. USA. Haemophilia 2006;12(3):205–11
33. Kaplan M, Waisman D, Mazor D et al. Effect of vitamin K1 on glucose-6-phosphate dehydrogenase deficient neonatal erythrocytes in vitro. Arch Dis Child Fetal Neonatal Ed 1998;79:F218–F220
34. http://www.crnusa.org/pdfs/CRN_G6PDDeficiency_0305.pdf
35. Marlar RA, Montgomery RR, Broekmans AW. Diagnosis and treatment of homozygous protein C deficiency. Report of the Working Party on Homozygous Protein C Deficiency of the Subcommittee on Protein C and Protein S, International Committee on Thrombosis and Haemostasis. J Pediatr 1989;114(4 Pt 1):528–34

36. Payne SD, Resnik R, Moore TR et al. Maternal characteristics and risk of severe neonatal thrombocytopenia and intracranial hemorrhage in pregnancies complicated by autoimmune thrombocytopenia. Am J Obstet Gynecol 1997;177(1):149–55

37. Molad Y. Systemic lupus erythematosus and pregnancy. Curr Opin Obstet Gynecol 2006;18(6):613–17

38. Buyon JP, Clancy RM. Neonatal lupus syndromes. Curr Opin Rheumatol 2003;15(5):535–41

39. Escamilla SA, Pettersen MD. Transient heart block in a neonate associated with previously undiagnosed maternal anti-Ro/SSA and anti-La/SSB antibodies. Pediatr Cardiol 2007;28(3):221–23

40. Askanase AD, Friedman DM, Copel J et al. Spectrum and progression of conduction abnormalities in infants born to mothers with anti-SSA/Ro-SSB/La antibodies. Lupus 2002;11(3):145–51

41. Ades AE, Parker S, Walker J et al. HCV prevalence in pregnant women in the UK. Epidemiol Infect 2007;125:399–405

42. Yeung LTF, King SM, Roberts EA. Mother-to-infant transmission of hepatitis C virus. Hepatology 2001;34:223–29

43. Ruiz-Extremera A, Salmeron J, Torres C et al. Follow-up of transmission of hepatitis C to babies of human immunodeficiency virus-negative women: the role of breast-feeding in transmission. Pediatr Infect Dis J 2000;19:511–16

44. Davison SM, Mieli-Vergani G, Sira J et al. Perinatal hepatitis C virus infection: diagnosis and management. Arch Dis Child 2006;91:781–85

45. UK: British HIV Association. http://www.bhiva.org

46. USA: CDC guidelines. http://www.cdc.gov/hiv/resources/guidelines

47. Siegel. M. Congenital malformations following chickenpox, measles, mumps, and hepatitis. Results of a cohort study. JAMA 1973;226(13):1521–24

48. St Geme JW Jr, Peralta H, Farias E et al. Experimental gestational mumps virus infection and endocardial fibroelastosis. Pediatrics 1971;48(5):821–26

49. Rivera MN, Kim WJ, Wells J et al. An X chromosome gene, WTX, is commonly inactivated in Wilms tumor. Science 2007;315:642–45

50. Roth KS. Medium-chain acyl-CoA dehydrogenase deficiency. e-medicine 2007. www.emedicine.com/ped/topic1392.htm

51. Hamosh A, Johnston MV, Valle D. Non-ketotic hyperglycinaemia. In: Scriver CR, Beaudet AL, Sly WS, Valle D (eds) The metabolic and molecular bases of inherited disease, 7th edn. Vol. 1. McGraw-Hill, New York, 1995

52. D'Alton ME, Simpson LL. Syndromes in twins. Semin Perinatol 1995;19:375

53. Pharoah PO, Adi Y. Consequences of in-utero death in a twin pregnancy. Lancet 2000;355:1597

54. Bacon CJ, Hall D, Stephenson TJ et al. How common is repeat sudden infant death syndrome? Arch Dis Child published online 2007; 12 June, e pub ahead of print

55. Wilhelm A, Holbert JM. Situs inversus. e-medicine 2003. www.emedicine.com/radio/topic639.htm

56. Abribandi M, Bazan C. Corpus callosum agenesis. e-medicine 2004. www.emedicine.com/radio/topic193.htm

57. Rajab A, Yoo S, Abdulgalil A et al. An autosomal recessive form of spastic cerebral palsy (CP) with microcephaly and mental retardation. Am J Med Genet 2006;140A:1504–10

58. Bethune M. Management options for echogenic intracardiac focus and choroid plexus cysts: a review including Australian Association of Obstetrical and Gynaecological Ultrasonologists consensus statement. Australas Radiol 2007;51:324–29

59. www.healthsystem.virginia.edu/UVAHealth/peds_genetics/multi.cfm

60. Harper CM. Congenital myasthenic syndromes. Semin Neurol 2004;24(1):111–23

61. Fielder AR, Posner EJ. Neonatal ophthalmology. In: Rennie JM (ed) Roberton's textbook of neonatology, 4th edn. Churchill Livingstone, Edinburgh, 2005

62. Ihalainen A. Clinical and epidemiological features of keratoconus genetic and external factors in the pathogenesis of the disease. Acta Ophthalmology Supplement 1986;178:1–64

63. Wang Y, Rabinowitz YS, Rotter JI et al. Genetic epidemiological study of keratoconus: evidence for major gene determination. Am J Med Genet 2000;93(5):403–9

64. Moll AC, Imhof SM, Schouten-van Meeteren AYN et al. At what age could familial screening for familial retinoblastoma be stopped? A register based study 1945–98. Br J Ophthalmol 2000;84:1170

65. Bialik V, Bialik GM, Blazer S et al. Developmental dysplasia of the hip: a new approach to incidence. Pediatrics 1999;103(1):93–99

66. Kokavec M, Bialik V. Developmental dysplasia of the hip. Prevention and real incidence,. Bratisl Lek Listy 2007;108(6):251–54

67. Dare CJ, Clarke NMP. Orthopaedic problems in the neonate. In: Rennie JM (ed) Roberton's textbook of neonatology, 4th edn. Churchill Livingstone, Edinburgh, 2005.

68. Godward S, Dezateux C. Surgery for congenital dislocation of the hip in the UK as a measure of outcome of screening. Lancet 1998;351:1149–52

69. Dogruel H, Atalar H, Yavuz OY. Clinical examination versus ultrasonography in detecting developmental dysplasia of the hip,. Int Orthop 2007, Mar 1 e pub a head of print

70. Cardy AH, Barker S, Chesney D et al. Pedigree analysis and epidemiological features of idiopathic congenital talipes equinovarus in the United Kingdom: a case-control study. BMC Musculoskeletal Disorders 2007;8:62

71. Boyer O, Gagnadoux MF, Guest G et al. Prognosis of autosomal dominant polycystic kidney disease diagnosed in utero or at birth. Pediatr Nephrol 2007;22:380

72. Onal B, Kogan BA. Natural history of patients with multicystic dysplastic kidney-what follow-up is needed? Journal of Urology 2006;176:1607–11

73. Aslam M, Watson AR. Trent & Anglia MCDK Study Group. Unilateral multicystic dysplastic kidney: long term outcomes. Arch Dis Child 2006;91(10):820–23

74. Kuller JA, Coulson CC, McCoy MC. Prenatal diagnosis of renal agenesis in a twin gestation. Prenat Diagn 1994;14(11):1090–92

75. Carter CO. The genetics of urinary tract malformations. J Genet Hum 1984;32(1):23–29

76. Roodhooft AM, Birnholz JC, Holmes LB. Familial nature of congenital absence and severe dysgenesis of both kidneys. N Engl J Med 1984;310:1341–45

77. Blumenthal I. Vesicoureteric reflux and urinary tract infection in children. Postgrad M J 2006;82:31–35

78. Thomas DFM. Urological disease in the fetus and infant. Diagnosis and management. Butterworth Heinemann, Oxford, 1997

79. Eber E. Antenatal diagnosis of congenital thoracic malformations: early surgery, late surgery, or no surgery? Semin Respir Crit Care Med 2007;28:355–66

80. Baraitser M, Winter RM. Colour atlas of congenital malformation syndromes. Mosby-Wolfe, London, 1996

81. Jones KL. Smith's recognizable patterns of human malformation. Saunders, New York, 2006

82. National Institute of neurological disorders and stroke. Tourette syndrome fact sheet. Http://www.ninds.nih.gov/disorders/tourette/detail_tourette.htm#96273231

83. Granata T, Freri E, Caccia C et al. Schizencephaly: clinical spectrum, epilepsy, and pathogenesis. J Child Neurol 2005;20:313–18

84. Oh KY, Kennedy AM, Frias AE et al. Fetal schizencephaly: pre- and postnatal imaging with a review of the clinical manifestations. Radiographics 2005;25:647–57

Chapter 2

Problems at birth and resuscitation

Paediatric assistance is requested at around a quarter of all deliveries and some form of support is required in 40% of these cases. Intensive resuscitation, respiratory support at least, is required at 3% of all deliveries. This chapter will cover the commoner problems that may lead to difficulties at delivery and in the early postnatal period and will emphasise the standard approach to resuscitation that is taught on the Resuscitation Council Neonatal Life Support Course.[1] With the current quality of antenatal imaging many problems can be detected in pregnancy (60–80% of major and 35% of minor abnormalities by routine screening at 18–20 weeks) and an appropriate early management plan can be initiated. However, unexpected problems will always occur and it is thus essential that all staff have the skills necessary to deal with these situations.

Neonatal Life Support Algorithm

Dry and wrap
↓
Assess – breathing, heart rate, colour, tone
↓
Open airway
↓
Re-assess
↓
Inflation breaths – 5 breaths; 2–3 seconds; 30 cmH$_2$O
↓
Re-assess
↓
Ventilation breaths – for 30 seconds: 30/minute; 25 cmH$_2$O
↓
Re-assess
↓
Cardiac compressions – (assuming good chest movements and no improvement in heart rate) 3 compressions to one breath
↓
Re-assess after 30 seconds
↓
Drugs

If the chest fails to move

Check head position
↓
Single person jaw thrust
↓
Two person jaw thrust
↓
Clear airway under direct vision
↓
Guedel airway

QUESTION 1

You are called to a delivery of a term baby where profound decelerations have been seen on the CTG. The baby is born in poor condition and there is thick meconium in the liquor and on the baby's skin.

i) Which of the following manoeuvres are appropriate? Give one answer.
- **a.** Perineal suction
- **b.** Clamping the chest
- **c.** Tracheal lavage with normal saline
- **d.** Immediate intubation and tracheal suction
- **e.** Dry and wrap.

The baby is not breathing and is white and hypotonic with a heart rate is 30 bpm. Initial T-piece ventilation fails to obtain chest movement.

ii) What two forms of immediate treatment are appropriate?
- **a.** Start cardiac compressions immediately
- **b.** Repeat inflation breaths
- **c.** Continue with ventilation breaths
- **d.** Prepare for drug administration through the umbilical vein
- **e.** Immediate intubation
- **f.** Check head position
- **g.** Visualise the oro-pharynx.

Following tracheal suction, chest movement is obtained. After 30 seconds of ventilation, the heart rate remains at 30 bpm.

iii) What two immediate actions are indicated?

The baby is transferred to the neonatal unit and requires ventilation. Initial ventilatory settings are:

Pressures 30/4, FiO_2 1.0, rate 40, Ti 0.4 s, flow 4 L/min

His initial arterial gas is as follows:

pH	7.03
PCO_2	10.6 kPa
PO_2	4.5 kPa
BE	−10.6 mmol/L
Bicarbonate	17.5 mEq/L

iv) How would you describe the gas? Give one answer.
- **a.** Respiratory acidosis
- **b.** Respiratory alkalosis
- **c.** Metabolic acidosis
- **d.** Metabolic alkalosis
- **e.** Mixed respiratory and metabolic alkalosis
- **f.** Mixed respiratory and metabolic acidosis
- **g.** Normal.

v) What ventilation manoeuvres could you do to improve the gas?

    a. Increase PIP

    b. Increase Ti

    c. Increase PEEP

    d. Increase oxygen

    e. Decrease Te

    f. Increase flow

    g. Decrease flow.

vi) What additional treatments could be considered?

At 2 hours of age, the baby develops a tension pneumothorax. Following drain insertion, the following chest X-ray is obtained.

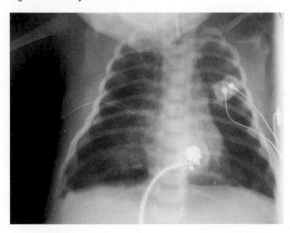

Figure 2.1

vii) List five abnormalities on the chest X-ray.

At 6 hours the following gas is obtained:

pH	7.18
PO_2	2.8 kPa
PCO_2	8.3 kPa
BE	−9.6 mmol/L
Bicarbonate	22.1 mEq/L

Ventilatory settings are:

    Pressures 35/5 cmH$_2$0, MAP 17, FiO$_2$ 1.0, Ti 0.4 s, rate 60

viii) What is the oxygenation index?

ix) What is the most likely diagnosis?

x) List four possible treatments.

QUESTION 2

You are asked to review a baby on the postnatal wards 12 hours of age after a difficult delivery. The baby is said to be fractious and is not feeding. As part of a septic screen, a chest X-ray is carried out.

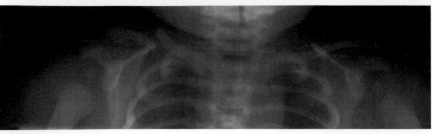

Figure 2.2

What abnormality does this X-ray show?

QUESTION 3

On a first day check, a baby is noted to have an absent red reflex.

i) What is the most likely diagnosis?
- **a.** Retinoblastoma
- **b.** Cataract
- **c.** Glaucoma
- **d.** African race.

ii) What is the most important action and why?

QUESTION 4

You are called urgently to the postnatal wards to see a baby. He was born at term by normal vaginal delivery with good Apgars and was feeding well for the first 2 days. Since this morning his mother has noticed that he is floppy, and not interested in feeds. The midwife has just been called to see him as his mother has tried to wake him for a feed and cannot rouse him. He is pale with cold peripheries, capillary refill time is 7 seconds, respiration is shallow, pulses are weak and heart rate is 180 bpm.

i) What are the two most likely diagnoses?
- **a.** Intracranial haemorrhage
- **b.** Sepsis
- **c.** Inborn error of metabolism
- **d.** Hypoglycaemia
- **e.** Hypernatraemia
- **f.** Hypocalcaemia
- **g.** Duct-dependent congenital heart disease
- **h.** Hypoxic–ischaemic encephalopathy.

ii) What two immediate actions would you undertake?

iii) What three investigations would be most useful in directing early management?

iv) What three investigations would be most helpful in establishing the differential diagnosis?

v) What would be the most appropriate immediate treatments? List four.

vi) The following blood count is obtained:

Haemoglobin	18.6 g/dL
WBC	25×10^9/L
Neutrophils	15×10^9/L
Lymphocytes	8.5×10^9/L
Monocytes	1.1×10^9/L
Eosinophils	0.4×10^9/L
Platelets	155×10^9/L

With this information what is the most likely diagnosis?

vii) While waiting for an echocardiogram you obtain the chest X-ray shown below.

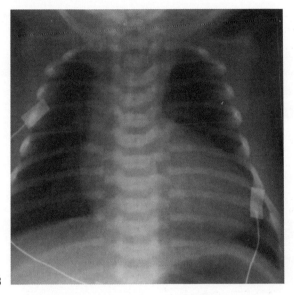

Figure 2.3

Describe the abnormalities.

viii) With this information what is your diagnosis and action?

ix) Parents are anxiously waiting for further information. What are you going to tell them?

QUESTION 5

i) Give three indications for postnatal administration of BCG.

ii) Give three contraindications for postnatal administration of BCG.

QUESTION 6

A baby is born following a ventouse delivery. Mother has noticed a swelling on the side of the head. Choose four features that would allow you to discriminate between a caput, cephalhaematoma and a subgaleal haematoma (subaponeurotic haematoma).

a. Location
b. Demarcation
c. Jaundice
d. Clinical time course
e. Petechiae
f. Bruising
g. Erythema
h. Time of presentation
i. History of instrumental delivery
j. Coagulation
k. Blood count.

QUESTION 7

You are asked to see a baby who has the obvious features of a brachial plexus injury.

i) How do you differentiate between an Erb and a Klumpke palsy?

ii) The parents want to know why it happened, how common it is, what treatments are available and what the long-term outcome is likely to be.

QUESTION 8

A baby has been born by difficult instrumental delivery. You are asked to review the baby and skull imaging is performed. The following picture is obtained.

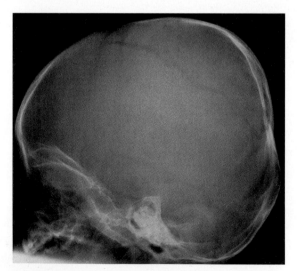

Figure 2.4

i) What does the X-ray show?

ii) What management is indicated and why?

QUESTION 9

A baby is born by normal vaginal delivery. A right sided facial palsy is noted and the right eye cannot be fully closed.

i) What is the most likely cause, and what immediate action would you consider?

ii) Which of the following syndromes are associated with a facial palsy? Choose three.
  a. Cardiofacial syndrome
  b. Edwards syndrome
  c. CHARGE syndrome
  d. Möbius syndrome
  e. Poland sequence
  f. Goldenhaar syndrome.

iii) The palsy persists and appears unchanged at an outpatient appointment two weeks later. What course of action would you recommend?

On more detailed examination in clinic, the infant is noted to have an inability to abduct the left eye. In addition there is mild talipes equinovarus and what appears to be a lack of chest wall bulk on the right side. There is also mild micrognathia and microtia.

iv) What syndrome is most likely?

v) What medication used in pregnancy is associated with this syndrome?

vi) What is the most likely long-term outcome if this diagnosis is correct?

QUESTION 10

A term baby presents with an intracranial bleed and gastrointestinal bleeding. He has not had vitamin K prophylaxis. Which of the following coagulation results will confirm the diagnosis of vitamin K deficiency bleeding? Choose three.

i) Normal PT, Normal APPT, Normal Fibrinogen, Normal Platelets

ii) Prolonged PT, Normal APPT, Normal Fibrinogen, Normal Platelets

iii) Prolonged PT, Prolonged APPT, Low Fibrinogen, Low Platelets

iv) Normal PT, Normal APPT, Normal Fibrinogen, Low Platelets

v) Very prolonged PT, Moderately prolonged APPT, Normal Fibrinogen, Increased Platelets

vi) Very prolonged PT, Moderately prolonged APPT, Increased Fibrinogen, Normal Platelets

vii) Normal PT, Prolonged APPT, Decreased Fibrinogen, Normal Platelets

viii) Normal PT, Very prolonged APPT, Normal Fibrinogen, Normal Platelets.

QUESTION 11

A 37 week gestation infant is admitted following an elective caesarean section. She has become tachypnoeic and a radial artery line has been inserted. She is noted to have a bruise on her left leg and a clotting screen is sent. The following result is obtained:

PT	17 seconds
APPT	84 seconds
Fibrinogen	2.5 g/L
Platelets	449×10^9/L

i) What does this coagulation result show?

ii) What abnormal conditions may explain it?

iii) What other explanation is possible?

iv) How would you distinguish between the possible causes?

QUESTION 12

A woman is admitted on to delivery suite at term. The CTG is abnormal with marked decelerations to 40 and a baseline bradycardia. She is taken immediately to theatre for an emergency caesarean section, and the baby is born 15 minutes later. At delivery the baby is white, floppy, and the heart rate is very slow.

i) What are your first actions? List four.

There is no respiratory effort, the heart rate is 20 bpm, and the baby is white and floppy.

ii) What are your next four steps?

The chest is seen to move well; however the heart rate remains at <20 bpm, and the baby is still white and floppy.

iii) What are your next actions? Suggest three.

The baseline heart rate remains at around 20 bpm. Good chest movement continues. You insert an umbilical venous catheter.

iv) What is the first thing you will do after successful placement?

v) Heart rate remains slow. You decide to give resuscitation drugs.
- **a.** What will you use?
- **b.** How much will you give?
- **c.** What order will you give them in and what is your rationale for doing so?

With the drugs you have administered, the heart rate rises to approximately 60 bpm but no further. Ventilation remains effective. The blood tests you send from umbilical venous blood are reported back as:

pH 6.8, BE −22 mmol/L, glucose 4.2 mmol/L

vi) What actions would you consider?

The heart rate rises a little further to 75 bpm. The baby remains very white and floppy. Further blood results come back with a haemoglobin from the umbilical venous sample of 15.2 g/dL. However, the obstetrician performing the C/S reports that there was 'an awful lot of blood about'.

vii) a. What else might you consider?
   b. What action would you take?

Following this action, the heart rate rises to >100 bpm but there is still no respiratory effort. The baby remains floppy and does not respond to stimulation. You admit the baby to the neonatal intensive care unit, and initiate positive pressure ventilation at pressures of 20/4, I:E ratio 0.3:0.8 seconds, FiO_2 0.21.

viii) What baseline monitoring would you consider? List six.

ix) What baseline investigations would you perform? List five.

Half an hour after admission, the following results are obtained from an arterial line:

pH 7.3, PCO_2 3.1 kPa, BE −15.5 mmol/L, lactate 9 mmol/L, Hb 10.2 g/dL

x) What three actions would you consider?

The nursing staff report oxygen desaturations on the monitor. They are uncertain as to whether there are associated abnormal movements. The baby remains extremely floppy.

xi) What further baseline investigations would you perform? Name six.

CFAM is commenced and the following trace is obtained.

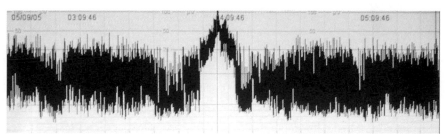

Figure 2.5

xii) a. Describe the trace. Is it normal?
   b. What key features have led to your conclusion?

xiii) What treatment modalities would you consider?

xiv) a. What is your first line medication for this condition?
   b. What dose would you prescribe (the baby weighs approximately 3.5 kg)?

Despite this treatment, there is no improvement in the baby's condition. The CFAM at this point is shown below.

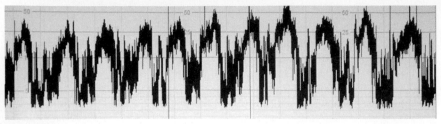

Figure 2.6

xv) Describe the trace.

xvi) What do you do now?

xvii) Following this treatment, the baby's clinical condition seems to stabilise, but the CFAM at this point is below.

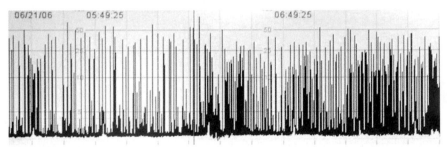

Figure 2.7

Describe the trace.

xviii) What other complications may this baby sustain and how would you assess them?

As part as a more detailed assessment, cranial ultrasonography is performed with Doppler studies of the anterior cerebral artery. The cerebral blood flow velocity is more than 3 SD from the mean and the PRI (Pourcelot Resistance Index) is 0.5.

xix) Explain the significance of these observations.

At 24 hours of age, the baby is anuric, urea 9.2 mmol/L, creatinine 165 μmol/L. Blood pressure is persistently low with a mean BP of 28–30 mmHg despite inotropic support. Echocardiography shows very poor myocardial contractility. Assessment of liver function shows markedly elevated transaminases and gamma-GT. The baby is profoundly hypotonic and unresponsive to painful stimuli. A formal EEG is performed and the following trace obtained.

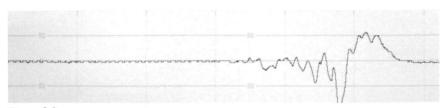

Figure 2.8

xx) What does this show?

xxi) What would be the main areas of discussion that you would have with the parents?

QUESTION 13

You are informed of the imminent delivery of a baby at 25 weeks gestation.

i) In the few minutes you have before delivery what specific areas of preparation will you concentrate on? List five.

ii) The infant is delivered and cries at birth. What immediate measure can be taken to minimise heat loss?

iii) What actions should you take to optimise ventilatory support immediately after birth?

QUESTION 14

You are called to see a baby boy on the postnatal wards who has had difficulty feeding. On examination the baby is noted to be floppy and has normal tendon reflexes. There are spontaneous anti-gravity movements. There is no fasciculation.

i) Is this central or peripheral hypotonia?

ii) What could be the likely cause? Choose two.
- **a.** Spinal muscular atrophy
- **b.** Prader–Willi syndrome
- **c.** Hypothyroid
- **d.** Congenital myotonic dystrophy
- **e.** Congenital myasthenia.

On further examination the baby is noted to have undescended testes and almond shape eyes.

iii) What is the most likely diagnosis?

iv) What test would confirm your diagnosis?

v) Which of the following endocrine problems is recognised as a characteristic finding in Prader–Willi Syndrome?
- **a.** Hypothyroidism
- **b.** Hypoinsulism
- **c.** Hypoparathyroidism
- **d.** Hypopituitarism
- **e.** Hypoaldosteronism.

The parents are keen to know the long-term developmental prognosis for their child.

vi) What will you tell them?

vii) The parents then ask about available treatment. What do you tell them?

ANSWER 1

i) **e.** Dry and wrap.

ii) **f.** Check head position.

  g. Visualise the oro-pharynx.

Many different treatment recommendations have been made in the past for meconium aspiration. Randomised controlled trials have failed to support any. Appropriate management of meconium aspiration should, as with all other scenarios, follow the normal resuscitation algorithm. There is evidence that suction on the perineum is ineffectual and this procedure cannot be recommended. Intubation and tracheal suction of all infants may be harmful to some and there is no evidence to support tracheal lavage. Clamping of the chest has no effect on a baby that is not breathing and may suppress respiration in an infant who is breathing effectively. The current recommendations therefore are to dry and wrap initially and then to assess respiration. If there is effective respiration, then no action is required, but close monitoring must be continued. If an infant shows no respiratory effort, then the airway must be opened, and cleared under direct vision, with inflation breaths thereafter if spontaneous respiration does not occur. An alternative strategy would be to attempt inflation breaths and only directly visualise if chest movement cannot be obtained, despite the use of appropriate airways opening manoeuvres.

iii) Continue effective ventilation and commence cardiac compressions. There is some debate as to whether cardiac compressions should be started immediately after inflation breaths or after 30 seconds of effective ventilation. Undoubtedly if there is no heart rate or profound bradycardia, then cardiac compressions should be started immediately after chest inflation has been obtained. However, if the infant is moderately bradycardic (60 bpm), it is reasonable to delay the commencement of compressions until a 30 second cycle of ventilation has been completed.

iv) Answer **f** is correct.

The pH is low (normal values 7.31–7.34 at 1–6 hours) showing an acidotic picture. The PCO_2 is raised (normal values 4.7–6.0 kPa at 1–6 hours) which could account for the low pH but the bicarbonate is also low (normal 20–26 mmol/L) which is also contributing to the acidosis. Thus it is a mixed acidosis.

v) Answers **a**, **c**, **e** and **f** are correct.

There are several ventilatory manoeuvres that could be tried to improve the gas and the baby's condition. Increasing the peak inspiratory pressure (PIP) would help oxygenation by increasing the mean airway pressure. Decreasing Te would increase the rate and thus decrease the carbon dioxide level. Increasing PEEP would again increase the mean airway pressure and might improve oxygenation. There is a possibility of gas trapping in meconium aspiration which may be worsened with a higher PEEP. Increasing the flow would increase the mean airway pressure and hopefully oxygenation. A standard flow would be 7 L/minute. Increasing the inspiratory time is not helpful with meconium aspiration as it can lead to air trapping and air leaks. We are unable to increase the oxygen any further as the baby is already in 100% oxygen. Decreasing the flow would lead to a decrease in mean airway pressure and thus worsen oxygenation.

vi) Additional treatments that could be tried are:
High frequency oscillation ventilation. This leads to improved gas exchange and can prevent up to 80% ECMO candidates requiring ECMO.

Surfactant. Meconium inactivates surfactant function and this may be important in the pathophysiology of meconium aspiration. Several studies including a Cochrane Review have shown a reduction in air leaks and a decreased need for ECMO.[2]

ECMO – see answer **x)** for details.[3]

vii) Five abnormalities on the chest X-ray:
   a. Partially drained pneumothorax
   b. Chest drain in situ
   c. Endotracheal tube in situ
   d. Transcutaneous monitor
   e. Patchy bilateral opacification.

viii) 80.

$$\text{Oxygenation index} = [(MAP \times FiO_2)/PaO_2] \times 100$$

The oxygenation index is an excellent measure of oxygenation in severe pulmonary disease. As the PaO_2 falls below 5–$6\,kPa$ ($kPa \times 7.6 = mmHg$), the denominator for the OI equation generates an exponential increase in OI. Studies during the introductory phase of ECMO suggested that an OI of greater than 40 on three out of five post-ductal arterial blood gases drawn within a 30-minute period defined a mortality greater than 80%.

ix) Persistent pulmonary hypertension. The gas in this case shows marked hypoxia, but with less severe hypercarbia. The high solubility of CO_2 means that the limited amount of blood entering the lungs is able to exchange CO_2 more effectively than oxygen.

x) a. Nitric oxide
     b. ECMO
     c. Tolazoline
     d. Prostacycline.

Nitric oxide is of proven benefit in term infants with established PPHN. It is a selective pulmonary vasodilator and there is evidence that a combination of HFOV and NO is better than either modality alone. In those infants who do not respond ECMO may be effective. If NO and HFOV are to be used it is advisable to discuss the individual patient with an ECMO centre early. There is evidence that delaying ECMO can lead to longer ECMO run times and poorer outcome. Prior to nitric oxide, vasodilators such as tolazoline and prostacycline were the available treatments. Vasodilatation was less selective and hypotension was a frequent side effect. If availability of nitric oxide is likely to be delayed, it is still appropriate to use these drugs. There are anecdotal reports of direct intratracheal administration of tolazoline and nebulised prostacycline. There is no evidence to support their use in this fashion.[3]

ANSWER 2

The X-ray shows a fractured right clavicle. Clavicle fractures occur in 0.2–5% of newborns. Large birth weight, technically difficult deliveries due to shoulder dystocia and the use of vacuum or forceps are associated with increased risk of clavicle fractures. However, some studies suggest that the majority occur with no reported difficulties during labour. Although these normally heal without complication, there are cases where an osteomyelitis has developed or there has been an associated brachial plexus injury. Re-fracture has been described in the literature, although this is rare. Clinical signs may be minimal movement of the affected limb with irritability, swelling with crepitus, absent Moro reflex or a palpable lump. Newborn fractures require no intervention apart from re-examination and possible repeat X-ray within 2 weeks to ensure healing is occurring. Early specialist intervention is recommended if there has been a brachial plexus injury.

ANSWER 3

i) Cataract is the most likely diagnosis to be picked up on day 1, although retinoblastoma and glaucoma do cause an absent red reflex. Cataracts occur in 2–3 per 10,000 live births. They are associated with congenital infection such as rubella, herpes simplex, toxoplasmosis and cytomegalovirus; syndromes, e.g. Lowes, Conradi's and Hallermann–Streiff; familial (the majority are autosomal dominant although autosomal recessive and X-linked have been described); and metabolic, such as hypocalcaemia, galactosaemia. Retinoblastoma does result in an absent red reflex but it is rare (the incidence is 1 in 20,000 live births) and average age for diagnosis is 18 months. Congenital glaucoma is infrequent but is a preventable cause of blindness. It presents with a cloudy cornea and progressive globe enlargement. It is sometimes difficult to see the red reflex in a baby of African race, but it is not absent. The corneas of darkly pigmented eyes reflect more light and appear cloudier than light eyes.

ii) Absent red reflex requires an urgent referral to ophthalmology. The best results are obtained when surgery and specialised ophthalmological support are initiated early, before amblyopia has developed. This may occur within six weeks from birth.

ANSWER 4

i) b. Sepsis.
g. Duct dependent congenital heart disease.
Sudden collapse at 2–3 days in a previously well baby, who has been feeding well and caused no concerns before, should raise the suspicion of a duct dependent heart lesion. Sepsis acquired at the time of birth usually presents earlier than this but cannot be excluded and appropriate treatment should be initiated while the diagnosis is clarified. Metabolic abnormalities may lead to sudden

collapse but in these conditions previous good health and good feeding is unlikely. Hypernatraemia is unlikely in a baby who is feeding well. Intracranial haemorrhage initiated at the time of delivery usually leads to a more gradual deterioration. Rarely a catastrophic bleed may lead to sudden collapse, normally shortly after birth. Hypoxic–ischaemic encephalopathy is unlikely to be a cause in a baby who has shown no abnormal signs in the first two days after birth.

ii) **a.** Secure airway and support breathing
   b. Obtain venous access.

Any seriously ill infant, irrespective of the cause, should be approached using the standard resuscitation algorithm. This infant has shallow respirations and obviously has impaired circulation, but A and B must come before C. This infant may well continue to deteriorate very rapidly and there is no doubt that vascular access will be needed. Peripheral venous access may well not be possible. The umbilical vein may be accessible but may not and if so intra-osseous access may be the only available option. It is important that access is obtained swiftly and repeated futile attempts for peripheral access should be discouraged.

iii) **a.** Blood glucose
    b. Blood gas
    c. Electrolytes

Any baby who has collapsed, irrespective of the cause, is likely to have an abnormal glucose (both low and high are possible). If the glucose is low, a bolus of 10% dextrose 2.5–5 mL/kg should be given intravenously and a continuous infusion started. A blood gas will allow assessment of ventilatory requirements and extent of acidosis. Electrolyte assessment is necessary as abnormalities may lead to collapse but may also be secondary to other causes. Irrespective of whether cause or effect, these must be treated.

iv) **a.** Septic screen
   b. Metabolic screen
   c. Echocardiogram

Ideally a full screen should be carried out on all babies who collapse, including a supra-pubic urine specimen, lumbar puncture, chest X-ray and these should be performed pre-antibiotic administration, provided this does not cause unnecessary delay. As antibiotics will be commenced before any results are available to support a diagnosis of sepsis, a septic screen will not influence early management but is essential to refine the diagnosis. The metabolic screen should include lactate, ammonia, acyl carnitines, amino and organic acids. A more detailed metabolic screen can be tailored to initial results after consultation with a biochemist. Although an alternative diagnosis may have become apparent before any results are available, it is important that these samples are sent early so that results become available relatively soon in the diagnostic process. An echocardiogram is most likely to give the definitive diagnosis of congenital heart disease and will allow assessment of the degree of cardiac compromise. Although chest X-rays may be helpful, even severe cardiac anomalies may have a relatively normal X-ray. An ECG is unlikely to be helpful in this case.

v) **a.** Ventilation.
   b. Antibiotics.
   c. Intravenous fluids.
   d. Prostaglandin E2.

This baby has collapsed and respiration is failing. Respiratory support is required and will be guided by blood gas analysis. Antibiotics should be commenced as soon as a septic screen has been performed and it is essential that there are no delays in starting therapy. The most likely organisms to cause postnatal collapse are Group B *Streptococcus* and *E. coli* and initial therapy should cover these organisms specifically.

This baby will need maintenance intravenous fluids. The need for a fluid bolus is contentious – the baby is showing signs of shock and a single fluid bolus would not be inappropriate. However, if a cardiac abnormality is responsible for the collapse, further fluid boluses may worsen the situation.

If the baby has collapsed following duct closure in a duct dependent heart lesion, the only effective therapeutic intervention is to re-open the duct using prostaglandin E2 or E1 (E2 is as effective as E1 and significantly cheaper). If an echocardiogram is immediately available, it may be appropriate to withhold treatment until the diagnosis is established. In practice this is often not the case and it is not acceptable to delay starting prostaglandin. In this situation, administration in itself may be diagnostic. The major side effects of Prostin are apnoeas, but as this infant is already ventilated for failing respiration it does not present a risk.

vi) Congenital heart disease. All these parameters are within the normal range for a newborn baby within the first week of life. A relatively high white cell count is normal ($10-26 \times 10^9$/L) and a high normal neutrophil count ($2.7-14.4 \times 10^9$/L) is more reassuring than worrying. Babies with severe sepsis leading to collapse are more likely to be neutropenic than have a neutrophilia. Similarly, severe infection is likely to be associated with marked thrombocytopenia rather than a low normal platelet count ($150-450 \times 10^9$/L). If overwhelming sepsis is excluded, heart disease becomes the most likely diagnosis in a previously well baby.

vii) **a.** Heart shape resembles egg on side.
   b. Narrow vascular pedicle.

viii) **a.** Transposition of the great arteries. Although these are the classical X-ray signs of a transposition, this diagnosis is possible with a relatively normal X-ray.
   b. Inform paediatric cardiologists. There is no doubt that this child will need to be managed within a specialised cardiac unit. In many centres early correction is performed and early transfer is indicated.

ix) It will be necessary to discuss the abnormal anatomy and the fact that surgery is required. Parents are likely to want to know why the diagnosis has been missed despite an apparently normal baby check and antenatal scans. It will be necessary to explain the contribution of the normal ductus and the fact that, prior to closure, there would have been no abnormal signs. Although antenatal scanning may detect some babies with this condition, it may not be detected in a significant proportion even with a very skilled ultrasonographer. Providing the baby did not suffer prolonged acidosis during the collapse, it should be possible to maintain stability with the Prostin infusion and successfully transfer to a specialist centre. The management thereafter will be determined by the particular practice of the specialist centre and is probably beyond the scope of your discussion with the parents.

An arterial switch is now the treatment of choice in most cases and operative survival has been reported in some centres to be 95–97% in infants with uncomplicated presentation. Long-term survival following the procedure is excellent, although complications happen in a significant number.

ANSWER 5

i) Current Health Protection Agency recommendations are that BCG should be given to:
  a. All infants in areas within the United Kingdom where the incidence of tuberculosis is greater than 40 per 100,000 population per year.
  b. Infants, wherever they live, with one or more parent or grandparent born in a country with a tuberculosis incidence of greater than 40 per 100,000.
  c. Previously unvaccinated new immigrants from high incidence countries.

Up-to-date prevalence of TB can be found at: http://www.globalhealthfacts.org.

ii) a. Maternal HIV.
  b. Mother has received continuous high dose steroids prior to delivery. In this case BCG should not be administered until adrenal function has been assessed in the infant.
  c. BCG should not be given to babies receiving corticosteroids or for at least 3 months after steroid therapy stopped.

ANSWER 6

  a. Location.
  b. Demarcation.
  d. Clinical time course.
  h. Time of presentation.

Caput succedaneum is the most common abnormality and is simply positional oedema due to pressure on the scalp at birth. A cephalhaematoma is bleeding between the skull and periosteum, most commonly seen over one or both parietal bones and rarely over the occipital or frontal bones. A subgaleal haematoma or subaponeurotic haematoma is bleeding between the epicranial aponeurosis that connects the frontal and occipital components of the occipitofrontalis muscle. Unconfined expansion allows wide spreading and it is vital to identify as early as possible, before circulatory collapse. The most important factors therefore in discrimination are as above.

A caput occurs on the scalp at point of contact with the cervix and can therefore extend across suture lines. It is vaguely demarcated, with pitting oedema that shifts with time under the influence of gravity. It is at its largest and firmest at the time of birth, softening progressively and usually disappearing within 48–72 hours.

Cephalhaematomas are most likely over the parietal bones and are discrete swellings with distinct margins, which do not cross suture lines. They are due to rupture of the diploic veins which are separate for each cranial bone. They usually increase in size after birth for the first 12–24 hours and then remain stable. They are usually smooth and firm on palpation. They normally resolve over the first 2–3 weeks but can remain for months and may calcify.

A subgaleal haematoma is not confined and therefore may be located across the scalp. It may present as a firm to fluctuant mass which may extend onto the forehead or the back of the neck and behind the ears. Crepitus may be felt particularly at the margins and a fluid wave may be palpable. It will progressively increase in size from birth and may be massive, particularly if associated with a consumptive coagulopathy.

ANSWER 7

i) Brachial plexus injuries occur in 1 in 2300 live births (UK 1998 figure) although figures as high as 4/1000 have been reported in the literature, with 90% being Erb's palsy (the most frequently affected regions C5, 6, less commonly also involving C7) and 10% Klumpke's (involvement of C8, T1). Clinical presentation of Erb's is typically the inability to abduct and externally rotate the shoulder, to flex the elbow and to supinate the forearm. When C7 is also involved neither the wrist nor fingers can be extended giving the classic Waiter's Tip sign. Involvement of the lower roots in Klumpke's palsy leads to involvement of the hand with a complete loss of grip, but preservation of movement elsewhere.

ii) In some cases it is thought that it is due to postural factors in utero although evidence for this is unclear. In most cases, it appears to be due to distraction at birth, i.e. pulling appears stretching leading to rupture, but this may be due to the birth process itself and does not have to be attributed to assistance. Risk factors are known to be shoulder dystocia (64% of cases), large birth weight, multiparity, assisted delivery, previous child with obstetric brachial palsy, prolonged labour and breech presentation. It is of interest to note that damage is most likely and prognosis worst in a small baby born by breech delivery, where C5/C6 avulsion occurs in approximately 80% of cases, and surgery is almost always required. Associated injuries are fractured clavicle (10%), fractured humerus (10%), subluxation of cervical spine (5%), spinal cord injury (5%), facial palsy (10–20%) and diaphragmatic palsy (5%).

Affected infants need to be followed up closely to assess the extent of recovery. Physiotherapy should be instigated early to maintain joint mobility and if recovery appears delayed or incomplete, surgery should be considered with referral to a specialist centre. In the absence of significant recovery, earlier referral is indicated. In a large UK study, about half of the infants had recovered fully at about 6 months of age but the remainder showed incomplete recovery, including 2% with no recovery. With appropriately timed surgery, substantial improvement may be reported but there is a significant long-term disability risk which should not be underestimated.[4]

ANSWER 8

i) The X-ray shows a linear skull fracture. Linear skull fractures are relatively common compared to depressed fractures and are usually in the parietal region. They commonly follow a forceps delivery or a prolonged, difficult labour. They have also been described following ventouse deliveries. Depressed fractures or ping-pong type fracture leads to an inward buckling of the bone where bone is depressed but not fractured. This injury is most commonly associated with forceps delivery and usually parietal bones are involved.[5]

ii) Uncomplicated linear fractures usually do not require treatment and heal within several months without sequelae. They can be associated with extra- and intracranial complications including haemorrhage, although these are rare. Another complication is tearing of the dura and the development of a leptomeningeal cyst. The fracture line may widen rapidly within weeks and infants therefore need a repeat X-ray at a few months of age to detect early widening of the fracture line.

For depressed fractures, some deformities resolve on their own, other reports include the use of digital pressure and use of suction from breast pump and obstetric vacuum extractors. Neuro-surgery is considered if other modalities are unsuccessful.

ANSWER 9

i) The most likely cause is birth trauma which accounts for approximately 80% of all cases. Forceps delivery is associated with approximately 75% of cases but it is of interest to note that in children with long-standing evidence of facial palsy there was no statistical association with the use of forceps and prenatal factors may be implicated.[6] Acutely, the only important aspect is to protect the exposed cornea and therefore artificial tears and patching may be indicated.

ii) **a.** Cardiofacial syndrome – **true.** This is also known as deletion 22q11.2 syndrome, velo-cardio-facial syndrome or Di George syndrome. There are abnormalities in the face and heart (as expected from the name) but there are also problems with mild learning difficulties, slender and hypotonic limbs with hyperextensible joints. Facial palsy is an occasional finding in this syndrome.

b. Edwards syndrome – **false.** There are characteristic facial features associated with trisomy 18, but facial palsy is not one of them.

c. CHARGE syndrome – **true.** The most common findings in this disorder are a colobomatous malformation, ear anomalies, cardiac defects, growth deficiency and mental retardation. Multiple cranial nerve abnormalities are also found, usually of I, VII, VIII, IX and X.

d. Möbius syndrome – **true.** The basic features of Möbius syndrome are mask-like facies with sixth and seventh cranial nerve palsies. Other cranial nerves can also be affected. See answer **iv**.

e. Poland sequence – **false.** Poland sequence is a unilateral defect of pectoralis major and syndactyly of the hand. Occasional hemi-vertebra occurs, as do renal anomalies and dextrocardia. Poland sequence has been grouped with Möbius syndrome because of a similar pathogenesis classified as the subclavian artery disruption sequence.

f. Goldenhaar syndrome – **false.** Also known as oculo-auriculo-vertebral spectrum, this abnormality occurs due to developmental problems with the first and second branchial arch. It is sometimes accompanied by renal, vertebral and ocular abnormalities hence the use of the word 'spectrum' in the name. Facial anomalies are marked but the majority of affected individuals are of normal intelligence. Facial palsy is not associated with Goldenhaar syndrome.

iii) Usually some recovery will be evident shortly after birth. In 90% of cases there is spontaneous recovery within four weeks of birth.[7] In infants with no evidence of resolution, referral to a surgeon with a specialised interest in this area is recommended. Surgical decompression is rarely needed but should be strongly considered if there is no recovery either on physical examination or electro-physiologically by five weeks of age.

iv) The combination of facial palsy with an abnormality of eye movement involving at least one cranial nerve is the minimum requirement for a diagnosis of Möbius syndrome. The sixth cranial nerve (abducent) is affected in approximately 75% cases. In approximately one-third of cases there may be defects affecting the lower limbs, facial structures and chest wall anomalies which are typical of Poland syndrome. It is for this reason that some reports suggest an association with facial nerve palsy and Poland syndrome. Experts in the field believe that these cases are Möbius syndrome variants.

v) An association between the use of misoprostol as an abortifacient has been reported to be associated with a 30-fold increase in the incidence of Möbius syndrome.

vi) During infancy, failure to thrive due to feeding problems and aspiration is not uncommon. Approximately 30% patients have mental retardation, which is commonly severe. Approximately one-quarter develop severe autistic symptoms. Speech impairment is very common.

ANSWER 10

Answers **ii**, **v** and **vi** are correct.

In all cases of vitamin K deficiency bleeding (previously haemorrhagic disease of the newborn), clotting studies show prolonged PT, normal platelets and normal fibrinogen. In a severe deficiency the APPT may also be prolonged and platelets and fibrinogen increased.

Other answers:

i) Normal.

iii) Compatible with disseminated intravascular coagulation with consumption of clotting factors and platelets.

iv) Thrombocytopenia – allo- or iso-immune with no other derangement of clotting.

vii) Need repeat sample – results do not match with clinical possibilities.

viii) Inherited deficiency of factor VIII, IX, XI, XII. Also consider heparin contamination.

ANSWER 11

i) The APPT is prolonged. PT is at the upper end of normal for a term infant immediately after birth. Fibrinogen is normal and platelets at the upper end of the normal range.

ii) This result could be explained by an inherited deficiency of factor VIII, IX, XI or XII. These conditions classically result in prolongation of APPT without affecting other parameters.

iii) If this coagulation screen had been performed on a sample taken through the arterial line the possibility of heparin contamination must be considered. This also may lead to prolongation of the APPT without affecting other clotting parameters.

iv) This could be differentiated from an inherited factor deficiency by use of the reptilase test. The reptilase time will be normal when the abnormality is due to heparin contamination but abnormal with inherited factor deficiencies. Assuming that heparin contamination could be discounted as a cause, further tests should be directed at differentiation between the different factor deficiencies. This will normally involve measurement of different factor levels but interpretation may be difficult in the newborn period and expert advice should be sought at the outset.

ANSWER 12

i) a. Dry and wrap. Despite the severity of the baby's condition, it is still vitally important to dry and wrap the baby.
   b. Call for help.
   c. Open the airway. The baby is extremely floppy and therefore airway opening manoeuvres are crucial in the early stage of resuscitation.
   d. Assess – colour, tone, heart rate and breathing.

ii) a. Inflation breaths. 5 at $30\,cmH_2O$ pressure, for 2–3 seconds each to see the chest rise.
   b. Ventilation breaths. 30 seconds comprising 15 ventilation breaths.
   c. External cardiac massage for 30 seconds.
   d. Re-assess – colour, tone, heart rate and breathing.

iii) Prepare to administer drugs, continue ventilation and cardiac compression, make sure help is available or on its way.

iv) Send blood for pH and blood gases, haemoglobin and blood glucose.

v) **a.** Adrenaline and sodium bicarbonate.
  b. 0.1 mL/kg 1 in 10,000 adrenaline.
  2–4 mL/kg of 4.2% sodium bicarbonate.
  c. There is as yet no consensus on the order of which drugs should be given. Adrenaline is frequently given first and followed by sodium bicarbonate when no or little response is observed. In an acidotic infant it is probably more sensible to administer bicarbonate before adrenaline as binding of adrenaline to its receptor is said to be less effective in an acidotic milieu.

vi) **a.** Further bicarbonate.
  b. Further adrenaline.

vii) **a.** Severe acute blood loss around the time of delivery. This baby has only shown partial response to appropriate resuscitation. It is therefore quite likely that there are further factors contributing. A haemoglobin of 15.2 g/dL is not unduly low but if blood loss is recent, this may well not represent the final haemoglobin once compensatory fluid shifts have occurred. The haemoglobin may well drop to very significant lower levels.
  b. Emergency transfusion with O negative CMV negative blood. This should be stored in a fridge on labour ward in Pedipacks.

viii) **a.** Heart rate.
  b. Respiratory rate.
  c. Oxygen saturation.
  d. Blood pressure.
  e. Urine output.
  f. Temperature.

There is already evidence to suggest that this baby has suffered a severe antepartum/peripartum injury. There may be considerable physiological instability, and thus all parameters normally measured in a sick infant should be recorded.

ix) **a.** Repeat blood gas (including lactate).
  b. Repeat haemoglobin.
  c. Baseline coagulation.
  d. Baseline U + E.
  e. Repeat blood glucose.

If there has been severe blood loss and a major ischaemic event, there may be rapid changes in haemoglobin and other measures. However, gas exchange may be minimally affected.

x) **a.** Blood transfusion.
  b. Reduction of ventilation to treat respiratory alkalosis.
  c. Treatment of metabolic acidosis.

On first impression a pH of 7.3 appears acceptable. However this is obtained through a combination of a metabolic acidosis and a respiratory alkalosis, neither of which are acceptable. In some cases, a moderately affected baby may spontaneously correct the metabolic acidosis, but it cannot be assumed that this will happen. Close monitoring and appropriate intervention is therefore essential.

xi) **a.** Glucose
b. Repeat gas
c. Calcium
d. Magnesium
e. Cerebral function monitoring (CFM)
f. Cranial USS

In this clinical scenario, seizure activity may be masked by the severe hypotonia. It is prudent in all cases of suspected seizures to check baseline electrolytes, especially glucose, calcium and magnesium. A repeat blood gas would help determine if there is a respiratory cause for the desaturations. A cranial USS would be useful to act as a baseline against which subsequent scans can be compared. Early scans may well show no significant abnormalities. CFM (cerebral function monitoring – integrated amplitude EEG) is a useful bedside test that is becoming widely available and easy to use with modern systems.

xii) **a.** The trace is abnormal.
b. The trace shows a normal upper limit (should be 10–40 μV) but the lower limit is depressed (should be >5 μV). There is absence of sleep–wake cycling which should normally be seen and there is a marked increase in activity with a narrowing of the width in the middle of the trace. This is clear evidence of seizure activity.

To illustrate these differences compare with the normal trace below.

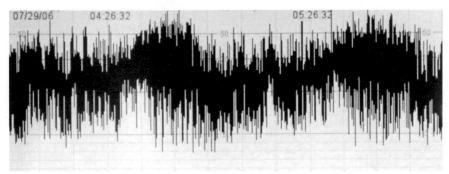

Figure 2.9

xiii) **a.** Anticonvulsants.
b. Fluid restriction.
c. Controlled hypothermia.

The CFM has shown clear evidence of fits. As there is evidence to suggest that uncontrolled seizure activity is associated with worse long-term outcome, this should be therefore be controlled. Anticonvulsant therapy remains the mainstay of treatment.

Cerebral oedema is likely to accompany a severe asphyxial episode and fluid restriction is normally commenced, although the evidence of a link between fluid intake and cerebral oedema has not been established. Renal compromise is likely in this case and fluid restriction would be a sensible part of management of this complication.

There is evidence to suggest that moderate hypothermia – either whole body or selective head cooling – may have a significant impact on outcome, particularly in moderate asphyxial injury. It is currently recommended that this should only be provided in specialist centres (within 6 hours in clinical trials), and in those without this facility care should be directed towards avoidance of active rewarming. The main UK trial (Total Body Hypothermia trial) finished recruiting at the end of 2006 with publication of provisional results of 18 month follow-up in abstract only at the end of 2008. As meta-analysis of the results of trials has shown a reduction in death or disability (RR 0.76; 95% CI 0.65–0.89) many centres are continuing to provide hypothermia for affected infants.[8]

xiv) **a.** Phenobarbitone remains the first-line agent for treatment of seizures in many centres. Although this is the case, there is no evidence base to support this.
b. Commonly phenobarbitone is commenced at 20 mg/kg – thus in this case a loading dose of 75 mg should be prescribed.

The current practice is to give further loads of 10 mg/kg to a maximum total of 40 mg/kg.

xv) The CFAM trace shows a lower baseline than normal and there is almost continuous seizure activity.

xvi) **a.** Further loading dose of phenobarbitone can be given up to total of 40 mg/kg.
b. Loading dose of phenytoin 20 mg/kg slowly over 30 minutes.
c. Consider other anticonvulsants – lignocaine, midazolam or lorazepam. There is much national variation in the second-line treatment of seizures if phenobarbitone does not control the seizures.

xvii) The CFAM shows severe depression of the baseline with burst suppression. This is suggested by very flat periods on the trace with intermittent short spikes. A continuous EEG would need to be examined to confirm this.

xviii) **a.** Renal failure:
Urine output
Dipstick urine for blood and protein
Urea and electrolytes
Urine electrolytes and osmolality.
b. Hepatic failure:
Liver function tests
Coagulation profile.
c. Bone marrow suppression:
FBC and differential.
d. Myocardial dysfunction:
Echocardiography
Ejection fraction calculation
Blood pressure.

Multi-system failure may follow a severe asphyxial insult and it is important that function of different systems is carefully assessed and treatments modified accordingly. Of particular importance is the use of aminoglycoside antibiotics in an infant whose renal function may be very poor.

xix) The use of cerebral ultrasound and Doppler assessment of cerebral haemo-dynamics has been shown to be of use in predicting the long-term outcome of these infants. A cerebral blood flow velocity above 3 SD from the mean is strongly associated with adverse outcome and is probably a more specific indicator than the Pourcelot Resistance Index (PRI = peak systolic-end diastolic/peak systolic pressure). A low PRI of <0.55 is strongly associated with poor outcome.

xx) Flat or low voltage trace with burst suppression.

xxi) This baby is showing signs of advanced multi-organ failure and an extremely high chance of death or of very severe brain damage if survival occurs. The combination of a low voltage EEG with burst suppression, low PRI on cerebral blood flow Doppler and severe multi-system failure firmly place this baby in this category. Discussion with parents should therefore be centred around the appropriateness of continuing intensive care. Should care be continued, all affected systems must be continuously monitored and a decision to continue care be constantly evaluated and re-assessed. All discussions and decisions should be clearly documented in the baby's notes, and records should be kept of all personnel involved in discussions.

ANSWER 13

i) **a.** Temperature control.
  b. Appropriate help.
  c. Surfactant.
  d. Ventilation.
  e. Discussion with parents.

Resuscitation should be well prepared for all infants. This is particularly the case for extremely immature infants. Temperature control is of vital importance and all equipment should be at working temperature well before delivery. Early surfactant is indicated and should be available and warm. Ventilation equipment, both on the resuscitaire and intensive care space the baby will occupy, should be prepared. If there is any chance, discussions with parents should be held, however briefly, before the baby is born.

ii) **a.** Plastic occlusive dressings, either in the form of a bag or a sheet, are now widely used to prevent evaporative heat loss. The limited amount of data available strongly supports this intervention.
  b. Use of a resuscitaire with a temperature probe. Although efforts must concentrate on prevention of even moderate hypothermia, care should be taken to avoid hyperthermia as well. Use of a resuscitaire on auto mode with measurement of the baby's temperature is a highly desirable means of optimising body temperature.
  c. Resuscitation in a warm ambient environment. Delivery suites are often relatively cool with air conditioning systems producing cold down drafts that may seriously impair the ability to maintain a stable thermal

environment. If this situation exists, the resuscitaire should be positioned in a location where external factors can be minimised.

    d. Maintenance of supportive environment during transfer to the intensive care unit. Although heaters on modern resuscitaires are extremely effective in maintaining satisfactory body temperature, this no longer works when the resuscitaire is disconnected from the main electrical supply. Transport over any distance should therefore be in a pre-warmed transport incubator. Transport over short distances can be performed on a disconnected resuscitaire, providing the infant is surrounded by an abundance of warmed towels. Heat loss from the head should be minimised by a hat.

iii) **a.** Prompt and appropriate resuscitation. It is generally felt that intervention to support respiration should commence immediately in very immature infants. There is no evidence to support an expectant policy and there is little doubt that allowing hypoxia and hypercarbia before resuscitation is commenced is likely to make subsequent resuscitation more difficult.

    b. Early surfactant. Randomised controlled trails have clearly shown that very early treatment with surfactant (within first 15 minutes) is associated with significantly better outcome than delaying surfactant until signs of respiratory distress develop. Some practitioners advocate a policy of surfactant administration before inflation breaths. Others recommend securing adequate lung inflation before surfactant administration. Currently available evidence suggests that there is no disadvantage from achieving adequate lung inflation prior to surfactant. Whichever policy is chosen, there is no question that delaying surfactant administration beyond the first few minutes cannot be recommended.

    c. Appropriate pressure for inflation and subsequent ventilation breaths. Resuscitation guidelines advocate the use of five prolonged relatively high pressure inflation breaths to recruit an appropriate degree of lung filling. However, these guidelines are specifically derived for resuscitation of term infants. Although adequate lung inflation must still be obtained in premature babies, there are concerns and limited evidence to suggest that early hyperinflation may be damaging to the lungs. To minimise this potential damage, pressure controlled T-piece delivery systems should be used instead of resuscitation bags with poorly controlled inflation pressure and normal breaths should be given. After adequate initial breaths, pressure must be decreased to continue with ventilation breaths. In some preterm infants, with hyaline membrane disease, chest movement may be difficult to ascertain, but a response in heart rate will be obtained.

    d. Avoidance of hyperoxia. Evidence for oxygen concentrations to be used in resuscitation of preterm babies is lacking. There is increasing evidence to suggest that there is no detriment from resuscitating term infants in air as opposed to 100% oxygen. Although there is currently no consensus as to the best oxygen concentration in which to initiate resuscitation, there is no reason to suppose that hyperoxia is desirable at this point when we know it is not at any other point. The commonest limiting factor determining management is the availability of an oxygen blender on the resuscitaire. Currently different practitioners are initiating resuscitation in air, or in an arbitrarily selected oxygen concentration and adjusting according to heart rate response. What is certain is that the routine use of 100% oxygen in the resuscitation of preterm infants cannot be recommended.[9]

e. Choice of appropriate ventilation strategy. Although there is general agreement that ventilatory support should be provided immediately in extremely premature infants, there are different schools of thought as to how this is best provided. Some practitioners advocate the use of CPAP from birth (some stipulating that the baby be intubated, surfactant administered and then extubated; some are strongly opposed to the destabilisation that an intubation/extubation policy may cause), others prefer to intubate and ventilate first and extubate to CPAP at a later date. The evidence to support any particular philosophy is inconclusive, and is to some extent dependent on the philosophy of an individual unit and the enthusiasm of staff in adhering to that philosophy.

ANSWER 14

i) Central. It is important to distinguish between central and peripheral hypotonia. Central hypotonia is caused by a problem above the lower motor neurone. The floppiness is much more severe than the weakness, and sometimes, despite being very floppy, infants can show strong movements on stimulation. Tendon reflexes are usually preserved and there is no fasciculation which is seen in peripheral hypotonia.

ii) **a. No** – SMA causes a peripheral neuromuscular hypotonia and presents with severe weakness as well as hypotonia. SMA also causes muscle fasciculation.

b. Yes – Prader–Willi syndrome could be the cause.

c. Yes – hypothyroidism is unusual in that it can cause both central and peripheral hypotonia.

d. No – congenital myotonic dystrophy causes peripheral hypotonia with marked weakness of respiratory muscles, feeding difficulties and facial diplegia.

e. No – congenital myasthenia occurs in 10–12% of infants born to mothers with myasthenia. The neurological features present are very dramatic and can evolve rapidly with feeding and respiratory problems. Generalised muscle weakness is present in 70% of cases.

iii) Prader–Willi syndrome. Babies with PWS have bitemporal narrowing and 'almond shaped' palpebral fissures (although this may become more evident postnatally as opposed to at birth). The hair and the skin can be lightly pigmented compared to the rest of the family. The genitalia are usually hypoplastic. Boys have cryptorchidism, and girls have small labia minora and clitoris.

iv) Chromosomal analysis should be requested looking specifically at the proximal long arm of chromosome 15 (15q11-q13). The majority of cases (about 75%) are caused by a deletion of the paternal copy of the appropriate region of chromosome 15 which can be picked up by fluorescence in situ hybridisation. Approximately 20% of cases are due to uniparental disomy, which occurs when both copies of the chromosomal region are inherited from a single parent, in this case the mother. These cases have a normal FISH study but an abnormal DNA methylation test. Uniparental disomy occurs sporadically, making the recurrence risk extremely low. A small minority of people have a translocation or imprinting irregularity involving chromosome 15. The recurrence risk is less than 1%.

v) Infants with PWS have hypothalamic hypopituitarism which leads to hypogonadism and growth hormone deficiency. The growth hormone deficiency leads to short stature and low muscle bulk. Other associated problems in later life are scoliosis, strabismus and osteoporosis.

vi) Infants with PWS have delayed milestones. The average age for walking alone is about 2 years although there is wide variation in this time. Hearing is normal but strabismus is common. Problems with speech, particularly articulation problems, are widely reported. Parents with babies with PWS describe them as being very quiet and placid babies. They sleep well and the main problems in the early postnatal period tend to be with feeding and weight gain, which persist up to 6 months or longer. Most children with PWS have borderline or moderate learning difficulties. The average IQ is about 70, although affected individuals may find it hard to perform at their IQ level, as emotional and social skills may be less well developed than in their peers. Writing and reading are usually considerably better than number skills and abstract thinking.

vii) In the early neonatal period, feeding and growth must be addressed. Many babies will need tube feeding with high calorie milks. The babies seem to tolerate nasogastric tubes and it is best to avoid gastrostomies as they can lead to significant areas of lipo-atrophy (predominantly abdominal) in later life. The most publicised complication of PWS is obesity. Between 2 and 6 years of age, children develop a hyperphagic phase which appears to be related to a hypothalamic problem affecting the satiety pathway. There has been much research into the specific defect, looking at neuropeptide Y, pro-opiomelanocortin, leptin and ghrelin. The hyperphagia is thought to be due to the decreased ability to feel satiated when the stomach is full. There have been many trials of treatment including appetite suppressant medication, surgery to decrease the gastric volume and behavioural therapy to decrease the feeding issues. Childhood obesity carries significant risk of morbidity including diabetes, heart failure and sleep apnoea. Dietary management is crucial during early childhood with dietetic input and mealtime routines. Growth hormone deficiency affects all individuals with PWS. Growth hormone is being used to improve linear growth and also improves amount of lean muscle mass compared to fat. Evidence shows that early treatment with growth hormone in the first year leads to improved growth and improved motor development. It has also been shown that facial and body appearance can normalise. Selective serotonin reuptake inhibitors can be helpful if the child shows obsessive–compulsive traits that are commonly seen along with other behavioural disorders.

Overall, the management of infants with PWS is best in a multidisciplinary team setting with paediatricians, endocrinologist, dieticians and psychologists. There are good support groups for parents (www.pwsa.co.uk).

REFERENCES

1. Resuscitation at birth. Newborn Life Support Provider Course Manual. Resuscitation Council (UK), London, 2006
2. Soll RF, Dargaville P. Surfactant for meconium aspiration syndrome in full term infants. Cochrane review 2000;(2):CD002054
3. Hintz SR, Suttner DM, Sheehan AM et al. Decreased use of neonatal extracorporeal membrane oxygenation (ECMO): how new treatment modalities have affected ECMO utilization. Pediatrics 2000;106(6):1339–43
4. Evans-Jones G, Kay SPJ, Weindling AM et al. Congenital brachial palsy: incidence, causes, and outcome in the United Kingdom and Republic of Ireland. Arch Dis Child Fetal Neonatal Ed 2003;88:F185–F189
5. King SJ, Boothroyd AE. Cranial trauma following birth in term infants. Br J Radiol 1998;71:233–38
6. Laing JHE, Harrison DH, Jones BM et al. Is permanent congenital facial palsy caused by birth trauma? Arch Dis Child 1996;74:(1)56–58
7. Smith JD, Crumley RL, Harker LA. Facial paralysis in the newborn. Otolaryngol Head Neck Surg 1981;89:(6)1021–24
8. Edwards AD, Azzopardi DV. Therapeutic hypothermia following perinatal asphyxia. Arch Dis Child Fetal Neonatal Ed 2006;91:F127–F131
9. Richmond S. ILCOR and neonatal resuscitation. Arch Dis Child Fetal Neonatal Ed 2007;92:F163–F165

Common postnatal problems

Every infant must have a thorough and detailed examination after birth, not only to exclude obvious congenital malformations but also to detect common post-natal conditions such as jaundice that may pose a risk to the baby and require treatment. The continuing provision of care for infants after birth allows us to complete screening that started before birth, and identify infants that require specific intervention after birth – the need for vaccination or imaging in the immediate postnatal period being typical examples. Many problems that are identified in the postnatal period do not require any treatment or intervention, but do mean that advice and reassurance must to be given to the parents.

This chapter aims to address the commoner problems that paediatricians are called to review on the postnatal ward. It is by no means an exhaustive list of the problems that may occur and a standard textbook of neonatology should be consulted for more detailed information.

QUESTIONS

1. The following are contraindications to the BCG vaccination. Choose two correct answers:
   a. Prematurity
   b. Down syndrome
   c. Babies born to HIV positive mothers
   d. Babies with chronic lung disease
   e. Family history of egg allergy
   f. Family history of inflammatory bowel disease
   g. Babies being treated with dexamethasone for chronic lung disease.

2. You are called to delivery suite to speak to some parents that have refused to let their baby have vitamin K. The father says that it is unsafe and causes cancer. Mum wishes to breast feed.
   a. What are you going to tell them?
   b. You find out that mother is on anticonvulsant medication. Does that affect what you say?
After you have discussed this with the family, the father then points out that there is a family history of glucose-6-phosphate dehydrogenase deficiency.
   c. What do you now tell the family?

aby is noted to have a sacral dimple on the postnatal check. On further examination, the dimple is found to be 2 cm above the anus and there is a small erythematous patch over the spine.

    a. Are there any investigations you would do?

    b. Why?

4. A mother was started on treatment for TB 7 days before delivery and her sputum for AFB is negative. Her baby is asymptomatic on examination. What management would be appropriate for the baby? Give two answers.

    a. Isolate the baby from the mother

    b. Encourage bottle feeding

    c. Treat with isoniazid, rifampicin and pyrazinamide

    d. Treat with isoniazid and rifampicin

    e. Treat with isoniazid

    f. Encourage breast feeding

    g. Vaccinate the baby with BCG at birth

    h. Vaccinate the baby with isoniazid-resistant BCG at three months

    i. Do nothing.

5. You are called to see a term baby who is now 28 hours old. The baby has not passed meconium. The parents want to take their baby home and are becoming quite agitated. How do you manage the situation? Choose the most appropriate action.

    a. Send baby home

    b. Send baby home with clinic review in one week

    c. Arrange urgent surgical review

    d. Arrange contrast studies

    e. Arrange plain abdominal X-ray

    f. Keep in for observation.

6. A baby is noted on routine postnatal check to have absent red reflexes. Which of the following diagnoses need to be considered?

    a. Congenital hypoparathyroidism

    b. Retinopathy of prematurity without plus disease

    c. Congenital hyperparathyroidism

    d. Hallermann–Streiff syndrome

    e. Persistence of the tunica vasculosa lentis

    f. Retinal haemorrhage

    g. Retinoblastoma

    h. Lowe syndrome

    i. Congenital glaucoma

    j. CHARGE syndrome.

7. On a routine review of a baby on the neonatal unit, you noticed the baby has purulent discharge from both eyes. The baby is 4 days old. What is the most likely organism to cause this? Choose the best answer.

    a. *Staphylococcus aureus*

    b. *Chlamydia trachomatis*

    c. *Neisseria gonorrhoea*
    d. *Haemophilus influenzae*
    e. *Streptococcus pneumoniae*
    f. *Pseudomonas aeruginosa*
    g. Herpes simplex.

8. i. Which of the following are risk factors for developmental dysplasia of the hip?
    a. Male
    b. Transverse lie
    c. Previous affected sibling
    d. Polyhydramnios
    e. Intra-uterine growth retardation
    f. First-born child
    g. Torticollis.
  ii. A mother reports that she required some form of harness when she was a baby. There have been two previous children who have been normal. The hips appear stable on examination. What action would you take?

9. A mother is known to have thyroid disease but has normal thyroid function tests. One of your SHOs organises for the baby to come back for thyroid function tests at 4 days of age. The results of these are as follows:

      Free T4   80 pmol/L
      Total T4   300 pmol/L
      TSH   2 mU/L

What action would you take?
    a. No action and discharge the child
    b. Repeat the tests in 2 weeks time
    c. Repeat the test in 2 days time
    d. Refer to paediatric endocrinology clinic
    e. None of the above.

10. A baby is noted on postnatal check to have an undescended testicle (UDT). Which of the following statements are correct?
    a. The majority of UDT will have descended successfully by 12 months of age
    b. If still not descended at 12 months, 75% will descend by 36 months of age
    c. Only a small minority are palpable
    d. Early orchidopexy will preserve fertility in the majority
    e. UDT requires orchidopexy to reduce the incidence of malignant change
    f. UDT requires urgent review because of the risk of torsion
    g. UDT usually responds well to hormonal therapy
    h. UDT may be associated with urinary tract abnormalities.

11. On postnatal examination, a baby is found to have talipes equinovarus. This cannot be corrected on manipulation.
    a. What is your management?
    b. The parents want to know what possibilities there are for long-term problems. What will you tell them?

12. The mother of a newborn baby girl informs you that her two previous babies, both boys, had pyloric stenosis, as did she. Which of the following statements are correct?

    a. The chance of pyloric stenosis in this baby is no different to that for a baby with no family history

    b. As this is a female infant, pyloric stenosis is less likely compared to a male infant

    c. A test feed and abdominal ultrasound should be performed

    d. Prophylactic pyloromyotomy is indicated

    e. The baby should be fed normally

    f. Treatment with anticholinergic drugs is now widely accepted as first-line management

    g. In up to 7% of cases of pyloric stenosis there may be associated malformations.

13. A term baby is two weeks old, breast fed and thriving, with normal urine and stool colour. Examination is unremarkable but she is noticed to be moderately jaundiced. The bilirubin is 180 μmol/L, conjugated 10. Which of the following investigations should you carry out as part of your initial assessment?

    a. Liver USS

    b. HIDA scan

    c. Haemoglobin

    d. DCT

    e. Urinalysis

    f. Clinitest

    g. Thyroid function tests

    h. Red cell fragility

    i. Blood cultures

    j. UDPGT

    k. Gene screen for Gilbert's.

14. How would your approach differ if the conjugated bilirubin had been 40 μmol/L but with normal urine and stool colour?

15. A liver ultrasound scan suggests that bile ducts are present, and shows what appears to be an abnormally large gall bladder. What is the most likely diagnosis? Choose one answer.

    a. Atypical biliary atresia

    b. Duodenal web with biliary reflux

    c. Normal variant

    d. Inspissated bile

    e. Diverticulum of the bile duct

    f. Cystic dilatation of the common bile duct

    g. Choledochocele.

16. A liver ultrasound examination is equivocal. A gall bladder is seen and the report states that the bile ducts were not clearly visualised but could have been obscured by the gall bladder. Which of the following is most appropriate? Choose one answer.

    a. Review in outpatients in 4 weeks time

    b. Repeat USS

c. Refer for immediate specialist opinion
d. Reassure and discharge
e. Arrange HIDA scan and review in outpatients.

17. A baby is born to a mother who was noted to have significant anti–D levels during pregnancy. A cord blood sample was sent and you have just been informed that the cord bilirubin level was 180 μmol/L. The baby is now 4 hours old. You send a repeat blood sample for group and crossmatch, and Coombs' test, and commence phototherapy. The following results are obtained within 2 hours:

Bilirubin   240 μmol/L
Hb   12.5 g/dL (fragments seen suggestive of
                       severe haemolysis)

Group A Rh positive
Coombs strongly positive

Blood bank informs you that there are very abnormal antibodies in addition to Rhesus antibodies, and there may well be a delay of a few hours until blood is available.

Which of the following should be considered?
a. Encourage frequent breast feeding
b. Immunoglobulin infusion
c. Phenobarbitone
d. Albumin
e. High intensity daylight fluorescent bulb phototherapy
f. Intravenous fluids
g. Metalloporphyrin treatment
h. Withhold vitamin K to reduce risk of added oxidative damage
i. Liver USS to exclude biliary atresia.

18. A midwife calls you to review a baby with the following. The parents are extremely anxious about the baby? What are you going to tell them?

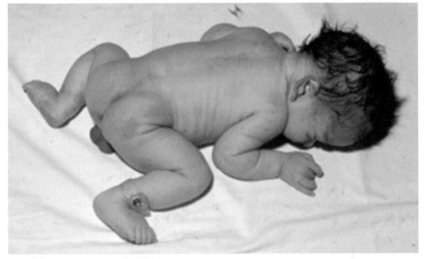

Figure 3.1

ANSWER 1

a. Prematurity is not a contraindication for immunisation. It is commonly thought that babies under a certain weight should not be immunised – this is also not the case.

b. Down syndrome (or any stable neurological condition) is not a contraindication for immunisation.[1]

c. Babies born to mothers with HIV must not be given BCG vaccine until the baby's serology is confirmed to be negative. There have been reports of dissemination of BCG in HIV positive individuals.[1]

d. Babies with chronic lung disease who are not receiving steroid treatment can receive the BCG vaccination.[1]

e. A family history of egg allergy is not a contraindication for BCG vaccination. Egg allergy is only a problem with yellow fever and influenza vaccines. There is increasing evidence that MMR vaccine can be given even to children with a history of previous anaphylaxis after egg ingestion.[1]

f. This is not contraindicated. There was previous speculation linking the MMR vaccine with inflammatory bowel disease but this evidence is not convincing.[1]

g. Babies who are receiving immunosuppressive doses of steroids, greater than 300 µg/kg/day of dexamethasone for at least one week (which is equivalent to 2 mg/kg/day prednisolone), should not receive live vaccines. Administration of live vaccines should be postponed for at least 3 months after immunosuppressive treatment has stopped.[1]

ANSWER 2

a. Vitamin K prevents vitamin K deficiency bleeding (VKDB – previously known as haemorrhagic disease of the newborn). Vitamin K is a fat soluble vitamin and humans have very low stores. Formula milk contains approximately 50 µg/mL which is more than 20 times higher than in breast milk. All babies have very low vitamin stores at birth and milk provides the only source until bacterial activity in the gut provides a secondary source. Deficiency is associated with a small but significant risk of serious bleeding in the newborn baby which can be prevented by postnatal administration of vitamin K. The incidence of classical (2–7 day) VKDB is 0.25–1.7% in infants who have not received postnatal vitamin K and is reduced to 2.7/100,000 infants given 1 mg orally at birth, 1 week and 1 month. Bleeding associated with vitamin K deficiency may be from mucosal surfaces, such as the gastrointestinal tract, and reversed by later vitamin K treatment. It may also be intracranial and associated with severe and irreversible brain damage. Early (first 24 hours) and late (2–8 weeks, although presentation 15 weeks after delivery has been reported) disease are classically manifest as intracranial bleeding.[2]

A paper published in 1992 suggested that babies who had received intramuscular vitamin K might be more likely to develop leukaemia.[3] Since then there have been more studies investigating the claim – a large analysis of data lead by the

Department of Health concluded that solid tumours were no commoner in children given intramuscular vitamin K at birth. The situation with regard to childhood leukaemia is less clear and it was felt that the situation was unlikely to be clarified by the collection of further data as all infants were now receiving prophylaxis. The increased risk, if real, is small (unadjusted odds ratio 1.25:95% CI 1.06–1.46), and this could be due to the fact that those selected for different modes of prophylaxis already had different risk factors for the later development of cancer. It must be acknowledged that it has not been possible to prove that no risk exists. This could only be proven by a controlled study that would not be possible either technically or ethically.

b. Yes it does. Maternal anticonvulsants, particularly phenobarbitone, phenytoin and carbamazepine, are reported to be associated with a significantly increased risk of VKDB, both early and classical. However, the risk appears relatively small. In a study measuring prothrombin times in 137 babies whose mothers were receiving phenobarbitone, phenytoin or carbamazepine, only 14 out of 105 babies born to mothers with therapeutic drug levels had prothrombin times above the normal range and none had an overt bleeding tendency. All reverted to normal within two hours of administration of 1 mg of parenteral vitamin K.[4] Sodium valproate does not appear to be associated with any coagulation abnormalities.

c. Infants with glucose-6-phosphate dehydrogenase (G6PD) deficiency may experience acute haemolytic episodes after exposure to identifiable pharmaceutical agents. Vitamin K1 has a potential as an oxidant substance and is frequently included in the list of drugs to be used with caution in this condition. However, a study observing the haemolysis rates in red cells incubated with a vitamin K1 preparation could show no difference in haemolysis between G6PD deficient and control red cells. The authors concluded that red blood cells in G6PD deficiency are not at increased risk of oxidative damage from vitamin K.[5]

ANSWER 3

a. Ultrasound of the spine and possible MRI.

b. Spinal dysraphism needs to be excluded.

Most infants with sacral dimples that fall within the natal cleft are healthy and have no associated abnormalities. 'High-risk' dimples are defined as those that are deep, larger than 0.5 cm, more than 2.5 cm from the anus or associated with other cutaneous markers, such as a fat pad, hairy patch or erythematous macule. One report shows that 40% of babies with atypical dimples have sacral dysraphism. Spinal dysraphisms are disorders of the caudal neural tube. They include a variety of anomalies ranging from tethered cord (commonest) to diastomatomyelia (a longitudinal cleft in the spinal cord which may be due to either a cartilaginous, fibrous or osseous bar). Symptoms are variable, and signs include sensory and motor deficits of the limbs, bladder and bowel dysfunction.

Ultrasound assesses the level of the conus of the spinal cord, and the presence of tethering. MRI is the superior investigation of choice and should be carried out if a baby is in the high-risk category.[6,7]

ANSWER 4

Answers **e** and **f** are correct.

Mothers only need to be separated from their newborn babies if they are considered to have infectious TB. This is unlikely unless the diagnosis was made very close to the date of delivery. There is no reason to recommend bottle feeding as the concentration of anti-tuberculosis drugs in breast milk is too low to constitute any problems, and therefore breast feeding should be encouraged. The child cannot be infected by the mother through breast milk but it must be noted that drugs in breast milk do not offer effective treatment for TB disease in a nursing infant.

Current recommendations are that infants should receive treatment if the mother has had less than two weeks of treatment herself, following confirmation of tuberculosis.[8] This should take the form of isoniazid 5 mg/kg and pyridoxine 5–10 mg daily in the first instance. Babies should not receive BCG initially but should have a tuberculin test at 6–12 weeks of age. If this is negative, medications may be discontinued and BCG given. If the skin test is positive, appropriate medication should be given for a total of six months. Isoniazid-resistant BCG is not required. BCG is said to be effective at reducing the chance of a child developing active disease by around 70–80%.

ANSWER 5

Answer **e** is correct.

Term infants pass meconium at or shortly after birth with sources quoting 95–98.5% passing the first stool within 24 hours after birth and 100% passage within 48 hours in normal infants. Of those who have not passed stool a relatively small proportion may have a significant underlying problem (Hirschsprung's disease affects around 1 in 5000 live births and these babies will represent approximately 1 in 250 of babies who have not passed meconium within the first 24 hours after birth).

The commonest cause of delayed passage of stool is meconium plug syndrome. In a radiological analysis of 133 infants with bowel obstruction, 66% had meconium plug syndrome, 20% had meconium ileus, and 18% had Hirschsprung's. Meconium plug syndrome is associated with a number of conditions all of which produce abnormal motility of the neonatal bowel. These conditions include pregnancy-induced hypertension, diabetes, magnesium sulphate or other tocolytic agents, prematurity, sepsis, hypothyroidism and other metabolic conditions.

Preterm infants are more likely to experience delay in passage of first stool. For those weighing less than 1500 g, just over 20% do not pass stool for 48 hours. For those weighing less than 1000 g, the median time for first passage is the third day, with 10% still not having passed stool at 12 days.[9,10]

Most people would advocate an abdominal X-ray, with review by a paediatric surgeon if there is any abnormality on the X-ray. Some people may delay this for 48 hours, provided the infant remains well.

ANSWER 6

a. Congenital hypoparathyroidism is one endocrine cause of an absent red reflex due to cataract.

b. Retinopathy of prematurity without plus disease does not cause an absent red reflex. Retinal detachment can cause loss of a red reflex but plus disease will have been present in this situation.

c. Congenital hyperparathyroidism does not cause an absent red reflex.

d. Hallermann–Streiff syndrome, also known as oculomandibulodyscephaly with hypotrichosis syndrome, is one of many syndromes in which cataract is either a common or occasional finding. Cataracts occur in 94% of cases of Hallermann–Streiff.

e. Persistence of the tunica vasculosa lentis will cause an abnormal red reflex.

Persistence of the tunica vasculosa lentis may be a normal finding reflecting delayed regression of a normal fetal vascular structure. In the majority of infants, regression of these vessels is usually complete by 34 weeks gestation. However, in a number of cases it may be associated with congenital infections including rubella and CMV, and it may also be found in premature infants with active ROP. All these infants should be referred for ophthalmological review.

Persistent hyperplastic primary vitreous is another congenital abnormality that leads to a white pupil. This is due to the embryonic vitreous failing to regress. At birth, a plaque of white tissue can be seen behind the lens. It may be associated with cataract, glaucoma and microphthalmia. Again urgent ophthalmological review is indicated for early surgery.

f. Retinal haemorrhages are variably reported to occur in 2.5–50% of all births. Approximately 50% of these occur unilaterally. When severe and widespread the red reflex may not appear normal. Limited data suggest these regress within 10 days and are not associated with any significant long-term problems.

g. Retinoblastoma presents with leukocoria, glaucoma and strabismus. This is the most common intraocular primary tumour of childhood with an incidence of 1 in 20,000 live births. Although the average age of diagnosis is 18 months, diagnosis has been made prenatally and in the early postnatal period. Retinoblastoma needs to be excluded as early treatment leads to a better outcome. Disease confined to the eye has a 98% 5-year disease-free survival.

h. Lowe syndrome consists of cataract, renal tubular acidosis, glaucoma, aminoaciduria and glycosuria. Therefore, the red reflex will be absent or abnormal.

i. Congenital glaucoma leads to epiphoria, photophobia and blepharospasm, and affected babies present with a cloudy cornea and enlargement of the eye. When corneal clouding is marked it may not be possible to elicit a red reflex. Again the prognosis depends on the age of onset and time to diagnosis.

j. CHARGE syndrome is classically associated with a coloboma. Retinal coloboma is the most common and again the red reflex will be abnormal.

Other causes of an absent red reflex are due to a cataract and there are many causes of this, ranging from viral (TORCH), metabolic (galactosaemia) and chromosomal (trisomy 13, 18 and 21) and Turner syndrome.

ANSWER 7

Answer **a** – *Staphylococcus aureus* is the most likely organism to cause conjunctivitis in this age group.

Conjunctivitis is a common neonatal infection occurring in 1–12% of all newborn infants and in a higher frequency in the developing world. The organisms responsible for causing conjunctivitis are isolated with a frequency given by the order of the organisms as listed in this question. *Staphylococcus aureus* is therefore the most common but may be present due to colonisation with no conjunctival reaction.

Chlamydia is becoming increasingly common and affects at least half of all infants born to a colonised mother. It is seen more often in the developing world. Infection may be associated with respiratory problems but is unlikely in this case as onset is usually 5–12 days after birth. It may start with one eye being affected and then becomes bilateral. Conventional cultures are negative and there is no response to usual treatment. The combination of these two factors usually prompts suspicion of Chlamydia. For the treatment of chlamydial ophthalmia or pneumonia, oral erythromycin and tetracycline eye drops for 2 weeks is recommended. However, in approximately 20–30% of infants, therapy will not eradicate the organism and the infant may require repeat treatment. There are a few published studies on the use of the new oral macrolide antibiotics, such as azithromycin, roxithromycin, or clarithromycin and these agents may be effective.[11,12]

Gonococcal conjunctivitis usually occurs earlier than four days, typically within 24 hours of delivery although late presentation has been reported. Copious purulent discharge is common and permanent damage may result. It is thus vital to make the diagnosis early and start treatment. A swab must be sent for both Gram stain and culture in enriched medium. Treatment used to be with systemic penicillin and penicillin eye drops, but now a single dose of intramuscular or intravenous ceftriaxone is used.[13]

Pseudomonal ophthalmia is a rare cause of neonatal conjunctivitis but can cause extreme damage to the eye. It causes a systemic infection along with conjunctivitis, and therefore requires intravenous antibiotics with review from ophthalmologists.

Herpes simplex is the commonest virus causing conjunctivitis but is a rare isolate. All purulent conjunctivitis need screening for the causative organisms and treatment with appropriate anti-microbial or anti-viral therapy. If not treated, neonatal conjunctivitis can have severe and permanent ophthalmological sequelae.

ANSWER 8

i. c, f and **g**

Risk factors can be identified in 40% of infants with DDH. Of these risk factors the most commonly documented are:

Positive family history. If there is one affected parent, there is a risk of 12% for the newborn infant. This rises to 36% if there has been a previous affected child as well as an affected parent.

Female sex. Girls are five times more likely to be affected than boys.

First-born child. There is an increased incidence in first-born Caucasian babies.

Oligohydramnios and macrosomia. These are both risk factors due to intra-uterine compression.

Breech presentation. The incidence is increased 10-fold if the breech presents with extended knees.

DDH is associated with other anomalies including talipes and torticollis.

ii. This infant should be referred for screening by an orthopaedic specialist due to the increased risk of DDH in the infant, as described above.

The finding of stable hips on examination is not a reassurance. Studies have reported up to 50% of cases of DDH being missed on routine examination and other reports have shown that very experienced senior personnel may be unable to detect DDH even when they know it to be present. All babies should therefore have their hips checked at any routine examination.

ANSWER 9

Answer **e** is correct.

This infant is thyrotoxic and requires urgent admission and treatment. Any other action may be too late as this is potentially an extremely dangerous condition. Free T4 is very high (normal range after day 3, 14–28 pmol/L) as is the total T4 (normal range 1–4 weeks, 106–214 pmol/L). TSH is still measurable and may be very difficult to interpret in the early neonatal period. The upper limit of normal may be as high as 120 mU/L on day 1 and then falls to lie within the normal range of 0.3–10 mU/L by 7 days. A value within these ranges cannot be taken to exclude hyperthyroidism within the neonatal period.

Transplacental passage of thyroid stimulating antibodies due to maternal Graves' disease is the commonest cause of neonatal thyrotoxicosis. When a mother is receiving thyroid suppressing drugs such as propylthiouracil, suppression of the features of hyperthyroidism may occur for several days following delivery. It is worth noting that symptoms may even develop when mothers have inactive Graves' disease or are hypothyroid on thyroid replacement therapy. Abnormalities of thyroid function have been detected in as many as 16.5% of babies born to mothers with Graves' disease, although a significantly smaller proportion are clinically thyrotoxic.

Severe hyperthyroidism is associated with significant mortality and these infants should therefore be referred for specialist treatment immediately. Propylthiouracil or carbimazole may be needed to suppress thyroid function and propranolol given to control peripheral stimulatory effects. Severely affected infants may require more intense treatment.

ANSWER 10

a. True – undescended testicle occurs in approximately 3% of babies born at term and in up to 33% of babies born prematurely. By 12 months, the incidence has fallen to around 1% (two-thirds will have resolved by this time). One-third are bilateral.

b. False – if undescended at 12 months, the testis is unlikely to descend after this time.

c. **False** – at least two-thirds of unilateral undescended testicles are palpable, usually within the inguinal canal or distal to the external ring.

d. **False** – the effect of orchidopexy on fertility is still debated but there is no doubt that impaired fertility may persist in some infants despite surgery. Biopsy of the testes at the time of orchidopexy shows abnormal histology, and abnormal testosterone levels have also been demonstrated in association with abnormal function of testicular cell lines. Patients with a history of UDT have subnormal semen analysis but equivalent paternity rates if unilateral. Fertility is severely impaired with bilateral UDT giving paternity rates of approximately 50%, unaffected by early surgical correction.

e. **False** – studies have demonstrated an increased risk of testicular malignancy of 7.4–60-fold; 15–20% of tumours arise in the normally descended contralateral testis. Orchidopexy does not appear to reduce this risk but does facilitate detection.

f. **False** – there is an increased incidence of torsion in undescended testes but this an uncommon complication.

g. **False** – hormonal replacement is controversial and is not a routine part of management. Trials combining buserelin and HCG have been associated with an increased descent rate but this remains an experimental treatment.

h. **True** – UDT is associated with a number of anomalies including epididymal abnormalities, hypospadias, posterior urethral vales and anomalies of the upper urinary tract. There is some evidence to suggest that both UDT and the anomaly may be due to abnormalities in fetal testosterone levels.

ANSWER 11

a. You need to refer this baby for specialist assessment. Talipes occur with an incidence of 1 in 1000 live births, with a male to female ratio of 2–4:1; 50% are bilateral. External compression in utero is responsible for postural talipes, but in these cases the neutral position can normally be obtained by manipulation. Abnormalities in ligaments and tendons, neural dysfunction, abnormal muscle development and defects in the development of bones of the foot have been associated with more severe forms of talipes and intervention is required in these cases. Treatment should begin as early as is practically possible and thus early referral is important. Stretching exercises should be commenced and continued. In more severe cases or those failing to respond to conservative treatment, serial plaster casts are required followed by tenotomy and prolonged splinting. Failure to respond to this treatment may require more complex surgical procedures.

b. In the long term, although functional recovery is good and only a small number require salvage surgery, the majority will have a foot that is not morphologically normal. It must be appreciated that the condition does not just affect the foot but the whole lower limb as a unit and a small calf and foot are normal features. There will commonly be some residual functional deficit, which only major surgery could possibly correct. This degree of surgical intervention is not felt to be warranted for the extra gain obtained.

ANSWER 12

a. **False** – pyloric stenosis occurs in 1–3% of live births. If a mother has had this condition, the incidence is 19% in male offspring and 7% in female offspring. It only occurs in 5% of boys and 2.5% of girls when the father was affected. It is 15 times more likely to occur in siblings of affected infants. It is frequently said to be commoner in first-born male offspring but this is disputed. The risk is lower with increased maternal age, higher maternal education and low birth weight.[14]

b. **True** – the male to female ratio of 4:1 remains constant despite varying estimates of incidence.

c. **False** – these are not indicated in the absence of symptoms.

d. **False** – this has never been described.

e. **True** – there is no evidence to suggest that manipulation of feeding regimes may influence onset of symptoms.

f. **False** – atropine treatment has been shown to be effective in small studies. Treatment results in a decrease in pyloric muscle thickness and in projectile vomiting. Although this has been reported in several studies, in both human and veterinary practice, it has not achieved widespread acceptance.[15]

g. **True** – major associations are malrotation, obstructive uropathy and oesophageal atresia. Other anomalies associated with pyloric stenosis include hiatus hernia and a deficiency in hepatic glucuronyl transferase activity similar to that seen in Gilbert's syndrome.

ANSWER 13

a. **False** – in the absence of a significantly elevated conjugated bilirubin, liver USS is not indicated.

b. **False** – as above.

c. **True** – assessment of haemoglobin with a full blood count and a screen would be a useful investigation at this stage.

d. **False** – this may be indicated in secondary assessment if haemolysis is thought to be a significant component.

e. **True** – to rule out infection which may present as prolonged jaundice.

f. **True** – to exclude galactosaemia.

g. **True** – this is normally recommended but every infant will have had a Guthrie test to rule out hypothyroidism. There is no evidence to suggest that this test misses infants who have developed unconjugated jaundice.

h. **False** – conditions such as elliptocytosis and spherocytosis can cause unconjugated hyperbilirubinaemia. However, both are rare, and unlikely to be relevant in the absence of other family history or evidence of haemolysis.

i. **False** – blood cultures are not indicated in the absence of other observations suggestive of sepsis.

j. **False** – UDPGT levels are used to exclude Crigler–Najjar syndrome, which even in its mild form is associated with severe jaundice and is difficult to treat.

k. **False** – although this test is possible, the condition is mild and self-limiting, and is generally not thought to warrant specific screening.

ANSWER 14

A conjugated bilirubinaemia greater than 25–30 μmol/L or 10% of total serum bilirubin is said to be significant.

Although pale stools and dark urine are characteristic of established conjugated jaundice, they may not be seen in the first 3–4 weeks after birth and therefore cannot be taken as definite indication of non-obstructive causes. Other causes of prolonged jaundice should be considered including alpha-1-anti-trypsin deficiency, cystic fibrosis, congenital infection, amino acidaemias, congenital hypopituitarism and biliary atresia.

ANSWER 15

Answer **f** is correct.

Cystic dilatation of the common bile duct, diverticulum of the bile duct and choledochocele with intrahepatic extension are all types of choledochal cyst. Of these, the commonest is cystic dilatation of the common bile duct. Choledochal cysts are four times more likely to found in girls compared to boys, and usually present within the first 10 years of life. In children, the features of abdominal pain, jaundice and abdominal mass only occur in one-third. In the case under discussion, the bile ducts are present and therefore the proximal biliary ductal system is either normal or enlarged. This is in contrast to the findings in biliary atresia where the bile ducts may be difficult to visualise. There may be substantial distal obstruction of the biliary tract in various forms of choledochal cysts.

ANSWER 16

Answer **c** is most appropriate.

This baby could have biliary atresia and there is very good evidence that the efficacy of surgical treatment decreases progressively with time. Biliary atresia involves progressive obliteration and sclerosis of bile ducts, and a major determinant of satisfactory outcome following porto-enterostomy is the patient's age at operation. In one series reporting outcome for 131 infants, long-term survival rate was 46% if operated on within the first 2.5 months after birth, compared with 24% for those where surgery was later than this.[16]

Other answers:

a. **False** – you have not excluded biliary atresia with these investigations and to leave for a further 4 weeks is not appropriate.

b. **False** – the ultrasound scan has failed to give you a diagnosis and repeating the scan may delay diagnosis further. The presence of a gall bladder on ultrasound does not exclude biliary atresia and may well be a persistent observation initially.

d. **False**.

e. **False** – though a HIDA scan is indicated, it would be more appropriate for referral to the specialist team who will continue the management of the baby, and organise further warranted investigations.

ANSWER 17

a. **False** – adequate hydration is essential and although breast milk is not contraindicated, it is not sensible to rely upon breast feeding to maintain this. Feed volumes during early postnatal breast feeding are very variable and hydration may be relatively poor. Furthermore, breast feeding will compromise phototherapy, which in this situation should be continuous and at maximum efficacy.

b. **True** – treatment of severe Rhesus or ABO isoimmunisation with high dose intravenous immunoglobulin has been shown to significantly reduce the need for exchange transfusion, duration of phototherapy and length of hospital stay. A single 0.5 g/kg dose on day one is effective.[17]

c. **False** – phenobarbitone may increase the rate of bilirubin conjugation by induction of hepatic enzymes. Treatment of mothers antenatally, and of babies postnatally, may result in a significant reduction in serum bilirubin levels. Since first reported in 1968, barbiturates have frequently been used in pregnancy and the neonatal period, but the lack of specificity of action and the significant risk of adverse side effects (depression of vitamin K clotting factors and respiratory depression) mean that current recommendations are that this form of treatment should only be used in exceptional circumstance when no other effective treatment modalities are available.

d. **False** – bilirubin is transported in the plasma tightly bound to albumin and the portion that is unbound, or loosely bound, can more readily leave the intravascular space and cross the intact blood–brain barrier. Elevations in the levels of unbound bilirubin (UB) have been associated with kernicterus in sick preterm newborns. Although it is acknowledged that albumin is important for bilirubin binding, there is no consensus as to whether routine administration of albumin is indicated in hyperbilirubinaemia. In infants who are hypoalbuminaemic, it seems prudent to make sure albumin levels are in the normal range to improve bilirubin binding and thus potentially decrease the passage of bilirubin across the blood–brain barrier causing damage. However, there is no evidence that raising albumin levels into a supra-normal range has added benefit.

The American Academy of Pediatrics states that the risk of bilirubin encephalopathy is unlikely to be a simple function of the total serum bilirubin level or the concentration of UB but is more likely a combination of both.[18]

e. **False** – daylight fluorescent bulbs provide suboptimal benefit. Light of a wavelength between 425 and 475 nm is thought to be most effective, and light in the blue region of the spectrum is thus most commonly used. Daylight tubes emit light at wavelengths of 300–700 nm but do not have a higher output in the blue spectrum. Green light may also be effective. Although the wavelength of green light is outside the optimal range, it penetrates further into the skin and may be more efficient at conversion of bilirubin to lumirubin than blue light. These bulbs are available but are not widely used. The minimal effective irradiance of phototherapy is 5 microwatts/cm^2/nm with reported increase in effectiveness up to 40 microwatts/cm^2/nm. This will be influenced by the nature of the phototherapy unit and by the distance from the infant.

f. **True** – adequate hydration is essential in the early postnatal period, and intravenous fluids may be the only way of ensuring this occurs.

g. **False** – the use of synthetic metalloporphyrins has been shown to be extremely effective in the management of jaundice in both preterm and term infants. These act through competitive inhibition of haem oxygenase and have been shown to reduce the need for exchange transfusion and the length of phototherapy. Although efficacy has been demonstrated, data on long-term safety is awaited. These products are not currently available in the UK but are available in the USA.

h. **False** – vitamin K should be given immediately after birth.

i. **False** – at this stage no radiological investigations are indicated unless the conjugated bilirubin is extremely high. This is unlikely in Rhesus disease.

ANSWER 18

Mongolian blue spots are flat birthmarks with blue-grey pigmentation, usually on the base of the spine, the buttocks and back and even sometimes on the ankles or wrists. The distinctive skin discoloration is due to the deep placement of the pigment and results from entrapment of melanocytes in the dermis during their migration from the neural crest into the epidermis

They are extremely common especially in Asian, East Indian, African and Latino heritage. They may be seen in about 10% of Caucasians and up to 90% of African–Americans. They typically disappear spontaneously within four years but can persist for life. No sex predilection is reported.

They commonly appear at birth or shortly after birth and look like bruises. They must therefore be documented well in the notes and parents should be made aware that they are present and that they are of no consequence. However they should be aware that others may still see them as bruises and raise concerns.

Several associations have been documented, e.g. cleft lip, melanoma, Hunter's syndrome. There is no long-term morbidity or mortality associated with them when an isolated finding.

REFERENCES

1. Department of Health. The Green Book – Immunisation against infectious disease. DoH, London, 2006
2. Hey E. Vitamin K – what, why, and when. Arch Dis Child Fetal Neonatal Ed 2003;88:F80–F83
3. Golding J, Greenwood R, Birmingham K et al. Childhood cancer, intramuscular vitamin K, and pethidine given during labour. BMJ 1992;305:341–46
4. Hey E. Effect of maternal anticonvulsant treatment on neonatal blood coagulation. Arch Dis Child 1999;81:F208–F210
5. Kaplan M, Waisman D, Mazor D et al. Effect of vitamin K1 on glucose-6-phosphate dehydrogenase deficient neonatal erythrocytes in vitro. Arch Dis Child Fetal Neonatal Ed 1998;79:F218–F220

6. Kriss VM, Dessai NS. Occult spinal dysraphism in neonates: assessment of high-risk cutaneous stigmata on sonography. Am J Radiol 1998;171:1687–92

7. Higgins JC, Axelsen F. Simple dimple rule for sacral dimples. Am Fam Phys 2002;65(12):2435

8. Health Protection Agency. Pregnancy and tuberculosis, guidance for clinicians. HPA, London, 2006

9. Fletcher MA. Physical diagnosis in neonatology. Lippincott-Raven, New York, 1998

10. Ashcroft K. Pediatric surgery. WB Saunders, Philadelphia, 2000

11. Darville T. *Chlamydia trachomatis* infections in neonates and young children. Semin Pediatr Infect Dis 2005;16(4):235–44

12. Zar HJ. Neonatal chlamydial infections: prevention and treatment. Paediatr Drugs 2005;7(2):103–10

13. Centers for Disease Control and Prevention. MMWR Recommendations and Reports. 2002;51:1–78

14. Applegate MS, Druschel CM. The epidemiology of infantile hypertrophic pyloric stenosis in New York State, 1983 to 1990. Arch Pediatr Adolesc Med 1995;149:1123–29

15. Kawahara H, Imura K, Nishikawa M et al. Intravenous atropine treatment in infantile hypertrophic pyloric stenosis. Arch Dis Child 2002;87:71–74

16. Grosfeld JL, Fitzgerald JF, Predaina R et al. The efficacy of hepatoportoenterostomy in biliary atresia. Surgery 1989;106:692–701

17. Gottstein R, Cooke RW. Systematic review of intravenous immunoglobulin in haemolytic disease of the newborn. Arch Dis Child Fetal Neonatal Ed 2003;88:F6–F10

18. Subcommittee on Hyperbilirubinemia. Management of hyperbilirubinemia in the newborn infant 35 or more weeks of gestation. Pediatrics 2004;114:297–316

Chapter 4

Fluid and electrolytes

Problems with fluid and electrolyte balance are common in the neonatal population. After birth there are rapid changes in the physiology of newborn infants which are essential if they are to cope with the change from an intra-uterine to an extra-uterine environment. The infant's renal system is susceptible to maternal drugs and may be influenced by changing conditions in the first few days of postnatal life. After birth, sodium and water balance can be problematic as the newborn infant has a limited ability to excrete sodium in the first days after birth, followed by an inability to retain sodium later on. This is compounded by problems with insensible water loss which occur due to a variety of factors including transepidermal loss due to skin immaturity, respiratory losses, and evaporative losses due to exposure to radiant heaters. Such losses may be very difficult to estimate accurately. Preterm infants frequently require medications during their stay on the neonatal unit and several of the more commonly used drugs can affect renal function and can lead to electrolyte imbalance.

This chapter covers the common problems of fluid balance and management of infants with electrolyte disturbances that are faced on a daily basis. Other topics covered in this chapter are problems with glucose metabolism and inborn errors of metabolism.

QUESTION 1

The following maternal drugs cause acute renal failure in a baby (answer true or false):
- **i)** Ibuprofen
- **ii)** Aspirin
- **iii)** Losartan
- **iv)** Celecoxib
- **v)** Gentamicin
- **vi)** Captopril.

QUESTION 2

A baby born at 24 weeks gestation is being nursed on a platform with an overhead radiant heater. His birth weight is 600 g and he is receiving a total fluid of 1.5 mL/h. He is now 24 hours old and his blood results are as follows:

Na	149 mmol/L
K	4.5 mmol/L

Urea	9.4 mmol/L
Creat	91 μmol/L
SBR	85 μmol/L
CRP	10 mg/L

His urine output has been 3.5 mL since birth.

    i) What is the most likely cause for this result?

        a. Postnatal diuresis

        b. Inappropriate ADH secretion

        c. Inadequate water intake

        d. Excessive water losses

        e. Acute renal failure

        f. Sepsis.

    ii) What action would you take to improve the situation? Give two answers.

The next day, his blood results are as follows:

Na	145 mmol/L
K	3.7 mmol/L
Urea	8.4 mmol/L
Creat	80 μmol/L
SBR	160 μmol/L

At this point the baby is on 120 mL/kg/day of 10% dextrose. His urine output has been 8 mL over the last 24 hours.

    iii) Which of the following actions do you take next? Choose one answer.

        a. Restrict fluid intake

        b. Increase fluid intake to 150 mL/kg/day

        c. Add additional sodium

        d. Challenge with fluid bolus and diuretics

        e. Observe and repeat U+E in 12 hours.

The next day his fluids are increased to 180 mL/kg/day. A loud systolic murmur becomes audible and pulses are bounding. Echocardiography shows evidence of a large ductus.

Urine output has been 18 mL over the last 24 hours. The following electrolytes are obtained:

Na	139 mmol/L
K	3.9 mmol/L
Urea	6.4 mmol/L
Creat	70 μmol/L

    iv) a. What changes would you make to his fluid regime?

        b. Would you add sodium and potassium to his fluids?

Over the next 24 hours the baby's respiratory condition deteriorates. A chest X-ray suggests moderate enlargement of the heart and a degree of pulmonary oedema. It is felt that the PDA is contributing significantly and the decision is made to commence indomethacin 0.6 mg/kg for 3 days. 24 hours later, the baby is thought to be more oedematous and the urine output has fallen to 0.4 mL/kg/hour with the following electrolytes:

Na	130 mmol/L
K	4.2 mmol/L
Urea	8.1 mmol/L
Creat	92 μmol/L

v) What do you think the most likely cause is for the current results?

vi) What action would you take?

vii) Which of the following measures of renal function could be helpful in distinguishing between prerenal and ischaemic acute renal failure?

    a. Sodium
    b. Potassium
    c. Urea
    d. Creatinine
    e. Urine output
    f. Urine osmolality
    g. Urine microscopy
    h. Urine sodium
    i. Fractional excretion of sodium.

viii) At the age of 72 hours, you notice that his urine output is now 2.7 mL/kg/hour and his ventilation has significantly improved. Why is this?

QUESTION 3

You are asked to review a baby on the postnatal wards who is now 3 days old. Mum has had a caesarean section for failure to progress and is breast feeding the baby. The midwives are concerned that the baby is jaundiced. Birth weight 3.6 kg. On examination the baby is obviously jaundiced and is quiet.

i) What investigations/observations would you request?

The midwife has performed a test feed and thinks that a reasonable feed intake was achieved. She has weighed the baby before and after the feed.

ii) Does this help?

The investigations from a capillary blood sample reveal:

Na	157 mmol/L
K	5.6 mmol/L
Urea	12.8 mmol/L
Creat	95 μmol/L
SBR	286 μmol/L (unconjugated 6)
CRP	8 mg/L
WBC	11.6 × 10^9 (neutrophils 9.1)

Platelets	242×10^9
Hb	21.5×10^9
Film	normal
HCT	68%
Weight	2.9 kg

iii) What is your first action?

Venous sample has comparable results with an HCT of 68%.

iv) What is the most important immediate action? Choose one answer.

    a. Dilutional exchange transfusion

    b. Glucose and insulin

    c. ECG monitoring

    d. Lumbar puncture

    e. Intravenous fluids

    f. NG feed.

v) How would you treat the baby? Which fluids would you consider using in immediate rehydration?

    a. 10% dextrose

    b. 5% dextrose

    c. 0.9% saline

    d. 0.45% saline

    e. 0.18% saline / 5% dextrose.

vi) What complications can occur if this is not treated? List four.

QUESTION 4

You are called to see a baby on transitional care who was born at 36 weeks gestation, weighing 1.8 kg. The baby is now 4 hours old and had a bottle feed of 40 mL of formula milk an hour ago. The blood glucose is 1.8 mmol/L.

i) What action would you take?

    a. Do nothing and reassure mum

    b. Give another bottle feed and repeat blood glucose measurement

    c. Carry out true laboratory glucose

    d. Carry out full hypoglycaemia screen

    e. Give bolus of intravenous dextrose

    f. Give intramuscular glucagon.

Another bottle feed is offered and the infant takes a further 30 mL. A repeat blood glucose an hour later is 1.4 mmol/L.

ii) What action would you take?

You are unable to establish an intravenous infusion. The infant starts to vomit and repeat blood glucose is 0.8 mmol/L.

iii) What action could you take to improve blood glucose while you are waiting for senior help?

iv) What action must you ensure happens within the next hour?

v) What other action should have been taken when the blood glucose was 0.8 mmol/L?

The baby is admitted to the neonatal unit and an infusion of 12.5% dextrose at 120 mL/kg/day is required to maintain the blood glucose above 2.6 mmol/L.

vi) What practical action should you take in regard to the baby's high concentration of dextrose solution?

vii) Is this glucose infusion rate abnormally high?

viii) What is the most likely reason for this infant's hypoglycaemia?

QUESTION 5

A term baby has suffered an asphyxial episode requiring full resuscitation at birth. Spontaneous respiration was not seen for 36 hours after birth although the heart rate had returned within 8 minutes of resuscitation.

A markedly abnormal CFAM was recorded and fits were treated with phenobarbitone, phenytoin and a midazolam infusion. The baby is now semi-comatose and breathing spontaneously and fitting has stopped. The baby has both a UVC and a UAC in situ.

Initial fluid replacement was 40 mL/kg/day of 10% dextrose with no additives and has been increased on day 3 to 90 mL/kg/day. Routine U+E analysis gives the following results.

Na	124 mmol/L
K	3.6 mmol/L
Urea	4.1 mmol/L
Creat	35 μmol/L

i) What explanation may account for this result? Choose the best answer.
- **a.** Acute renal failure
- **b.** Iatrogenic fluid overload
- **c.** SIADH
- **d.** Diabetes insipidus
- **e.** Iatrogenic electrolyte depletion
- **f.** Abnormal maternal electrolytes.

ii) What in the history supports your favoured diagnosis?

iii) Which of the following observations would be most helpful? Choose three answers.
- **a.** Urine output
- **b.** Blood pressure
- **c.** ECG
- **d.** Capillary refill time
- **e.** Skin turgor
- **f.** Heart rate
- **g.** Temperature
- **h.** Toe–core temperature differential.

iv) Which of the following investigations would be most helpful? Choose two.

    a. Urinary sodium

    b. Urinary osmolality

    c. Fractional excretion of sodium

    d. Serial plasma sodium

    e. Renin-angiotensin-aldosterone measurements

    f. Renal ultrasound

    g. Serum ADH levels

    h. Plasma osmolality.

QUESTION 6

A 2-day-old term baby has a total plasma calcium of 1.7 mmol/L; ionised calcium is 0.65 mmol/L. The baby is well.

i) Which of the following is the most likely? Choose one answer.

    a. Normal phenomenon

    b. Pseudohyperparathyroidism

    c. Infant of diabetic mother

    d. Maternal elevated vitamin D intake

    e. Exchange transfusion

    f. Diuretic therapy

    g. Hypoalbuminaemia

    h. Maternal hypoparathyroidism

    i. Low calcium intake

    j. Perinatal asphyxia

    k. PTH resistance

    l. Hypoparathyroidism

    m. IUGR

    n. Maternal anticonvulsants

    o. Maternal anti-TB therapy.

ii) Explain why you feel the other diagnoses are less likely.

iii) How do you treat the baby?

QUESTION 7

A preterm infant born at 28 weeks received one week of diuretic therapy following diagnosis of a PDA. The clinical course thereafter was uneventful. A renal ultrasound performed at 36 weeks corrected gestational age (as part of the screen for suspected UTI) revealed bilateral nephrocalcinosis.

The parents want to know how this has happened and what the long-term consequences are for their baby. What will you tell them?

QUESTION 8

A term baby is born following a severe antepartum haemorrhage and requires full resuscitation. A diagnosis of hypoxic–ischaemic encephalopathy is made. At 48 hours the baby is still ventilated because of a lack of respiratory effort. The following ECG is obtained.

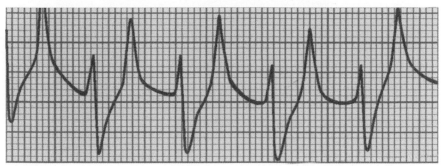

Figure 4.1

i) What does this show?

ii) What is the underlying cause?

iii) What is the treatment? Give six key elements.

QUESTION 9

A baby suddenly collapses on the postnatal ward at the age of 36 hours. Prior to collapse, his feeding had deteriorated and he had started to vomit. On examination the baby is lethargic and tachypnoeic. Examination is unremarkable.

i) What is your differential diagnosis? Give four possibilities.

You bring the baby round to the neonatal unit and commence intravenous fluids and start antibiotics. Basic investigations are performed and results are as follows:

CXR	Normal
Hb	17.4 g/dL
WCC	9.4×10^9/L
Plat	351×10^9/L
CRP	11.3 mg/L
Blood glucose	3.2 mmol/L

The baby deteriorates and becomes more lethargic and drowsy.

ii) What urgent investigations would you now consider? Give four.

While awaiting the results of these investigations the baby becomes more tachypnoeic with marked recession. There is a sudden dramatic deterioration. Oxygen saturations fall to <40% and heart rate to <30.

iii) What differential diagnoses do you consider?

The following chest X-ray is obtained.

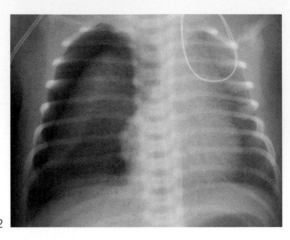

Figure 4.2

iv) What does it show and what would you do?

While dealing with this problem the results of your other investigations return; the results obtained are as follows:

Echocardiogram	Normal
Ammonia	350 μmol/L
Lactate	3.4 mmol/L
Capillary blood gas	pH 7.48
PCO_2	2.1 kPa
PO_2	3.2 kPa
BE	−8.0 mmol/L
Bic	15.5 mEq/L

v) What is the most likely diagnosis? Choose one answer.

    a. Sepsis
    b. Transient hyperammonaemia of the newborn
    c. Organic acid defect
    d. Fatty acid oxidation defect
    e. Urea cycle defect
    f. Congenital heart disease.

vi) What would be the basis of your management? Explain your decisions.

vii) What would you say to the parents?

QUESTION 10

A baby is found to have an anion gap of 27 mmol/L with an acidosis. Which two of the following are likely causes?

    a. Propionic acidaemia
    b. Phenylketonuria
    c. Renal tubular acidosis
    d. MCAD

e. Maple syrup disease

f. Total villous atrophy.

QUESTION 11

Which of the following could cause an elevation in lactic acid in a term baby?

a. Hypoxia

b. Cardiac disease

c. Infection

d. Convulsions

e. Breath holding

f. Pyruvate dehydrogenase deficiency

g. Fructose-1,6-bisphosphatase deficiency

h. Mitochondrial defects

i. Urea cycle defect

j. Ornithine transcarbamylase deficiency.

QUESTION 12

A term baby weighing 5.2 kg is born by caesarean section. Hairy ears are noted and the infant appears macrosomic. Blood glucose is measured and is 0.1 mmol/L one hour after birth.

The baby is brought round to the neonatal unit for further management. Several attempts are made at siting a peripheral cannula with no success.

i) What action do you take?

ii) There is a suggestion to give a bolus of 10% dextrose. Should you give this?

After one hour of the dextrose infusion, the blood glucose is checked again and is still 0.1 mmol/L. The baby remains asymptomatic.

iii) What do you do now?

By the age of 4 hours, the baby is on 15% dextrose at a rate of 7 mL/kg/hr and the blood glucose remains low at 0.5 mmol/L.

iv) What action do you take? Give three answers.

v) What other medications may help?

vi) What is the most likely diagnosis in this baby?

ANSWER 1

i) **True** – non-steroidal anti-inflammatory drugs are known to cause acute renal failure in neonates secondary to vascular damage.

ii) **False** – Aspirin is the most commonly ingested drug in pregnancy either as a single drug or in combination with other drugs. It may cause problems with increased perinatal mortality, intrauterine growth restriction and decreased albumin binding capacity, and can also affect the clotting ability of the newborn with reports of increased incidence of intracranial haemorrhage. There are however no data reporting renal failure in neonates after use in the mother.

iii) True – losartan is an angiotensin II receptor antagonist that has many similar properties to those of ACE inhibitors. It is used for the treatment of hypertension. Unlike ACE inhibitors, it does not inhibit the breakdown of bradykinin and other kinins which cause the persistent dry cough which commonly complicates ACE inhibitor therapy.

iv) True – COX-2 inhibitors are newly developed drugs for inflammation that selectively block the COX-2 enzyme. Blocking this enzyme impedes the production of prostaglandins. During renal development, immunoreactive COX-2 is first observed in mid-gestation embryonic stages, notably in cells undergoing induction and/or morphogenesis and for the duration of nephrogenesis.

It has been shown in animal models of the postnatal kidney that COX-2 expression is relatively low at birth, increases in the first two postnatal weeks, and then gradually declines to low levels. This expression pattern of COX-2 in the developing kidney is of interest because of the evidence that COX metabolites play important functional and developmental roles in the fetal kidney. Although a full set of glomeruli is achieved by 34 weeks of pregnancy, glomerular and tubular maturation goes on up to 2 months into postnatal life. COX-2 inhibitors used in the last part of pregnancy can adversely affect the maturation of tubules and cause renal failure which can be irreversible.

v) False – although gentamicin can be nephrotoxic in the neonatal period, requiring monitoring of levels, no problems have been reported as a result of maternal gentamicin. Gentamicin is an aminoglycoside antibiotic that can cross the placenta and enter the fetal circulation. No toxicity has been seen in newborns whose mothers received gentamicin, and there have been no links with congenital defects.

vi) True – captopril, which is an angiotensin-converting enzyme inhibitor, also causes ARF. Use of ACEIs during the second and third trimesters of pregnancy has been associated with a pattern of defects known as ACEI fetopathy. The predominant feature of the fetopathy is renal tubular dysplasia. Other associated conditions include intra-uterine growth retardation (IUGR) and patent ductus arteriosus (PDA). These features may be related to fetal hypotension secondary to ACEI-induced decreases in fetal angiotensin or increased bradykinin.

ANSWER 2

i) Inadequate water intake is the most likely explanation for these results. The majority of babies become oliguric in the early postnatal period and a diuresis is unlikely in the first 24 hours. This urine output is less than 0.25 mL/kg/h, signifying oliguria. Normal value would be greater than 1 mL/kg/h. Inappropriate ADH secretion does occur but is an uncommon phenomenon and usually is found in association with other significant problems (see below). A fluid intake of 60 mL/kg/day is insufficient for a preterm baby who has high insensible losses. Nursing on a platform is almost certainly the most serious contributory factor in this baby. Insensible losses will be extremely high and impossible to quantify. Transepidermal water loss may be as high as $60 g/m^2/h$ in a baby born at 24 weeks' gestation.

Acute renal failure may well develop in this infant if fluid balance is not corrected but is unlikely to be the primary cause at present. Sepsis is always a possibility but most preterm babies would be on prophylactic antibiotics in view of preterm delivery.

ii) a. Nursing the baby in an incubator with high humidity is the best method of reducing insensible losses.
b. Increasing daily fluid intake to 80–100 mL/kg/day or higher, with frequent monitoring of electrolytes, urine output and, wherever possible, weight.

iii) Answer **b** is correct. The baby's urine output is still low and his electrolytes suggest that he is still receiving an inadequate amount of water. Further restriction of fluid intake will almost certainly precipitate acute prerenal failure. Adding additional sodium would exacerbate the hypernatraemia that is already present. Although a fluid bolus might be beneficial in this situation, the combination with a diuretic would be likely to further exacerbate renal problems. Action must be taken at this stage and waiting for 12 hours to repeat the electrolytes will almost certainly show a further increase in the sodium levels.

iv) It is likely that this baby is starting to enter the polyuric phase that many preterm babies have after their initial oliguria. Urine output is reasonable at 1.4 mL/kg/h; urea and electrolytes are normalising. Appropriate management would be to maintain the same fluid intake but carefully monitor urine output and U+E. It is likely that sodium and potassium will continue to fall and it would therefore be appropriate to commence supplementation at 1–2 mmol/kg/day.

v) This baby was already in a degree of heart failure which will have compromised renal perfusion. Indomethacin may well have lead to a marked decrease in renal perfusion and has precipitated acute renal failure. It is however also possible that this baby has become dehydrated because urine losses during the polyuria were not being matched by replacement.

vi) It would be prudent to discontinue indomethacin as there is a strong possibility that this is responsible for the deterioration. However, if it was felt that cardiac function was being seriously compromised by the PDA, the alternatives of low dose indomethacin or ibuprofen could be used.

Urine output has decreased almost certainly due to poor renal perfusion and it would therefore be sensible to reduce fluid intake to prevent further haemodilution.

vii) Sodium, potassium, urea and creatinine are unlikely to help differentiate between the prerenal and ischaemic acute renal failure. All may reflect a variable combination of dilution and impaired renal function.

A more detailed assessment of renal function may help differentiate between the two causes:

Urinalysis is usually normal in prerenal failure and although it may be normal in established acute renal failure, cellular debris and granular casts may be seen.

Urine volume is always decreased in prerenal failure and is likely to change from decreased to normal or even raised as acute renal failure becomes established.

Urine sodium is normally low (<20 mmol/L) in prerenal failure and may increase above this in established renal failure.

Fractional excretion of sodium is less than 2% in prerenal failure and greater than 2–3% in acute renal failure.

Urine osmolality is elevated to above 350 mOsmol/L in prerenal failure and is reduced due to water retention in established renal failure.

These observations reflect the fact that the renal tubules are still functioning in prerenal failure and are able to retain some salt and excrete some water. In acute renal failure these functions are lost and therefore sodium losses will be higher and haemoconcentration will be poor. In a very premature baby, these results may be more difficult to interpret as the underlying renal function may well have been poor before renal failure intervened.

viii) Premature infants often enter a diuretic phase associated with an increase in GFR and a transient increase in the fractional excretion of sodium. The polyuric phase usually starts between 24 and 48 hours although a range of 12–100 hours has been quoted. This is then followed by an adaptive phase during which the GFR decreases and urine output parallels fluid intake.[1]

The surfactant-deficient lung, with damaged epithelial and endothelial barriers, is susceptible to water accumulation. Lung gas exchange in babies with hyaline membrane disease is further compromised when total body water intake exceeds renal and insensible losses. The onset of diuresis heralds an improvement in lung function and oxygenation.

ANSWER 3

i) U + E, SBR (split), CRP, FBC and film, blood glucose and blood cultures would be the investigations of choice. The weight should also be requested to compare with birth weight.

ii) No, this does not help. In the past, this was a frequently performed practice. It is now no longer widely used and there are reports suggesting accuracy and precision are such that it cannot be relied upon.[2] This has been disputed however, and there are authorities who claim that the use of accurate scales may provide reliable information.[3]

iii) Repeating the blood test urgently with a venous sample. A capillary sample may give misleadingly high values particularly if there is a degree of dehydration.

iv) This baby is suffering from hypernatraemic dehydration and is at considerable risk of developing problems. This is a serious complication of breast feeding and results from the combination of inadequate fluid intake and persistence of high milk sodium concentrations secondary to poor milk drainage from the breast.[4] A recent paper has shown an incidence of 1.9% in term or near term babies that was increased in primiparous women.[5] The most common presenting symptom was jaundice in over 80% of cases, and lethargy and fever are also common. It can be difficult in these babies to pick up dehydration clinically as hypernatraemic dehydration leads to better preservation of extracellular volume and therefore less pronounced signs of dehydration. Weight loss is a much easier way to pick up inadequate feeding and dehydration. Although a dilutional exchange transfusion may be warranted for an elevated haematocrit, particularly if the infant is symptomatic, it is appropriate to increase fluid intake first and reassess the effect on the haematocrit.

v) Rehydration should commence with normal saline. The elevated plasma sodium in the baby will have been accompanied by natriuresis and elevated urinary sodium. Although plasma sodium is high, the baby will be sodium deficient. Electrolytes should be monitored closely and the amount of sodium chloride in the resuscitation fluid adjusted accordingly. Rehydration with fluids without sodium chloride will lead to hyponatraemia that may be sudden in onset. Fluid replacement should not be performed at an abnormally high rate as this may precipitate cerebral oedema due to rapid shifts in extracellular water. A resuscitation volume of 20–30 mL/kg of normal saline over 60 minutes should be used. Subsequent rehydration should be with either normal saline or a saline/dextrose mixture so as to reduce the serum sodium at a rate that should not exceed 12 mmol/L/day.[6]

vi) Seizures, intracranial haemorrhage, vascular thrombosis, death.

ANSWER 4

i) Answer **b** is correct.

ii) It is unlikely that the baby will take any more milk as he has just taken 70 mL. Therefore the best treatment would be to give a bolus of intravenous dextrose. Commence intravenous 10% dextrose at a rate of at least 3 mL/kg/hr.

iii) Give glucagon 100 µg/kg intramuscularly.

iv) Establish intravenous access and start a dextrose infusion. The glucagon will result in utilisation of whatever glycogen is available and once this is used, profound hypoglycaemia will occur. Glycogen stores are extremely limited.

v) Samples should have been taken for the investigation of severe hypoglycaemia. Blood should be sent to confirm the hypoglycaemia, pH and lactate should also be measured and samples should be stored for intermediary metabolites, ketone bodies and fatty acids, insulin, c-peptide, glucagon, catecholamine, corticosteroids and growth hormone. The next urine sample should be stored for amino and organic acids profiles. Although these investigations may not be required at present, samples should be stored for later analysis when indicated. Different laboratories may have different protocols for the samples to be taken.

vi) To maintain a high concentration dextrose infusion, central access should be obtained, either by a peripheral long line or an umbilical venous catheter.

vii) Yes. Normal glucose infusion rates providing 4–6 mg/kg/min will usually maintain normoglycaemia. In this infant the infusion is giving 10.4 mg/kg/min (120 mL/kg of 12.5% dextrose = 15 g glucose/24 hours/kg = 15,000 mg/day = 10.4 mg/kg/min).

viii) This infant has a weight of 1.8 kg which is on the 2nd centile at 26 weeks. Infants who are significantly growth retarded may have transient hyperinsulinism in combination with reduced glycogen stores, and may develop severe hypoglycaemia that persists for several days. It is normally manageable by glucose infusion and additional treatment is rarely needed.

ANSWER 5

i) Answer **c** is the best answer – SIADH. This infant has significant hyponatraemia. This, in combination with the other results, also supports the possibility of haemodilution. Iatrogenic fluid overload is particularly unlikely in this situation where there has been fluid restriction as part of the management. If anything, one would expect an elevated sodium in this situation. Diabetes insipidus would lead to hypernatraemia and although this has been reported in infants, it is exceptionally rare. Failure to adequately replace electrolytes may lead to significant hyponatraemia but again is unlikely in this particular situation in view of the postnatal age and fluid restriction. Acute renal failure would lead to hypernatraemia, with an elevation in both urea and creatinine.

ii) The most relevant part of the history is the clinical evidence of a significant brain injury. The principle associations of SIADH are pneumothorax, positive pressure ventilation, acute brain injury and central nervous system infection. It has also been reported following maternal substance misuse.[7]

iii) Answers **b**, **d** and **h** are correct – blood pressure, CRT and temperature differential. SIADH is characterised by hyponatraemia in the presence of normovolaemia, normal blood pressure, and normal renal and cardiac function. Blood pressure would be a useful observation but although a normal BP is suggestive of a good circulating volume, the range of normal BP is wide and correlates poorly with circulating blood volume. It is essential that you establish some other measure of circulating volume in combination with BP measurements such as core–toe differential, capillary refill time and Doppler echocardiography. ECG will offer little additional help and urine output will be of limited assistance as both oliguria and polyuria could be due to a variety of different complications. Skin turgor is notably unreliable as a clinical sign in neonates.

iv) The two most helpful investigations would be **b** (urinary) and **h** (plasma) osmolality. SIADH results from an elevation of anti-diuretic hormone that is inappropriate for osmolality, extracellular fluid volume and blood volume (the factors that normally regulate ADH secretion). SIADH is manifested by hyponatraemia and corresponding hypo-osmolality and a concentrated urine. The urinary osmolality is generally greater than the plasma osmolality in SIADH. Plasma osmolality less than 280 mOsm/kg is abnormally low and the urine osmolality will be inappropriately high for this value. Urine osmolality will usually be greater than 100 mOsm/L but may be difficult to interpret in extremely premature babies.

i) Answer **a** is correct. This baby has early hypocalcaemia. The definition of hypocalcaemia varies widely, because of the lack of clinical signs in many babies and the lack of consensus of a lower limit of normal (values of 1.75–2.0 mmol/L have been quoted). It is therefore better to use a level of ionised calcium, as this is the metabolically active form of calcium and changes in the ionised component are more likely to have a physiological effect. Hypocalcaemia is defined as an ionised calcium of less than 1.22–1.4 mM.[8]

Early hypocalcaemia is defined as a low calcium level in the first 4 days of life. Exaggeration of the normal physiological fall of serum calcium within the first 3 days is a common occurrence. At birth, maternal calcium supply ends, and the infant's level is maintained by a flux of increased calcium from trabecular bone or increased gut absorption from good oral intake. In term infants, there is a physiological decline in serum calcium after birth usually reaching a nadir within 24–48 hours. It then rises again over the following few days. Approximately 3% of healthy term infants have a total calcium below 2 mmol/L at 24 hours of age.[8]

ii) Pseudohypoparathyroidism is a rare cause of hypocalcaemia in infancy due to peripheral lack of response to the action of PTH. It has not been documented in infancy but minimal adult data describes it to cover both ectopic hyperparathyroidism and the more commonly encountered non-parathyroid humoral hypercalcaemia of malignancy, metastatic breast cancer being the classic example.

Hyperparathyroidism is associated with hypercalcaemia, not hypocalcaemia.

Hypocalcaemia is well described in infants of diabetic mothers, and is a combination of an exaggerated normal postnatal fall, a degree of PTH resistance and increased calcium demands due to the high metabolic rate in these infants. The hypocalcaemia appears to be related to hypomagnesaemia which is secondary to maternal urinary loss of magnesium. The extent of hypocalcaemia in these infants is influenced by the severity of maternal disease.

Maternal vitamin D deficiency may lead to vitamin D deficiency and hypocalcaemia in the newborn infant. This is commoner in certain ethnic groups and reflects maternal diet and exposure to sunlight.

Exchange transfusion has been associated with hypocalcaemia and appears to be due to the use of calcium-chelating anticoagulants. Newer anticoagulants do not have this effect and this complication is now very unlikely.

Diuretic therapy may induce hypercalciuria and thus hypocalcaemia, but is unlikely in this situation as the infant is well.

Hypoalbuminaemia may be associated with a low total calcium, as in this case, but ionised calcium should be within the normal range.

Maternal hyperparathyroidism may be associated with significant neonatal hypocalcaemia, but hypoparathyroidism leads to neonatal hyperparathyroidism and a normally self-limiting hypercalcaemia.

Low calcium intake may be associated with hypocalcaemia but would normally reflect a prolonged period of poor dietary intake rather than a coincidental finding soon after birth.

Birth asphyxia or any perinatal stress causes an exaggeration in the normal postnatal fall in calcium levels.

iii) Although hypocalcaemia is self-limiting, infants with symptoms or an abnormal ECG with prolonged QTc should be treated with oral or intravenous calcium. The baby in this question is asymptomatic and well, and therefore no treatment is indicated, but calcium levels should be monitored to ensure that they return to normality.

ANSWER 7

Nephrocalcinosis is a common finding in preterm infants with an incidence of 16–64% in infants with a birth weight below 1500 g. There are many sources, including text books, which suggest a strong association with diuretic therapy, but this association does not appear so clear cut when detailed analysis of risk factors has been performed. Studies suggest that it is only seen in those with severe respiratory disease who have been ventilated and progress to develop chronic lung disease (CLD). Other factors which appear associated are gestational age, male sex, duration and frequency of gentamicin therapy, gentamicin and vancomycin toxicity and postnatal dexamethasone. Interestingly, in one study, diuretic therapy did not appear relevant and duration of oxygen was found to be the strongest clinical indicator of renal calcification. It is possible that the much quoted association between nephrocalcinosis and diuretics is only a reflection of the presence of CLD.[9]

Preterm infants with lung disease are reported to have decreased urinary citrate, which may predispose them to nephrocalcinosis because citrate is a known inhibitor of renal calcification in adults and children. Follow-up studies have shown that progressive resolution of nephrocalcinosis occurs in the majority of cases (with figures quoted between 85% by 30 months and 75% at a median of 6.75 years). In one paper, in the 25% of patients in whom nephrocalcinosis persisted, there was no evidence to suggest an association with renal dysfunction or long-term symptoms or persisting abnormalities in calcium metabolism or excretion.[10] Renal function does not appear to be adversely affected into childhood. There is no reliable information on the consequence of neonatal nephrocalcinosis persisting into adult life. Although the natural history of nephrocalcinosis is that it resolves, some infants will develop renal calculi although it is not proven that this is a direct result of the nephrocalcinosis.

ANSWER 8

i) The ECG shows tall peaked T waves, and widening of the QRS complexes.

ii) The cause is hyperkalaemia due to acute renal failure secondary to perinatal asphyxia.

iii) The treatment options are:
  a. Maintenance of normocalcaemia using 10% calcium gluconate, 0.1–0.2 mL/kg. Hypocalcaemia and hypomagnesaemia potentiate the toxic effect of hyperkalaemia on the heart.
  b. Intravenous salbutamol, 4 μg/kg over 5 minutes. Salbutamol promotes intracellular transport of potassium thus lowering the blood levels.

c. Intravenous glucose and insulin infusion (5 mL/kg of a solution of 12 units insulin in 100 mL 25% glucose given over 30 minutes). This also promotes influx of potassium into cells and has an additive effect with salbutamol.

d. Intravenous sodium bicarbonate 1 mmoL/kg. This also may result in a shift of potassium from extracellular to intracellular compartments.

e. Oral/rectal calcium-chelating agents such as resonium will help to remove potassium from the body. They are, however, associated with bowel obstruction and perforation, and should therefore only be used where there are no concerns about gut integrity.

f. Dialysis. Potassium can be effectively removed by dialysis and should be considered early if aggressive management is thought to be appropriate.

ANSWER 9

i) With the amount of information available at this moment it is difficult to give specific diagnoses. However, given the age and history the following possibilities should be considered:

a. Sepsis – this must always be top of the list
b. Congenital heart disease – not uncommon to present in this way at this age
c. Inborn error of metabolism – rare but very important to detect
d. Hypoglycaemia
e. Intra-abdominal pathology – volvulus for example
f. Electrolyte disturbance
g. Endocrine problem – congenital adrenal hyperplasia for example.

ii) As all the 'routine' bloods have been unremarkable it is appropriate to start screening for some of the less likely but serious possibilities. Further investigation should include an echocardiogram to exclude congenital heart disease, electrolytes to exclude acute disturbances and a capillary or arterial blood gas. Lactate is essential and should be requested separately if it is not a part of the routine blood gas analysis. Plasma ammonia should be measured urgently as hyperammonaemia is suggestive of a narrow range of serious conditions that will require urgent intervention.

iii) Common things are common. In a baby who is struggling to breathe and showing marked recession before, during and after the deterioration, a pneumothorax must be top of the list. Babies with congenital heart disease may show sudden deterioration but rarely as acutely as this. Although metabolic conditions may lead to babies who are very unwell it would be rare to deteriorate as rapidly as this. Babies with severe hypoglycaemia can deteriorate very quickly, but in this case a blood glucose within the normal range has been recorded already. Fits may lead to a sudden alteration in conscious state and are not always accompanied by obvious seizure activity but the respiratory signs in this case are not usually associated with fits.

iv) Tension pneumothorax with midline shift to the left. Insertion of a chest drain is essential. The pneumothorax must be drained before assessing the need for ventilation. Commencing positive pressure ventilation pre-drainage of an air leak may worsen the tension effect due to alterations in the intra-thoracic pressure, while at the same time detracting from the urgency of chest drain insertion.

v) Answer **e** is the most likely. Normal ammonia concentrations in neonates should be less than $65\,\mu mol/L$, but research has frequently shown concentrations of up to $180\,\mu mol/L$ in sick newborns who do not have a primary metabolic disturbance. Higher ammonia concentrations warrant thorough investigation for metabolic causes. A level greater than $150\,\mu mol/L$ (or persistently greater than $100\,\mu mol/L$) is an inborn error of metabolism until proven otherwise. If hyper-ammonaemia is not recognised and treated, the illness progresses rapidly to coma, seizures and death.

The onset of hyperammonaemia 24 hours after birth is characteristic of the primary urea cycle defects and several of the organic acidaemias (propionic, meth-ylmalonic and isovaleric acidaemia) defects. In either case respiratory alkalosis may be the initial acid–base disturbance. In the absence of a severe acidosis, ketosis or hypoglycaemia, a provisional diagnosis of a urea cycle defect should be made.

Urea cycle defects are generally associated with a respiratory alkalosis in response to the increased respiratory rate because of the hyperammonaemia. They can be associated with a mild acidosis, but the acidosis is rarely the main present-ing feature. Acidosis may subsequently develop as decompensation occurs.

vi) Management.[11,12]

   a. Resuscitate as for any collapsed infant. Management of respiratory prob-lems as appropriate and establish vascular access. All feeds should be discontinued.

   b. Discuss with regional metabolic expert immediately. These conditions have very poor outlook with or without treatment and involvement of a specialist from the outset is essential.

   c. Discuss with local paediatric intensive care facility. Haemofiltration or haemodialysis may be required and it is important that the availability of such treatment is established early on. Haemodialysis is reported to be the most efficient treatment but peritoneal dialysis and haemofiltration are options. Exchange transfusion can be used but is much less efficient and should only be regarded as a temporary treatment when access to dialysis is not immediately available.

   d. Intravenous dextrose should be administered to restore hydration as the majority of these infants are dehydrated as a consequence of vomiting and poor intake. Maintenance electrolytes should be added and adjusted according to frequent biochemical monitoring. Tissue perfusion increases with adequate hydration and catabolism is reduced.

   e. Arginine. The use of other elements in management (see below) reduces available nitrogen and there is thus a decrease in arginine synthesis. Arginine thus becomes an essential amino acid in all urea cycle defects except arginase deficiency.

   f. Sodium phenylbutyrate and/or sodium benzoate at a dose of 250–500 mg/kg/day. These compounds help excrete nitrogen waste through alternative pathways. If benzoate is used amino acid nitrogen is excreted as hippuric acid. If phenylbutyrate is used phenyl glutamine is excreted.

g. Carnitine. This enhances fatty acid oxidation by transport into the mitochondria. This is most appropriate for organic acid disorders and is normally given until the diagnosis is established.

vii) Parental discussion. The prognosis for babies with urea cycle disorders should be guarded. Without treatment they will die. Even with treatment many will die and the long-term outcome for survivors is largely unknown. Growth and development are likely to be affected and there may be recurrent life-threatening metabolic crises. Liver transplant is an option but there is little information on long-term quality of life. Gene therapy may be the ultimate treatment but is not a possibility at present.

ANSWER 10

Answers **a** and **b** are correct. A normal anion gap is 12–16 mmol/L and is calculated by the following formula (all units mmol/L):

$$\text{Anion gap} = (Na + K) - (Cl + HCO_3)$$

In reality, the total cations and total anions in a solution balance exactly. The gap is therefore due to unmeasured anions, mainly albumin, phosphate and small amounts of organic anions including lactate. In patients with acidosis, the calculation of the anion gap can be particularly useful. If the anion gap is increased, there must be either an increase in one of the 'normal' unmeasured anions (e.g. lactate) or a substantial increase in the level of an organic anion, which is normally only present in tiny amounts (e.g. ketoacids, complex organic anions). This helps determine whether the metabolic acidosis is caused by an accumulation of organic acids or a decrease in bicarbonate.

A normal anion gap with acidosis is likely to be due to renal tubular acidosis or intestinal bicarbonate loss. If the anion gap is increased, an organic acidaemia is very likely.

a. Propionic acidaemia is an organic acid disorder and presents with severe metabolic acidosis, poor feeding and drowsiness. There is hyperammonaemia and hypoglycaemia. A high anion gap is present.

b. Phenylketonuria leads to accumulation of phenylalanine which does not add to the anion gap.

c. Renal tubular acidosis leads to a metabolic acidosis with a normal anion gap. This is due to a hyperchloraemic metabolic acidosis secondary to renal loss of bicarbonate.

d. Medium chain acyl-CoA dehydrogenase deficiency leads to accumulation of medium-chain fatty acids or partially degraded fatty acids in tissues and these may cause liver and brain damage. As medium-chain fatty acids from food and from fats stored in the body cannot be metabolised they are not converted into energy, leading to characteristic signs and symptoms such as lethargy and hypoglycaemia. A high anion gap is present.

e. Maple syrup disease is a defect in the metabolism of the branched chain amino acids (valine, leucine and isoleucine) due to a deficiency of one of three enzyme systems, of which the commonest is branched chain 2-ketoacid dehydrogenase complex. Babies develop severe ketoacidosis and are often hypoglycaemic. Although ketosis is prominent, metabolic acidosis is not often present until later in the course of disease. It usually presents at the end of the first week of extra-uterine life with vomiting, seizures and dystonia. It derives its name from the characteristic sweet, burnt-sugar smell of the urine.

f. Total villous atrophy does not lead to an increased anion gap. It leads to a metabolic acidosis with a normal anion gap due to gastrointestinal loss of bicarbonate.

ANSWER 11

All are correct. Infants with lactic acidosis present a difficult diagnostic problem. A high plasma lactate can be secondary to hypoxia, cardiac disease, infection or convulsions. Although the lactate may be elevated it is normally not to the same levels as seen in the more worrying congenital lactic acidoses.

Primary lactic acidosis may be caused by inborn errors of metabolism (IEM), e.g. disorders of pyruvate metabolism (leading to inability to convert lactic acid back to pyruvate to enter the Krebs cycle), gluconeogenesis disorder (leading the body to scavenge pyruvate which is converted to lactic acid with ATP production), respiratory chain defects (causing inability to produce ATP during the Krebs cycle), or a mitochondrial disorder (e.g. error in oxidative phosphorylation).

Venous obstruction by tourniquet for blood sampling, crying or breath holding may increase plasma lactate concentrations and it is therefore wise to obtain an arterial blood sample to confirm the lactic acidosis.

As a rule of thumb, a persistent increase of plasma lactate above 3 mmol/L in a non-asphyxiated infant who has no evidence of multi-organ failure, should lead to further investigations for an IEM.

As discussed earlier, other IEMs (fatty acid oxidation disorders, organic acidaemias and urea cycle defects) may be associated with a lactic acidosis, although this is usually mild and not the presenting feature.

ANSWER 12

i) Establishing central access in a macrosomic baby, as in this case, is crucial. It is notoriously difficult to get a peripheral cannula sited and an umbilical venous catheter would be easy and quick to insert. In the rare occurrence where this is not possible, it would be more appropriate to use an intra-osseous route rather than continue to strive to achieve venous access. With access secured an infusion of 10% dextrose should be started at 3 mL/kg/h.

ii) Boluses of concentrated dextrose solution should be avoided because of the risk of rebound hypoglycaemia and cerebral oedema. They should only be required if the infant is symptomatic and should be 3–5 mL/kg given slowly followed by an infusion.

iii) The rate of infusion should be increased according to the blood glucose measurements. If there are other factors that mean that fluid intake should be restricted, the concentration of the dextrose solution should be increased.

iv) a. As severe hypoglycaemia is persisting, investigations must be carried out to ascertain the cause. This will include pH and lactate, and blood samples should be stored for intermediary metabolites, ketone bodies and fatty acids, insulin, c-peptide, glucagon, catecholamines, corticosteroids and growth hormone. The next urine sample should be stored for amino and organic acid profiles.

b. Specialist advice should be sought at an early stage in these cases as hyperinsulinism, which is not self-limiting and is resistant to very high glucose concentration, has a risk of precipitating heart failure, especially if there is co-existing hypertrophic cardiomyopathy

c. Diazoxide should be given at a dose of 10–20 mg/kg/day. This suppresses pancreatic insulin release. It is usually given with chlorthiazide, which enhances the hyperglycaemic effect and may help prevent the fluid retention which is one of the side effects of diazoxide.

v) Octreotide could be given. This is an analogue of somatostatin, the hypothalamic release-inhibiting hormone. It also suppresses insulin release and can be given either by subcutaneous or intravenous injection at a dose of 10 μg/kg/day. There are some concerns about long-term tolerance and the possible effects on other hormones. To reduce this risk, glucagon is also given at the same time.

Glucagon has been used to treat hypoglycaemia as it has glycogenolytic properties. It should however only be used when a brief period of hypoglycaemia needs to be prevented, e.g. when a drip needs re-siting, as prolonged use may cause further release of insulin, thus worsening the situation.

Nifedipine has also been used to treat hyperinsulinism. In 30–40% of cases of persistent hyperinsulinaemic hypoglycaemia of infancy (PHHI) there are gene mutations leading to functional loss in K^+-ATP channels leading to disregulation of calcium fluxes and unregulated insulin release. Blood pressure monitoring is crucial.

vi) This baby is likely to have persistent hyperinsulinaemic hypoglycaemia of infancy (previously known as nesidioblastosis). PHHI leads to recurrent and persisting hypoglycaemia which can be difficult to treat. It occurs in macrosomic babies with extremely high insulin levels and high glucose requirements. The risk of neurological damage is high and thus treatment must be initiated immediately. There are several different histological forms, focal and diffuse, and several different underlying pathologies. Early referral and treatment in a specialist centre is essential.

Self-limiting hyperinsulinism may occur in infants born to mothers with poorly controlled diabetes, or where there has been antenatal administration of thiazide diuretics. It is also encountered in Beckwith–Wiedemann syndrome where it is a common feature – in this case there are normally other abnormalities detected. In these cases the hypoglycaemia is usually less severe and easier to manage.[13]

REFERENCES

1. Bidiwala KS, Lorenz JM, Kleinman LI. Renal function correlates of postnatal diuresis in preterm infants. Pediatrics 1988;82:50–58

2. Savenije OEM, Brand PLP. Accuracy and precision of test weighing to assess milk intake in newborn infants. Arch Dis Child Fetal Neonatal Ed 2006;91:F330–F332

3. Meier PP, Engstrom JL. Test weighing for term and premature infants is an accurate procedure. Arch Dis Child Fetal Neonatal Ed 2007;92:F155–F156

4. Morton JA. The clinical usefulness of breast milk sodium in the assessment of lactogenesis. Pediatrics 1994;93(5):802–6

5. Moritz ML, Manole MD, Bogen DL, Ayus JC. Breastfeeding-associated hypernatremia: are we missing the diagnosis? Pediatrics 2005;116(3):e343–e347

6. Laing IA, Wong CM. Hypernatraemia in the first few days: is the incidence rising? Arch Dis Child Fetal Neonatal Ed 2002;87:F158–F162

7. Winrow AP, Kovar IZ, Jani BR, Gatzoulis M. Early hyponatraemia and neonatal drug withdrawal. Acta Paediatrica 1992;81:847–48

8. Hsu SC, Levine MA. Perinatal calcium metabolism: physiology and pathophysiology. Semin Neonatol 2004;9(1):23–36

9. Narendra A, White MP, Rolton RA et al. Nephrocalcinosis in preterm babies. Arch Dis Child Fetal Neonatal Ed 2001;85:F207–F213

10. Porter E, McKie A, Beattie TJ et al. Neonatal nephrocalcinosis: long term follow up. Arch Dis Child Fetal Neonatal Ed 2006;91:F333–F336

11. Chakrapani A, Cleary MA, Wraith JE. Detection of inborn errors of metabolism in the newborn. Arch Dis Child Fetal Neonatal Ed 2001;84:F205–F210

12. Chakrapani A, Wraith JE. Principles of management of the more common metabolic disorders. Curr Paediatr 2002;12:117–24

13. Rahier J, Guiot Y, Sempoux C. Persistent hyperinsulinaemic hypoglycaemia of infancy: a heterogeneous syndrome unrelated to nesidioblastosis. Arch Dis Child Fetal Neonatal Ed 2000;82:F108–F112

Chapter 5

Problems with prematurity

The problems of prematurity are varied and can be complex. This chapter works through many of the problems that preterm infants face after delivery from difficult ventilation and hypotension through to the later problems of chronic lung disease, retinopathy of prematurity, and apnoea of prematurity.

Although there are separate chapters in the book for X-rays and other images, some pictures of scans are included in this chapter to help build up a more realistic representation of the difficulties that commonly accompany the day-to-day management of the premature infant.

QUESTION 1

A 27 week baby is brought to the neonatal unit. He was born in good condition, requiring minimal resuscitation and is put on to nasal CPAP in 25% oxygen. Over the next four hours, his condition deteriorates. Oxygen requirement increases, there is obvious recession and he is having recurrent apnoeas. A capillary gas at this point shows a mixed acidosis.

i) Which of the following actions would you consider? Choose the three most appropriate answers.
   a. Continue and reassess in an hour
   b. Increase CPAP pressure
   c. Intubate and give surfactant, and extubate back onto CPAP
   d. Intubate, give surfactant, and ventilate
   e. Give antibiotics
   f. Load with caffeine
   g. CXR
   h. Change to trigger assist CPAP.

A CXR is obtained.

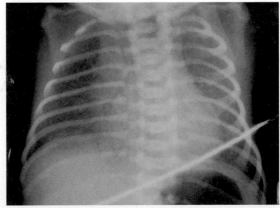

Figure 5.1

ii) Describe the CXR.

The baby is given surfactant and antibiotics and is ventilated but pressures and oxygen requirement continue to increase. Arterial blood gases are just acceptable at pressures of 26/4 in 80% oxygen. The baby suddenly becomes profoundly bradycardic and oxygen saturations fall to below 50%.

iii) What four options would you immediately investigate?

Transillumination shows a very bright hemithorax, and there is some improvement following insertion of a chest drain. Two hours later, there is further deterioration and a pneumothorax is detected on the opposite side. A chest drain results in re-inflation but the clinical condition does not improve significantly.

12 hours after the first pneumothorax he is in 100% oxygen, with pressures 32/4 and an arterial blood gas shows the following:

pH	7.18
PO_2	2.4 kPa
PCO_2	9.8 kPa
BE	−4 mEq/L
HCO_3	28 mmol/L

CXR shows relatively solid lungs with an air bronchogram. The pneumothoraces are well drained.

iv) Which of the following actions would you consider?
    a. Increase PIP
    b. Increase PEEP
    c. Repeat surfactant
    d. HFOV
    e. Nitric oxide
    f. Discuss palliative care with parents
    g. Diuretics
    h. Tolazoline.

The baby stabilises on HFOV over the next few days and returns to conventional ventilation when MAP falls to 12. He remains on conventional ventilation for the next 21 days, at the end of which pressure is 20/4 and he is in 60% oxygen. A CXR is obtained (Figure 5.2).

v) Describe the CXR.

vi) Which of the following treatments would you consider? Choose two answers.
    a. Antibiotics
    b. Diuretics
    c. Aminophylline
    d. Dexamethasone
    e. Indomethacin
    f. Inhaled corticosteroids
    g. Inhaled bronchodilators
    h. Disodium cromoglycate.

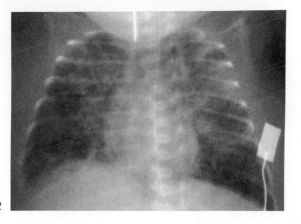

Figure 5.2

As part of the assessment of this infant, an echocardiogram has been performed which shows a large and clinically significant duct. The infant is now 4 weeks old (CGA 31 weeks).

vii) Which of the following interventions would you consider?
- **a.** Fluid restriction
- **b.** Digoxin
- **c.** Indomethacin
- **d.** Ibuprofen
- **e.** Surgical ligation
- **f.** Diuretics
- **g.** Expectant treatment
- **h.** Prostacycline
- **i.** ACE inhibitors.

After duct ligation and a course of dexamethasone, the baby is weaned off all ventilation and progresses onto low flow oxygen. He is ready to go home, gaining weight but still requiring 0.5 L low flow oxygen.

viii) What advice would you give the parents and what extra medication might you consider?

QUESTION 2

Which of the following are risk factors for the development of retinopathy of prematurity?

a. Race

b. Vitamin E

c. Alkalosis

d. Hypercarbia

e. Surfactant

f. Oxygen

g. Exchange transfusions

h. Postnatal steroids.

QUESTION 3

Proliferative retinopathy of prematurity (ROP) has developed and the ophthalmologists feel laser therapy is essential. Which of the following statements are correct?

i) Laser therapy prevents progression of ROP in more than 75% cases.

ii) Laser therapy is necessary if there are 5 continuous or 8 cumulative clock hours of stage 3 ROP in zones 1 or 2 in the presence of plus disease.

iii) Immediate laser therapy is essential for any stage of ROP with plus disease in zone 1.

iv) Laser therapy is essential for any stage of ROP in zone 1 whether or not plus disease is present.

v) Laser treatment can be performed up to 4 weeks after detection of threshold criteria.

vi) Laser therapy is more effective than cryotherapy at prevention of proliferative ROP.

vii) Laser therapy is preferred to cryotherapy for treatment of ROP.

viii) Laser therapy must be done under general anaesthetic.

ix) In infants where laser therapy has successfully treated retinopathy, long-term visual prognosis is excellent.

QUESTION 4

A 29 week infant is now 2 weeks old and has been off CPAP for five days. He is noticed to have bradycardias which are often associated with a fall in oxygen saturations. He has had several apnoeas and recently has required brief respiratory support (mask ventilation) until he started to breathe again. Caffeine was started 8 days ago and is being continued. Which of the following statements are correct?

i) Apnoea of prematurity is uncommon after 30 weeks' gestation and further investigation is essential.

ii) There should be a low threshold for septic screen and antibiotic treatment.

iii) There is a strong association between apnoea and gastro-oesophageal reflux (GOR).

iv) Central and obstructive apnoea are easily distinguishable and equally common.

v) The fact that this infant is receiving caffeine makes central apnoea unlikely as a diagnosis.

vi) Infants with repeated apnoeas that are difficult to treat are at increased risk of sudden infant death following discharge.

vii) Doxapram is useful as a first-line agent for the treatment of apnoea.

viii) Kinaesthetic stimulation may be useful in infants with troublesome apnoeas.

ix) Blood transfusion may be helpful in the treatment of apnoea if haemoglobin is low.

x) Recent immunisation could well be a precipitating event.

QUESTION 5

Which of the following statements are true about hypotension and its management?

i) Infants with RDS are often hypotensive.

ii) Infants whose mothers have received antenatal steroids are more likely to be hypotensive.

iii) A pneumothorax may cause an increase in the cerebral blood flow velocity and systemic hypotension.

iv) Hypotension is a risk factor for germinal matrix haemorrhage.

v) Dopamine works on alpha-adrenergic receptors only.

vi) Dobutamine works on alpha-adrenergic receptors only.

vii) Dopamine is more effective alone than dobutamine alone.

viii) Adrenaline increase the blood pressure by peripheral vasoconstriction.

ix) Adrenaline has a similar effect on the blood pressure to dopamine.

QUESTION 6

A chest X-ray is performed.

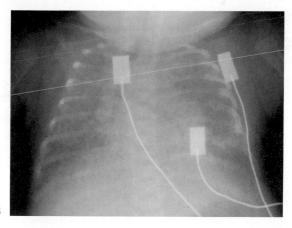

Figure 5.3

i) Describe four abnormalities on the chest X-ray.

As a consequence of what you see a skeletal survey is also carried out. The X-ray of the legs as part of the skeletal survey is shown in Figure 5.4.

ii) Describe four abnormalities on the X-ray of the legs.

iii) What is the most likely diagnosis?

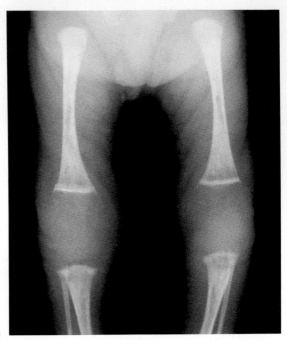

Figure 5.4

iv) Which of the following are likely to be associated with the diagnosis?

    a. Indomethacin

    b. Caffeine

    c. Furosemide

    d. Dexamethasone

    e. Immobilisation

    f. Alkaline phosphatase >500 IU/L

    g. Urine calcium:phosphate ratio >1

    h. Serum calcium level <2 mmol/L.

QUESTION 7

A 26 week gestation infant requires ventilation from birth for moderately severe respiratory distress syndrome. He is moderately stable in 40% oxygen, pressures 22/4, and dopamine has been needed to maintain a satisfactory blood pressure. A routine ultrasound scan performed on day 2 is shown in Figure 5.5.

    i) What abnormality is shown?

   ii) What is the likely prognosis?

  iii) The parents want to know how common this is and why this has happened. What do you tell them?

QUESTION 8

A 25 week gestation baby has been ventilated for 4 days during which ventilatory requirements did not exceed a peak pressure of 20 cmH$_2$O. Blood pressure is stable

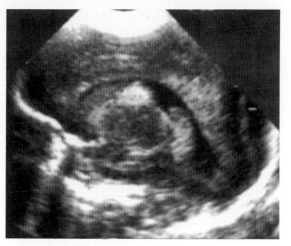

Figure 5.5

and inotropic support was not required. Bilateral small GMHs were noted on day one, which did not appear to increase in size on subsequent scans although there was thought to be a small amount of free blood within the ventricles. After 4 days of weaning ventilation, the baby is stable on CPAP.

On day 13, some abnormal movements are noted, and the baby is thought to have had a seizure. A repeat cranial ultrasound is performed, the first for five days. The scan is shown below.

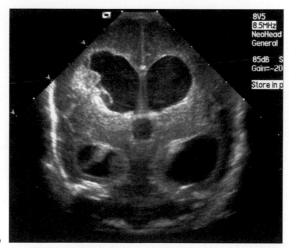

Figure 5.6

i) What does the scan show?

ii) Why has it happened?

iii) What will you tell the parents?

iv) The parents have been studying the internet and have found reports on the use of acetazolamide, repeated ventricular taps and ventriculostomy, in the management of PHVD. What will you tell them about these treatment options and then explain to them what your plan will be?

QUESTION 9

A 26 week gestation infant has suffered from moderately severe respiratory distress and has required high frequency oscillation ventilation, requiring a mean airway pressure of 16 mmH$_2$0. A significant GMH/IVH is noted on day two with a smaller haemorrhage on the left. Despite the use of both dopamine and dobutamine blood pressure has remained unstable. The baby developed a tension pneumothorax on day three but responded well to prompt drainage. On day five, the baby deteriorates further with increasing ventilation requirements, coagulopathy, sudden fall in haemoglobin and marked hypotension. Sepsis is suspected and antibiotics are commenced. A cerebral ultrasound is performed 24 hours later.

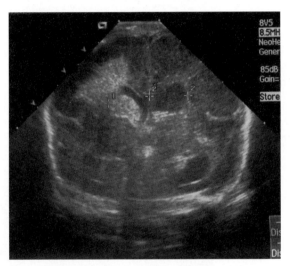

Figure 5.7

i) Describe the scan.

ii) Why has this happened?

iii) What will you tell the parents?

iv) What is your next step in managing this baby?

QUESTION 10

A 28 week gestation baby was born following prolonged rupture of membranes. Mother had developed a pyrexia which had not responded to 24 hours of antibiotics and an emergency section was performed. pH at birth was 6.95 and prolonged resuscitation was required. Surprisingly, the baby stabilised relatively quickly and only a short period of ventilation was required. Initial cerebral ultrasound showed no evidence of GM-IVH but there was some debate over increased periventricular echogenicity. At 6 weeks postnatal age, a routine ultrasound scan was performed and is shown in Figure 5.8.

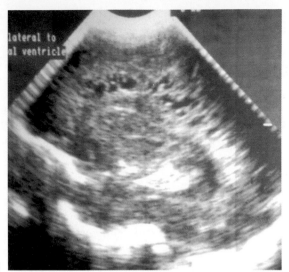

Figure 5.8

i) Describe the scan.

ii) Why has this happened?

iii) What will you tell the parents?

iv) What is your next step in managing this baby?

ANSWER 1

i) d, e and **g** are most appropriate.

  a. This would not be advisable. An infant becoming progressively more symptomatic is extremely unlikely to show spontaneous improvement at this gestation.

  b. If there is widespread atelectasis, increased CPAP pressure may help by recruiting more lung, but would not be a sensible first-line option. It should not be considered unless the CXR confirms the atelectasis, and unless surfactant replacement has been given.

  c. Practice differs with respect to this option. There are some who believe this is appropriate and others who feel disturbance caused to the baby is likely to jeopardise stability and it is far more rational to continue gentle ventilation for some hours after administration. Some fairly strong opinions are held in the face of an extremely limited evidence base.

  d. As mentioned above practice varies but this is probably the safest option. It is important that surfactant is given properly and that the most minimal ventilation possible is provided, and the infant is weaned as quickly as possible.

  e. As a rule most units have a policy of antibiotic administration to preterm babies with respiratory distress as sepsis cannot be ruled out immediately after birth and it is known that infection does contribute to a proportion of preterm deliveries.

f. This might be appropriate in due course but a lack of respiratory drive is unlikely to be the main component of this infant's respiratory difficulties.

g. A CXR is essential in this situation as, although respiratory distress syndrome is the most likely diagnosis, other possibilities cannot be excluded, such as a pneumothorax.

h. Newer advanced CPAP modes, e.g. trigger assist and pressure trigger assist, are becoming increasingly popular. However, the exact circumstances in which use is most beneficial are unclear. In this particular situation, surfactant would seem to be the most important component of immediate management.

ii) The chest X-ray shows changes which are consistent with moderate respiratory distress syndrome. There is a homogeneous ground-glass appearance with an air bronchogram. The air bronchogram is more prominent behind the heart which can be a normal observation. The X-ray is slightly rotated making comments about heart size unreliable.

iii) In the case of any sudden deterioration in an infant, think DOPE:

Displacement – although much can be done to optimise the stability of endotracheal tubes, this still remains a common reason for deterioration.

Obstruction – many babies produce copious secretion of variable viscosity and tube obstruction is not uncommon.

Pneumothorax – although the incidence of pneumothorax has fallen significantly since the advent of surfactant replacement therapy, it is still an important and potentially lethal reason for sudden deterioration.

Equipment – equipment failure may be a cause with tube disconnection being the commonest mechanical problem.

iv) a. Although increasing PIP may improve oxygenation, it is unlikely to be highly effective while continuing to ventilate conventionally as the elevated pressure is not sustained for long enough to recruit atelectatic alveoli.

b. Increasing PEEP may help recruit alveoli but very high pressure may be needed in a very sick infant. Research has shown this may be effective but the pressures required are usually outside the comfort zone for many practising neonatologists. Increasing PEEP will improve mean airway pressure but at the cost of decreased tidal volume, and the acidosis may worsen.

c. This may be worth a trial, particularly if insufficient treatment has been given previously. Although randomised controlled trials do not show any evidence of benefit from more than two doses, it must be remembered that this refers to a large group with heterogeneous conditions, and does not preclude the possibility of a response in selected individuals. Surfactant is inactivated by the inflammatory exudate that develops in RDS, and it may therefore be necessary to use higher than normal doses.

d. Those who use HFOV would argue this would be the most appropriate intervention at this moment (in fact they would almost certainly suggest that it should have been commenced earlier).

There still remains some debate about the most appropriate use of HFOV but there is good evidence to support its use for rescue ventilation, when the higher sustained MAP will assist in the recruitment of alveoli, but may require several hours in which to do so.

    e. Although it is tempting to try nitric oxide when oxygen requirements are high, the currently available evidence does not support use in preterm infants. Nitric oxide is indicated when there is evidence of pulmonary hypertension. In this case the primary problem is alveolar collapse.[1]

    f. Discussions should be held with the parents throughout the baby's admission and they should be aware that their baby is very sick. It is rare for practitioners to consider palliative care when the problems are primarily respiratory and further treatment options exist. It might be appropriate to discuss this as a future option, but would not seem an appropriate action at present.

    g. There is no role for diuretics in the acute management of severe respiratory distress syndrome.

    h. Tolazoline is a vasodilator thought to act through H2 histamine receptors. Over the years, it has gained a reputation as a drug that may be effective in persistent pulmonary hypertension. On rare occasions, administration may be associated with a dramatic improvement in oxygenation. This has led people to associate the use of tolazoline with poor oxygenation for other reasons. As with nitric oxide, administration is unlikely to be effective unless pulmonary hypertension is the principle problem, and the associated hypotension that it causes may be problematic.

v) The chest X-ray shows:
    Endotracheal tube in situ
    Hyperinflated lung fields – upward sloping ribs, compressed heart and bulging pleura
    Widespread patchy opacification
    Flattened diaphragm on the left
    Early cystic change, particularly at bases.

vi) b and **d**.

    a. Antibiotics. Unless there is evidence of intercurrent infection there is no particular indication for antibiotic therapy. Antibiotics are not infrequently given, as the changes on CXR frequently involve patchy opacification which is difficult to distinguish from areas of infection.

    b. Diuretics. Administration of diuretics may be associated with a rapid increase in compliance and a reduction in airway resistance. However, there is no published evidence of long-term benefit. Furosemide is often administered initially followed by maintenance therapy with a thiazide diuretic and spironolactone. Side effects are not uncommon, particularly nephrocalcinosis (see Chapter 4, question **7**), and a strong case can be made for limiting the use of this therapy, particularly in long courses.

c. Aminophylline. Small reports have suggested that intravenous and oral methylxanthines may be associated with some benefit. Evidence is limited and there is no proof of long-term benefit.

d. Dexamethasone. There is considerable debate about the use of dexamethasone in preterm infants. A decade ago there was wide usage, and steroids were often given to extubated babies simply because they required oxygen. Evidence suggests that corticosteroid administration may be associated with earlier extubation, reduced duration of supplementary oxygen, and, in some groups, with a small increase in survival. However, long-term studies have suggested there may be a significant association between dexamethasone therapy and later neurodevelopmental problems, particularly cerebral palsy. At the time of writing, there is no clear consensus as to the most appropriate use of this therapy, and indeed whether it should be used at all. In practice, dexamethasone is still used – usually in infants who have been ventilated for a considerable period and have made little progress. There is some interest in the use of regimes that use a much lower total dose of steroids than were administered in the past and there is limited evidence that total dose is relevant with respect to complications.

e. Indomethacin has no role in this situation. It is however essential that cardiac function is assessed in any infant who appears to be making no progress on the ventilator. Significant PDAs should be treated to optimise weaning from the ventilator.

f. Inhaled corticosteroids, such as betamethasone or fluticasone, have been used in a number of trials, and meta-analysis has been performed. Although some short-term benefit maybe be seen (smaller in magnitude and slower in onset when compared to systemic steroids), there is no evidence of sustained benefit.

g. Inhaled bronchodilators (both salbutamol and ipratropium) may be associated with improvements in airway resistance, compliance and blood gases. There is no evidence of long-term benefit. Infants with chronic lung disease will often show evidence of both reversible and irreversible airway constriction in the months and years after discharge, and bronchodilator therapy is frequently used in this situation.

h. Disodium cromoglycate may have an anti-inflammatory action; in a small number of studies use has been associated with some improvement in ventilated infants. This treatment has never attained widespread use in this population.

vii) a. Fluid restriction is unlikely to help at this time due to the age of the baby. The evidence that fluid restriction is beneficial in the management of a ductus arteriosus is very limited and probably stems from the fact there has been a reported association between the development of the ductus arteriosus and higher fluid intake in the immediate postnatal period. The suggestion therefore that later restriction of fluid may be helpful in closing the ductus is not necessarily a logical one. There are some who counsel against fluid restriction because of the associated nutritional deficit that this causes. Most people would consider fluid restriction if there was evidence of heart failure but, in the absence of this complication, opinion is divided.

b. Digoxin has been advocated for use in heart failure in babies but is not widely used. It has no role in this situation.

c. Indomethacin has an established role in the closure of the ductus arteriosus and is discussed in more detail in Chapter 4. Efficacy is reduced in infants who are particularly immature and if administered at a postnatal age of more than 2 weeks.[2] Despite this known fact, many people will still attempt a course of indomethacin in older infants.

d. Ibuprofen may be effective in closing a duct but there is no information about the age at which it is maximally effective. It is likely to be similar to that for indomethacin.

e. Surgical ligation will be the only guaranteed effective treatment if there is a significant ductus, treatment is felt to be necessary and indomethacin has been ineffective or is contraindicated. Data suggest that the rate of surgical closure is highly dependent on the availability and proximity of surgical expertise. Although this procedure is normally well tolerated, and effective, mortality as high as 10% has been reported and other significant complications may develop. Manipulation of the mediastinum may be associated with the development of chylothorax requiring prolonged drainage and nutrition with medium chain triglycerides (Monogen milk). Ventilation requirements can increase significantly in the postoperative period and acute and severe exacerbation of chronic lung disease can ensue.

f. Diuretics may be indicated if heart failure is present, but have no specific role in ductal closure. There is some evidence that furosemide may, by an effect upon renal prostaglandin production, keep the duct open.

g. Expectant treatment. If an infant appears stable and making progress, this may be a very appropriate course of action. No treatment of the ductus is without possible complication, and should not be started without careful consideration. The presence of a ductus, does not, by itself, mean treatment is needed. However, in this case, the ductus is likely to be contributing to the infant's condition.

h. Prostacyclin (epoprostenol) is a vasodilator that may be effective in persistent pulmonary hypertension. It has no effect upon the ductus.

i. ACE inhibitors are occasionally indicated in heart failure and hypertension, and anecdotally in a small number of babies with established chronic lung disease who have episodes of profound desaturations thought to be due to vascular instability. There is no published evidence of benefit in this situation, nor is there any evidence of effect upon the ductus.

viii) Advice is to avoid contact with upper respiratory tract infections wherever possible, and consider palivizumab prophylaxis.

A substantial proportion of infants with chronic lung diseases are re-admitted to hospital within the first 2 years after birth (median of two admissions per baby). The majority of admissions are with upper respiratory tract infections and a number of infants may be extremely unwell requiring intensive care and ventilation. There is a significant mortality in this group. Parents should therefore be advised to avoid, wherever possible, unnecessary exposure to people with respiratory tract infections, for instance in shopping centres, on public transport and in GP surgeries.

Infants with CLD who contract RSV-positive bronchiolitis may develop severe infection and there has been interest in the use of palivizumab prophylaxis. A course of treatment with this monoclonal antibody must run throughout the bronchiolitis season and is very expensive; it consists of five monthly injections. Evidence shows that this can reduce the incidence of RSV but does not appear to influence the incidence of RSV-related death or requirement for ventilation. It may reduce the proportion of infants with longer-term respiratory morbidity, and decreases the health care expenditure for an individual. However, the cost of the prophylaxis programme for potentially susceptible infants would far exceed the health care savings for the relatively small number of individuals who would benefit. A number of cost–benefit analyses from different countries have failed to prove economic benefit. Currently many support prophylaxis for infants who go home in oxygen within 3 months of the beginning of the RSV season. There is more debate over the use in infants who do not. Current recommendations also suggest that prophylaxis should be used in infants with severe cyanotic heart disease and infants with immunodeficiencies. In both cases it is recommended that this is at the discretion of a specialist.

ANSWER 2

There have been many studies looking at the incidence and risk factors for ROP. Over the years there has been no real change in incidence despite advances in neonatal care and it is still up to 68% in babies <1250 g.[3]

- a. Race. There is no difference in the incidence of ROP in white or black babies. There are data to show that more severe ROP occurred more commonly in white babies.[3]

- b. Vitamin E is a naturally occurring anti-oxidant and it has been postulated that it may be protective against the development of ROP. This remains unproven despite a number of studies. It is thought that vitamin E may have an effect on the severity of ROP.[4]

- c. Alkalosis is not a risk factor for the development of ROP. Acidosis on the other hand has been shown to be a risk factor.

- d. Hypercarbia. Recent data have shown that this is not a risk factor for the development of ROP.[5]

- e. Surfactant. Despite surfactant decreasing the severity of respiratory distress syndrome and chronic lung disease, it does not appear to affect the incidence of ROP.[6]

- f. Oxygen. Studies over 50 years ago showed that high oxygen levels were a risk factor for developing ROP. After these studies, practice in the 1960s was to decrease oxygen usage, which led to a decrease in ROP but an associated increase in both morbidity and mortality. More recently there have been several large studies which have demonstrated a link between high inspired oxygen concentrations and the incidence and severity of ROP. It has also been shown that arterial oxygen levels are critical within the first few weeks after delivery. The BOOST-2 trial is currently under way which will look at the safe upper and lower limits of oxygen saturations.[7]

g. Exchange transfusions. There are conflicting data regarding exchange transfusions as a risk factor for ROP. They may be an independent risk factor or may be an indicator of a sick and therefore high-risk baby.

h. Postnatal steroids. There is some evidence from RCTs to suggest increased severity of ROP in infants who have received postnatal steroids. Animal studies have suggested that a combination of postnatal steroids and postnatal hyperoxia results in marked inhibition of retinal vascular development.[8,9]

ANSWER 3

i) False – exact figures for the efficacy of laser therapy are difficult to find from published literature. However, it is reported to be as equally effective as cryotherapy, which is associated with good outcomes in approximately 50% of treated infants.

ii) True – current recommendations are that these are the threshold criteria at which ROP should be treated.

iii) False – any stage of ROP with plus disease in zone 1, stage 3 with or without plus disease in zone 1, or stage 2 or 3 with plus disease in zone 2 are classified as type 1 prethreshold criteria. This is regarded as highly active ROP where close monitoring and early treatment are recommended.

iv) False – stage 1 or 2 without plus disease in zone 1 or stage 3 without plus disease in zone 2 is classified as type 2 prethreshold criteria. Conservative management is indicated but close follow-up should be continued.

v) False – laser treatment should be performed within 2–3 days of detection of threshold criteria. A maximum window of 2 weeks has been suggested, although some authorities suggest this is too wide.

vi) False – limited data suggest that laser therapy is equally as effective as cryotherapy.

vii) True – laser therapy has almost completely replaced cryotherapy in the treatment of ROP. It appears to be better tolerated as a procedure and as it does not involve all layers of the eye (unlike cryotherapy) it is less likely to have wide ranging effects on vision.

viii) False – laser therapy is frequently performed with sedation and analgesia only.

ix) False – there are very limited data on long-term follow-up of infants who have been treated for ROP. In one study following infants up to 10 years after cryotherapy, 45% of eyes had a visual acuity of 6/60 or less.[10] In another study, comparing laser treated versus naturally regressed eyes, there was no difference in near acuity, colour vision, contrast sensitivity or refraction but significantly worse visual acuity.[11]

ANSWER 4

i) False – apnoea occurs in over 80% of infants born at <30 weeks, in about 50% born at 30–31 weeks, and 14% at 32–33 weeks gestation. Although there should be a low threshold for investigation, the condition is so common that it would be inappropriate to investigate all episodes.

ii) True – of all the possible causes of an increasing frequency of apnoeas, sepsis is the one with the most serious implications. Careful evaluation is therefore essential and screening and treatment should be commenced in any infant with clinical suspicions of infection.

iii) False – although associations between GOR and apnoea are often claimed, this has been difficult to prove as studies have not been able to demonstrate a temporal relationship between episodes of GOR and presence of apnoeas.

iv) False – central apnoea is the most common observation with relatively short apnoeic episodes, while a mixture of obstructive and central is more common with prolonged apnoea. Pure obstructive apnoea is reported to be responsible for 6–10% of apnoeic episodes. It is difficult to distinguish between these types without relatively complex monitoring devices.

v) False – methylxanthines appear to have a central stimulant effect on respiration and also are reported to increase contraction of the diaphragm. There is a surprising lack of evidence from large trials on methylxanthine administration but small studies have suggested it may lead to a significant reduction in the number of apnoeas. Even if caffeine is being given, this does not mean that therapeutic levels are being attained and, furthermore, evidence does not suggest that treatment will completely abolish apnoeas.

vi) False – there is currently no evidence to link the presence or severity of apnoeas with later sudden infant death.

vii) False – doxapram acts as a non-specific central nervous system stimulant and is thus associated with significant side effects which may be severe, e.g. seizures. There is some limited evidence to suggest that it may be effective but it cannot be proposed as first-line treatment.

viii) False – kinaesthetic stimulation in the form of rocking cots, oscillating mattresses or inflating rubber gloves positioned beneath the infant has been used but evidence of efficacy is lacking.

ix) True – there is evidence that transfusion is beneficial if haemoglobin is low.

x) False – although immunisation may be associated with significant reactions in preterm babies, including profound apnoea requiring ventilatory support, it certainly should not be the case in this infant who is only two weeks old. If this infant had received immunisation, it would strongly suggest that correct immunisation protocols have not been followed.

i) True – and this is associated with a worse prognosis.

ii) False – these infants are less likely to be hypotensive. There is a suggestion that antenatal steroids are likely to cause not only maturation of the respiratory system but of other systems as well. They may also result in earlier maturation of the circulatory system and it has been reported that infants born between 23 and 27 weeks gestation whose mothers had received steroids were less likely to receive inotropic support for blood pressure in the first 48 hours after birth.[12]

iii) False – a pneumothorax has been shown to be associated with a decrease in the pulsatility index which correlates with an increase in cerebral blood flow velocity. An increase in the diastolic blood pressure can also be seen with narrowing of pulse pressure.[13]

iv) True – hypotension is a common complication of respiratory distress syndrome. Preterm infants have not fully developed the auto-regulation that usually protects the brain against pressure swings. Auto-regulation is also impaired by acidosis and hypoxia which are most likely to be present in respiratory distress syndrome.

v) False – dopamine has different actions at different doses. At low doses, up to 2 μg/kg/min, it dilates renal, mesenteric and coronary arteries. At higher doses, 2–10 μg/kg/min, myocardial contractility is increased by both alpha- and beta-adrenergic actions. At doses above 10 μg/kg/min, it shows alpha-adrenergic activity and is a vasoconstrictor of all vascular beds.

vi) False – dobutamine is an isoprenaline analogue with primarily beta-adrenergic effects on the myocardium. It has no effect on renal arteries.

vii) True – dopamine is more successful than dobutamine in increasing the MAP to >30 mmHg in infants born at <34 weeks gestation. Dopamine seems to be preferred by most neonatal clinicians as it is relatively safe to use and because of its ability to preserve renal and mesenteric perfusion at low doses. It increases the blood pressure by inotropic and vasoactive mechanisms. Dobutamine is more likely to increase cardiac output and, unlike dopamine, does not have to rely on the release of endogenous catecholamines for activity. This may be of relevance in stressed or asphyxiated babies whose catecholamine stores are depleted.[14]

viii) True – adrenaline works by not only increasing myocardial contractility but by peripheral vasoconstriction.

ix) True – there is no difference in rate of treatment failure or need for rescue therapy in babies given either adrenaline or dopamine. Adrenaline, however, has more short-term adverse effects, e.g. higher plasma lactate, lower bicarbonate levels requiring correction and higher blood glucose levels requiring treatment with insulin.[15]

ANSWER 6

i) The CXR shows:
   a. Fractures of multiple ribs with callus formation
   b. Patchy opacifications in both lung fields
   c. Thin ribs with reduced bone density
   d. Tracheal shift to the right.

ii) a. There is cortical thinning.
   b. The end of the bone has an irregular 'frayed' appearance.
   c. There is a band of denser ossification in the metaphysis with comparative lucency behind.
   d. The distal end of the femur shows widening of the metaphysis with a degree of cupping.

iii) Osteopenia of prematurity.

iv) a. False – indomethacin does not increase the risk of osteopenia.

   b. True – caffeine, a methylxanthine, increases renal calcium excretion in preterm infants and thus increases the risk of osteopenia of prematurity.[16]

   c. True – long-term furosemide therapy can lead to secondary hyperparathyroidism and bone disease.[17]

   d. True – dexamethasone impairs calcium regulation and reduces bone mineralisation.[18]

   e. True – osteoblasts increase in activity in response to mechanical loading. Without stimulation, i.e. in periods of immobility, bone resorption and urinary calcium loss increase and bone mass is reduced.[19]

   f. True – there is conflicting evidence as to whether ALP is a marker for metabolic bone disease in preterm infants. One study suggests that an ALP of greater than five times the upper adult limit of normal is an indicator of the risk of rickets. Other authors, using DEXA (dual energy X-ray absorptiometry scan) as a screening tool, suggest no association between bone mineral content and ALP.[20]

   g. False – a urinary ratio of excretion of calcium:phosphate of <1 shows that the infant is phosphate replete and thus excretes more phosphate than calcium in the urine, and is therefore at low risk of developing osteopenia of prematurity.

   h. False – serum calcium is not a useful screening test as infants can maintain a normal calcium level at the expense of bone calcium loss. The level can also increase with phosphorus depletion and hypophosphataemia.

ANSWER 7

i) The ultrasound shows an isolated germinal matrix (subependymal) haemorrhage. There is no evidence of ventricular dilatation and the parenchyma is not affected.

ii) It is generally felt that uncomplicated GMH-IVH has a good prognosis and risks of disability in very low birth weight survivors with GMH have been quoted to be around 4%.[21] However, more recent studies have shown that extremely low birth weight infants with grades I–II IVH have poorer neurodevelopmental outcomes at 20 months corrected gestational age than infants with normal cranial ultrasound.[22,23] Another group report impaired cortical development after uncomplicated IVH associated with a 16% reduction in cerebral cortical grey matter volume at near-term age.[24] There has in the past been a tendency to with-hold this information from parents because of the belief that outcome would be normal. Recent evidence and a move away from medical paternalism would suggest that this is no longer appropriate. As with all preterm infants, these babies should have careful neurodevelopmental follow-up.

iii) Germinal matrix haemorrhage (GMH) is common in very low birth weight infants with rates between 20–30% being reported in a number of studies from different countries. Although incidence is related to illness severity, lesions may develop in infants who have been remarkably well, and conversely, may not occur in infants who have been very unstable. Around half of all lesions develop within the first 24 hours after birth and they are uncommon after 72 hours. Haemorrhage occurs in the subependymal germinal matrix, which is found on the inferior ventricular surface, and is particularly abundant in the region of the caudate nucleus. This layer is undergoing repeated division during neuronal and axonal proliferation. It therefore requires a high blood supply, and there is a dense plexus of both arterioles and draining veins in the subependymal region. In utero blood supply is probably fairly constant in this region, but may vary considerably following premature delivery due to a combination of fluctuations in blood pressure and a lack of cerebral autoregulation. Changes from a pressure passive circulation as autoregulation develops probably explains why these haemorrhages are only seen in the very early neonatal period.

ANSWER 8

i) The scan shows marked ventricular dilatation. In addition there appears to be blood on the inferolateral wall of the right ventricle and there may well be a small area of parenchymal involvement beneath. There is no apparent midline shift.

ii) Post-haemorrhagic hydrocephalus is normally regarded as being a combination of mechanical occlusion of drainage pathways, particularly in the cerebral aqueduct, and an obliterative arachnoiditis. In 1981, it was reported that about 30% of infants with GMH-IVH developed post-haemorrhagic ventricular dilatation.[25] It is quite possible that these figures are not applicable to today's practice and population of preterm infants. Data from 2002 showed 22% of all VLBW infants develop an IVH, with a mean gestational age of 26.8 weeks. A quarter of the infants exhibited post-haemorrhagic ventricular dilatation (PVD).[26]

Other sources have given figures between 5% association with a mild GMH-IVH, rising to in excess of 50% with severe GMH-IVH. The development of

PVD after IVH and adverse short-term outcome, such as the requirement for surgery, were predicted most strongly by the severity of IVH.[26]

iii) Ventricular dilatation regresses relatively quickly in approximately 50% of affected infants. In the remainder, the condition is either persistent or rapidly progressive. It is not necessarily easy to predict which path will be followed by each individual, although the likelihood of regression decreases with increasing severity of the original haemorrhage. The incidence of adverse neurodevelopmental outcome is much higher in this group of infants and figures of 50–80% have been quoted. In the large multi-centre ventriculomegaly trial, outcome was normal in only 11/112 infants enrolled.[27] However, these studies have tended to report on infants with the most severe ventricular dilatation and it is probably true to say that there is limited information on those with transient or mild dilatation. Studies have also shown that long-term sequelae are more common in the group where ventricular dilatation is associated with a degree of parenchymal involvement.

iv) Acetazolamide was routinely used in ventricular dilatation until the results of a randomised controlled trial in 1998, which demonstrated a significantly worse long-term outcome following this treatment.[28] A similar conclusion was reached when a randomised controlled trial evaluated routine ventricular tapping. This treatment, used for more than two decades, appeared significantly worse than expectant management.[29] Although there was interest in management by neuro-endoscopic third ventriculostomy (production of a temporary shunt in the floor of the third ventricle by laser ablation) the limited experience available to date does not appear to support use of this technique in this age group.[30]

Current management is based around regular measurement of head circumference and ventricular indices on cranial ultrasound scan, with early involvement of paediatric neurosurgeons. If head circumference velocity remains within normal limits, there is usually no indication for intervention. However, if head circumference is increasing rapidly, then formal surgical drainage may be required. The approach taken will be dictated to a large degree by the size of the infant. If large enough, a definitive ventriculo-peritoneal shunt may be inserted but, if too small for this procedure, a low profile reservoir will be inserted to enable regular tapping to be performed.

ANSWER 9

i) The ultrasound scan shows a large right-sided parenchymal infarct with midline shift. There is a large haemorrhage on the floor of the right ventricle and a small haemorrhage on the floor of the left. This could represent a GMH-IVH on the left side or possibly be due to free blood passing across from the IVH on the right.

ii) Current thinking is that the GMH-IVH compresses the venous plexus which drains blood from the periventricular cortex. As a consequence the area becomes ischaemic and the ischemia in turn leads to a haemorrhagic infarct. In some infants it is thought that the injury may primarily be a reperfusion injury following an ischaemic insult. Ultrasound cannot differentiate between the different pathological processes. Parenchymal lesions are reported to occur in 10–20%

of those infants with a GMH-IVH, and extension usually occurs within 24–48 hours of the initial bleed. Extension is more common when the initial bleed is large and is more likely in babies who remain unstable.

iii) Outcome following parenchymal involvement is more difficult to quantify as there are different pathological processes responsible and size, position, laterality and the presence of additional pathologies (PHVD for example) vary. There is no doubt that outcome is likely to be poor with extensive infarction, particularly bilaterally. However, for infants with unilateral and relatively small lesions a significant proportion of infants are normal at follow-up.[31,32]

iv) Damage cannot be reversed in this situation, but further damage may be avoided by concentrating on stabilisation. Although in this case sepsis was thought to be the reason for deterioration, this may have been attributable to the haemorrhage itself. Any treatable abnormalities in coagulation should be treated, blood pressure stabilised and circulating volume maintained. Serial scans are indicated and regular communication with the parents is essential.

ANSWER 10

i) The scan shows bilateral widespread periventricular cystic degeneration. The appearance is consistent with periventricular leukomalacia (PVL).

ii) In a relatively small number of infants a different pathological process may be observed where multiple cysts develop at the watershed zones between different cerebral vascular supplies. This condition, periventricular leukomalacia (PVL), is classically thought to be an ischaemia reperfusion injury although there is much debate as to the exact process. Alteration in perfusion due to hypocarbia has been implicated and damage due to oxygen free radicals is likely to contribute. These lesions are strongly associated with chorioamnionitis and it has been suggested that elevated inflammatory cytokines in the fetus may be responsible, at least in part, for the cystic degeneration.[33]

iii) Severe PVL affects approximately 5% of infants and milder PVL around 20%. It is less gestational age dependent than SEH-IVH. When bilateral and extensive there is a very strong association with cerebral palsy, more so than with any other lesion. When localised and unilateral, prognosis is difficult to predict with any certainty. In this specific case, the chance of severe neurodevelopmental impairment is very high.[34,35]

iv) Regrettably, there is little that can be done to influence the pathological process in this condition. Should an infant still be dependent upon intensive care when extensive PVL is diagnosed, there is an opportunity to discuss the appropriateness of continuing this level of care. However, many infants are in special care at the time of diagnosis. In these cases, early involvement of physiotherapists and speech and language therapists is advisable and regular communication and support for parents is essential. Following discharge, regular outpatient follow-up with appropriate specialist input is mandatory. As cure is not an option, prevention is the ideal. Close liaison with obstetric and midwifery services is crucial and formulation of management plans for high-risk mothers may help.

REFERENCES

1. Stark AR. Inhaled NO for preterm infants – getting to yes? N Engl J Med 2006;355:404–6
2. Norton ME, Merrill J, Cooper BA et al. Neonatal complications after the administration of indomethacin for preterm labor. N Engl J Med 1993;329(22):1602–7
3. Good WV, Hardy RJ, Dobson V et al. Early Treatment for Retinopathy of Prematurity Cooperative Group. The incidence and course of retinopathy of prematurity: findings from the early treatment for retinopathy of prematurity study. Pediatrics 2005;116:15–23
4. Raju TN, Langenberg P, Bhutani V et al. Vitamin E prophylaxis to reduce retinopathy of prematurity: a reappraisal of published trials. J Pediatr 1997;131(6):844–50
5. Gellen B, McIntosh N, McColm JR et al. Is the partial pressure of carbon dioxide in the blood related to the development of retinopathy of prematurity. Br J Ophthalmol 2001;85:1044–45
6. Pennefather PM, Tin W, Clarke MP et al. Retinopathy of prematurity in a controlled trial of prophylactic surfactant treatment. Br J Ophthalmol 1996;80:420–24
7. York JR, Landers S, Kirby RS et al. Arterial oxygen fluctuation and retinopathy of prematurity in very-low-birth-weight infants. J Perinatol 2004;24:82–87
8. Halliday H, Ehrenkranz RA, Doyle LW et al. Early postnatal (<96 hours) corticosteroids for preventing chronic lung disease in preterm infants. Cochrane Database Syst Rev 2003;(1):CD001146
9. Lawas-Alejo PA, Slivka S, Hernandez H et al. Hyperoxia and glucocorticoid modify retinal vessel growth and interleukin-1 receptor antagonist in newborn rabbits. Pediatr Res 1999;45(3):313–17
10. Cryotherapy for Retinopathy of Prematurity Cooperative Group. Multicenter trial of cryotherapy for retinopathy of prematurity: ophthalmological outcomes at 10 years. Arch Ophth 2001;119:1110–18
11. McLoone E, O'Keefe M, McLoone S, Lanigan B. Long term functional and structural outcomes of laser therapy for retinopathy of prematurity. Br J Ophthalmol 2006;90(6):754–59
12. Moise AA, Wearden ME, Kozinetz CA et al. Antenatal steroids are associated with less need for blood pressure support in extremely premature infants. Pediatrics 1995;95(6):845–50
13. Hill A, Perlman JM, Volpe JJ. Relationship of pneumothorax to occurrence of intraventricular hemorrhage in the premature newborn. Pediatrics 1982;69(2):144–49
14. Klarr JM, Faix RG, Pryce CJ, Bhatt-Mehta V. Randomized, blind trial of dopamine versus dobutamine for treatment of hypotension in preterm infants with respiratory distress syndrome. J Pediatr 1994;125(1):117–22
15. Valverde E, Pellicer A, Madero R et al. Dopamine versus epinephrine for cardiovascular support in low birth weight infants: analysis of systemic effects and neonatal clinical outcomes. Pediatrics 2006;117(6):e1213–e1222
16. Zanardo V, Dani C, Trevisanuto D et al. Methylxanthines increase renal calcium excretion in preterm infants. Biol Neonate 1995;68(3):169–74
17. Venkataraman PS, Han BK, Tsang RC, Daugherty CC. Secondary hyperparathyroidism and bone disease in infants receiving long-term furosemide therapy. Am J Dis Child 1983;137(12):1157–61
18. Weiler HA, Wang Z, Atkinson SA. Dexamethasone treatment impairs calcium regulation and reduces bone mineralization in infant pigs. Am J Clin Nutr 1995;61(4):805–11
19. Eliakim A, Nemet D, Friedland O et al. Spontaneous activity in premature infants affects bone strength. J Perinatol 2002;22:650–52
20. Kovar I, Mayne P, Barltrop D. Plasma alkaline phosphatase activity: a screening test for rickets in preterm neonates. Lancet 1982;Feb 6:308–10
21. Rennie J, De Vries L. Roberton's textbook of neonatology, 4th edn.Churchill Livingstone, Edinburgh, 2005
22. Lowe J, Papile L. Neurodevelopmental performance of very-low-birth-weight infants with mild periventricular, intraventricular hemorrhage. Outcome at 5 to 6 years of age. Am J Dis Child 1990;144:1242–45
23. Patra K, Wilson-Costello P, Taylor HG et al. Grades I–II intraventricular hemorrhage in extremely low birth weight infants: effects on neurodevelopment. J Pediatr 2006;149(2):169–73
24. Vasileiadis GT, Gelman N, Han VK et al. Uncomplicated intraventricular hemorrhage is followed by reduced cortical volume at near-term age. Pediatrics 2004;114(3):e367–e372

25. Levene MI, Starte D. A longitudinal study of post-haemorrhagic ventricular dilatation in the newborn. Arch Dis Child 1981;56:905–10

26. Murphy BP, Inder TE, Rooks V et al. Posthaemorrhagic ventricular dilatation in the premature infant: natural history and predictors of outcome. Arch Dis Child Fetal Neonatal Ed 2002;87(1):F37–F41

27. Ventriculomegaly Trial Group. Randomised trial of early tapping in neonatal posthaemorrhagic ventricular dilatation: results at 30 months. Arch Dis Child 1994;70:129–36

28. International PHVD Drug Trial Group. International randomised controlled trial of acetazolamide and frusemide in posthaemorrhagic ventricular dilatation in infancy. Lancet 1998;352:433–40

29. Ventriculomegaly Trial Group. Randomised trial of early tapping in neonatal posthaemorrhagic ventricular dilatation. Arch Dis Child 1990;65:3–10

30. Buxton N, Punt J. Failure to follow patients with hydrocephalus shunts can lead to death. Br J Neurosurg 1998;12:399–401

31. Guzzetta F, Shackelford GD, Volpe S et al. Periventricular intraparenchymal echodensities in the premature newborn: critical determinant of neurologic outcome. Pediatrics 1986;78:995–1006

32. de Vries LS, Roelants-van Rijn AM, Rademaker KJ et al. Unilateral parenchymal haemorrhagic infarction in the preterm infant. Eur J Paediatr Neurol 2001;5:139–49

33. Wu YW, Colford JM. Chorioamnionitis as a risk factor for cerebral palsy: a meta-analysis. JAMA 2000;284:1417–24

34. Trounce JQ, Rutter N, Levene MI. Periventricular leucomalacia and intraventricular haemorrhage in the preterm neonate. Arch Dis Child 1988;61:1196–202

35. Han TR, Bang MS, Lim JY et al. Risk factors of cerebral palsy in preterm infants. Am J Phys Med Rehab 2002;81:297–303

Chapter 6

Ventilation and blood gases

Problems with respiration provide a substantial proportion of the acute work-load of a neonatologist. Early respiratory problems lead to physiological instability, which in turn contributes to other pathological processes that lead to mortality and morbidity. The management of early respiratory difficulties itself contributes to subsequent problems, with severe chronic lung disease rarely occurring in infants that have not received mechanical ventilation. The knowledge that positive pressure ventilation may in itself be harmful has led to a quest for methods to reduce the need for such support. Different modalities of ventilation have been developed and are widely used – not necessarily with evidence to support their use or inform on the best methods of using that particular technique. Surfactant is widely used and continuous positive airway pressure is gaining wider acceptance as a primary means of providing respiratory support as opposed to a modality principally for weaning babies from positive pressure ventilation. Whatever the method used, the mode in which it is used and the adjuncts used in association with it (e.g. surfactant) there will be changes in respiratory status which may be rapid and potentially very serious. Central to effective monitoring of respiratory status is the measurement of blood gases and any individual responsible for the care of acutely unwell infants must be comfortable with the interpretation of blood gas results and with the impact of changes in ventilation on the different parameters being measured.

In this chapter a series of blood gas results are given. Where appropriate, ventilator settings and relevant history are also given. The results should be interpreted and a decision made as to what the result implies – acidosis or alkalosis, metabolic or respiratory. An explanation for the abnormality should be given where possible and a plan formulated for the action that needs to be taken to rectify the problem. On occasion you may conclude that the result is normal and therefore no action need be taken. Think carefully. Making no changes is not the same as doing nothing and a normal result does not necessarily mean that some action should not be taken to see whether a normal result can still be obtained when the amount of support is reduced. Neonatal care must always be proactive. Doing nothing is rarely the best option.

1. You are presented with the following blood gas result on a 31 week infant who is 2 hours old.

pH	7.35	HCO$_3$	20.4
PcO$_2$	3.10	BE	−4.2
PcCO$_2$	4.9	FiO$_2$	0.21

  a. What does this show?

  b. What further piece of information do you need to be able to interpret it correctly?

2. A 34 week infant is delivered by emergency caesarean section for fetal distress. At 4 hours she is settled and breathing spontaneously in room air. The following blood gas result is obtained from a capillary sample.

pH	7.37	HCO$_3$	24.5
PcO$_2$	4.2	BE	−0.4
PcCO$_2$	5.6	FiO$_2$	0.21

  a. What does this show?

  b. What further information would help you to decide what action to take?

3. A term infant has been born following a difficult delivery during which the CTG had shown frequent decelerations. She is quietly breathing room air. Respiratory rate is 48/minute and there is no recession and grunting. The baby responds appropriately to handling. A capillary blood sample is taken 30 minutes after birth and the following blood gas result obtained.

pH	7.26	HCO$_3$	21.8
PcO$_2$	2.8	BE	−5.5
PcCO$_2$	6.5	FiO$_2$	0.21

  a. What does this show?

  b. What factors in the history should be considered before taking action in response to this result?

4. An infant is born at 28 weeks gestation, has received surfactant and is on CPAP. An umbilical arterial line has been inserted and a blood sample is taken through it while an X-ray is awaited and sent for blood gas analysis. The following result is obtained.

pH	7.35	PIP	
PaO$_2$	3.5	PEEP	4
PaCO$_2$	5.7	TI	
HCO$_3$	23.7	TE	
BE	−1.6	Flow	8 L/min
FiO$_2$	0.34		

The infant is being monitored. Heart rate is 134 bpm, respiratory rate 50/minute, SaO$_2$ is 100%.

a. What do these results show?
b. What is the most likely explanation?
c. What two actions will you take?

5. A 37 week infant is born by emergency caesarean section after a haemorrhage due to a torn umbilical cord. The baby is moderately bradycardic and approximately one minute of cardiac compression is given. As the heart rate remains relatively slow a bolus of 10 mL/kg of 0.9% saline is given with some improvement. The infant is transferred to the neonatal unit. Monitoring is started and oxygen saturation is 97%. A blood sample is obtained by arterial stab 20 minutes after birth and the result of blood gas analysis is shown below.

pH	7.22
PaO_2	8.5
$PaCO_2$	5.0
HCO_3	15.2
BE	−11.7
FiO_2	0.25
Hb	13.2 g/dl

a. What does the blood gas show?
b. What must be done when such a result is obtained?
c. What is the most likely explanation in this case and what action should be taken?

6. A 29 week gestation infant is 2 hours old. He has a respiratory rate of 70 and there is mild recession. A soft end-expiratory grunt is audible. An arterial blood sample is taken and blood gas analysis is performed.

pH	7.32
PaO_2	6.5
$PaCO_2$	6.2
HCO_3	24.0
BE	−2.1
FiO_2	0.32

a. What does the blood gas show?
b. What two actions should be taken?
c. What three investigations might you want to be sure had been performed?

7. A 38 week gestation infant was well at birth. At 6 hours of age she is noted to be tachycardic and tachypnoeic. An end-expiratory grunt is heard. An arterial stab is performed and blood gas analysis performed.

pH	7.36
PaO_2	9.6
$PaCO_2$	4.8
HCO_3	20.5
BE	−3.8
FiO_2	0.21

a. What does blood the gas show?
b. What three investigations would you make sure had been done?
c. What therapy would you start?

8. A 29 week gestation infant has been given oxygen since birth. Inspired oxygen is steadily rising. The baby has had a number of bradycardias and one severe apnoea. An umbilical arterial line has been inserted and a blood sample is taken for blood gas analysis. The following result is obtained.

pH	7.30
PaO_2	5.4
$PaCO_2$	6.2
HCO_3	22.9
BE	-3.5
FiO_2	0.60

   a. What does blood the gas show?
   b. A septic screen and chest X-ray have already been performed. What further management would you consider?

9. A 27 week gestation infant is 12 hours old. She is grunting and there is obvious recession. Her respiratory rate is 90/minute and there are frequent bradycardias. The following result is obtained from an umbilical arterial line blood sample.

pH	7.35
PaO_2	4.4
$PaCO_2$	6.8
HCO_3	28.3
BE	2.05
FiO_2	0.55

   a. What does the blood gas show?
   b. What are the main problems that must be treated?
   c. What measures could be taken to address them?

10. A 32 week gestation infant is born to a mother whose membranes ruptured 60 hours before delivery. Group B streptococcus had been grown from an introital swab taken when mother was admitted at 20 weeks with some abdominal pains that subsequently resolved. Mother received no medication between rupture of membranes and delivery other than analgesia. At 4 hours of age the baby is grunting and appears poorly perfused. A capillary sample is attempted but perfusion is very poor and the sample clots before it is completed. After some discussion it is decided that a radial artery stab should be performed. The following result is obtained.

pH	7.20
PaO_2	9.9
$PaCO_2$	5.1
HCO_3	14.8
BE	-12.6
FiO_2	0.35

   a. What is the most important treatment to be commenced?
   b. Why?
   c. What investigations are urgently needed?
   d. What serious error in management has been made?

11. An infant has been born at 28 weeks gestation and weighs 1.3 kg. There was good respiratory effort initially and a decision was made to place him on CPAP at a pressure of 6 cmH$_2$O. Initial capillary gas was poor but thought to be due to poor perfusion. Over the last two hours the baby has become more symptomatic with obvious recession and occasional bradycardias and desaturation. An umbilical arterial line has been inserted and a blood sample is taken. The following result is obtained.

pH	7.18	PIP	
PaO$_2$	4.6	PEEP	6
PaCO$_2$	7.3	TI	
HCO$_3$	20.2	TE	
BE	−8.9	Flow	8 L/min
FiO$_2$	0.55		

a. What do these results show?
b. What is the most likely explanation?
c. What actions will you take?

12. Following on from question 11, the infant was intubated, given surfactant and positive pressure ventilation was commenced. Oxygen saturation has been above 95% and a further arterial blood gas sample is taken at three hours.

pH	7.5	PIP	18
PaO$_2$	12.5	PEEP	4
PaCO$_2$	2.6	TI	0.35
HCO$_3$	15 .5	TE	0.65
BE	−4.0	Flow	8.5 L/min
FiO$_2$	0.45		

MAP 8. 9 mBar, VT 10.4 mL, MV 0.62 L/min

a. What do these results show?
b. What is the explanation?
c. What actions will you take?
d. What errors in management have been made?

13. A 28 week gestation, 1.15 kg baby has been ventilated for respiratory distress syndrome. He has received surfactant and oxygenation has started to improve. He is now 6 hours old. An umbilical artery catheter has been inserted and an arterial blood gas taken. Arterial blood pressure is 32/18 with a mean of 24.

pH	7.2	PIP	22
PaO$_2$	7.7	PEEP	5
PaCO$_2$	4.8	TI	0.4
HCO$_3$	13.9	TE	0.6
BE	−13.2	Flow	8 L/min
FiO$_2$	0.29		

MAP 14. 6 mBar, VT 5.75 mL, MV 0.37 L/min

a. What do these results show?
b. What is the most likely explanation?
c. What actions will you take?

14. A 26 week, 800 g infant has been ventilated for severe respiratory distress syndrome. He is now 48 hours old and remains unstable. The following arterial blood gas is obtained.

pH	7.16	PIP	22
PaO_2	5.8	PEEP	5
$PaCO_2$	8.0	TI	0.35
HCO_3	21.1	TE	0.65
BE	−8.7	Flow	7.5 L/min
FiO_2	0.65		

MAP 10. 5 mBar, VT 2.4 mL, MV 0.15 L/min

   a. What do these results show?
   b. What is the most likely explanation?
   c. What actions will you take?

15. A 29 week gestation infant, birth weight 1.5 kg, has been ventilated for two days and has been stable and ventilation is weaning. He suddenly becomes bradycardic and remains with a heart rate below 60. At the same time his oxygen requirement rises sharply. The following arterial blood gas is obtained within two minutes of the bradycardia.

pH	7.28	PIP	18
PaO_2	2.5	PEEP	4
$PaCO_2$	10.9	TI	0.4
HCO_3	35.5	TE	0.9
BE	5.3	Flow	8.5 L/min
FiO_2	0.75		

MAP 8. 3 mBar, VT 3.2 mL, MV 0.14 L/min

   a. What do these results show?
   b. What is the most likely explanation?
   c. What actions will you take?

16. In the same infant the peak inspiratory pressure has been increased. The infant remains bradycardic and the oxygen saturation has fallen and is no longer measurable. A repeat arterial blood gas is obtained.

pH	7.06	PIP	26
PaO_2	1.2	PEEP	4
$PaCO_2$	11.8	TI	0.4
HCO_3	24.5	TE	0.9
BE	−8.7	Flow	8.5 L/min
FiO_2	1.0		

MAP 10. 8 mBar, VT 1.1 mL, MV 0.11 L/min

   a. What do these results show?
   b. What is the most likely explanation?
   c. What actions will you take?

17. In the same infant as question **16** a chest drain has now been inserted and good chest movement is seen. Oxygen saturation improves and inspired oxygen concentration can be reduced. The following arterial blood gas is obtained an hour later.

pH	7.48	PIP	22
PaO$_2$	10.1	PEEP	5
PaCO$_2$	3.5	TI	0.35
HCO$_3$	19.9	TE	0.65
BE	−1.1	Flow	7.5 L/min
FiO$_2$	0.55		

MAP 10. 7 mBar, VT 12.1 mL, MV 0.56 L/min

a. What do these results show?
b. What is the most likely explanation?
c. What actions will you take?
d. What basic error has been made?

18. A 26 week infant is 8 days old. He weighed 1.0 kg at birth. He was initially maintained on CPAP but changed to positive pressure ventilation on day two. He reached maximum pressures of 28/4 and inspired oxygen of 0.8. The following arterial gas is obtained.

pH	7.50	PIP	24
PaO$_2$	4.7	PEEP	4
PaCO$_2$	3.1	TI	0.4
HCO$_3$	18.5	TE	0.6
BE	−1.7	Flow	9.1 L/min
FiO$_2$	0.60		

MAP 11 . 5 mBar, VT 7.1 mL, MV 0.4 L/min

a. What do these results show?
b. What is the most likely explanation?
c. What actions will you take?

19. A 37 week gestation female infant weighing 2.8 kg is admitted following an elective caesarean section as the mother's two previous deliveries had also been by caesarean section. She develops quite severe respiratory signs and has a respiratory acidosis. She will not tolerate CPAP and gases deteriorate further. She is intubated and positive pressure ventilation is commenced. Oxygenation remains poor and an arterial blood gases obtained.

pH	7.28	PIP	24
PaO$_2$	5.1	PEEP	4
PaCO$_2$	6.7	TI	0.5
HCO$_3$	23.6	TE	0.5
BE	−3.5	Flow	3.0 L/min
FiO$_2$	0.71		

MAP 9. 2 mBar, VT 8.1 mL, MV 0.49 L/min

a. What do these results show?
b. What is the most likely explanation?
c. What actions will you take?

20. A 27 week infant has required ventilation from birth. She is active and making obvious respiratory movements. Her weight is 1.07 kg. An arterial gas is obtained.

pH	7.16	PIP	22
PaO$_2$	5.8	PEEP	4
PaCO$_2$	6.7	TI	0.6
HCO$_3$	17.7	TE	0.8
BE	−11.4	Flow	8.0 L/min
FiO$_2$	0.65		

MAP 11. 6 mBar, VT 4.4 mL, MV 0.18 L/min

    a. What do these results show?
    b. What is the most likely explanation?
    c. What actions will you take?

21. A 28 week infant has required ventilation following a difficult delivery. Initial ventilation was minimal but his condition has deteriorated over the first 36 hours despite three doses of surfactant. The lungs appear poorly aerated on X-ray and there are widespread inflammatory changes. The following arterial blood gas is obtained. He weighs 1.3 kg.

pH	7.17	PIP	24
PaO$_2$	4.9	PEEP	5
PaCO$_2$	9.9	TI	0.35
HCO$_3$	26.7	TE	0.65
BE	−4.2	Flow	9.0 L/min
FiO$_2$	0.85		

MAP 11. 2 mBar, VT 4.9 mL, MV 0.28 L/min

    a. What do these results show?
    b. What is the most likely explanation?
    c. What actions will you take?

22. A 34 week infant has developed severe abdominal distension and an ileal atresia has been diagnosed. Laparotomy is performed for which he requires ventilation. Postoperatively ventilatory requirements steadily increase and 48 hours after surgery the following arterial blood gas is obtained. Chest X-ray shows a ground-glass appearance and low lung volumes. His weight at birth was 2.1 kg.

pH	7.20	PIP	24
PaO$_2$	6.1	PEEP	4
PaCO$_2$	10.1	TI	0.4
HCO$_3$	29.3	TE	0.9
BE	−1.2	Flow	10.2 L/min
FiO$_2$	0.85		

MAP 10. 1 mBar, VT 6.3 mL, MV 0.29 L/min

    a. What do these results show?
    b. What is the most likely explanation?
    c. What actions will you take?

23. In the same infant surfactant has been given and some changes made to ventilation. The following gas is obtained 90 minutes later.

pH	7.38	PIP	24
PaO_2	14.6	PEEP	4
$PaCO_2$	4.1	TI	0.35
HCO_3	18.3	TE	0.35
BE	−5.0	Flow	10.2 L/min
FiO_2	0.55		

MAP 14. 0 mBar, VT 12.1 mL, MV 1.04 L/min

a. What do these results show?
b. What is the most likely explanation?
c. What actions will you take?

24. In the same infant some changes in ventilation are made. The following arterial blood gas is obtained two hours later.

pH	7.52	PIP	22
PaO_2	9.8	PEEP	4
$PaCO_2$	3.3	TI	0.35
HCO_3	21	TE	0.35
BE	1.11	Flow	10.2 L/min
FiO_2	0.35		

MAP 12. 5 mBar, VT 13.2 mL, MV 1.13 L/min

a. What do these results show?
b. What is the most likely explanation?
c. What actions will you take?

25. A 34 week gestation infant required air only at birth. Her condition has steadily deteriorated and she required ventilation 36 hours after birth. The following arterial blood gas is obtained at 72 hours of age. She weighs 2.1 kg.

pH	7.26	PIP	22
PaO_2	9.1	PEEP	5
$PaCO_2$	8.3	TI	0.4
HCO_3	27.8	TE	0.9
BE	−0.7	Flow	8.7 L/min
FiO_2	0.80		

MAP 10. 8 mBar, VT 12.2 mL, MV 0.56 L/min

a. What do these results show?
b. What is the most likely explanation?
c. What actions will you take?

26. In the same infant as question 25 the expiratory time has been reduced and the ventilator rate increased. The following arterial blood gas is obtained one hour after the change.

pH	7.38	PIP	22
PaO_2	11.4	PEEP	5
$PaCO_2$	6.1	TI	0.4
HCO_3	27.3	TE	0.6
BE	2.1	Flow	8.7 L/min
FiO_2	0.65		

MAP 11. 8 mBar, VT 12.2 mL, MV 0.3 L/min

a. What do these results show?
b. What is the most likely explanation?
c. What actions will you take?

27. A 27 week gestation infant weighing 0.98 kg has moderately severe RDS and has required ventilation from birth. Carbon dioxide is good but oxygenation is difficult. The following arterial blood gas is obtained.

pH	7.36	PIP	22
PaO_2	4.7	PEEP	4
$PaCO_2$	5.1	TI	0.3
HCO_3	21.7	TE	0.5
BE	−2.8	Flow	3.0 L/min
FiO_2	0.85		

MAP 7. 7 mBar, VT 4.4 mL, MV 0.33 L/min

a. What do these results show?
b. What is the most likely explanation?
c. What actions will you take?

28. Continuing with the case above. You have elected to increase the flow and have found that after setting 9 L/min you are able to get good chest movement and the ventilator display shows that you now have a good airway pressure curve. Oxygenation improves and you are able to reduce the inspired oxygen concentration. The unit is busy and you are unable to see the baby for a further six hours. However, a colleague performed a blood gas analysis after three hours and reassured you that the pH was acceptable and oxygenation was better. When you are able to return you check the arterial gas, which is shown below.

pH	7.35	PIP	22
PaO_2	8.9	PEEP	5
$PaCO_2$	2.1	TI	0.35
HCO_3	8.8	TE	0.65
BE	−13.4	Flow	7.5 L/min
FiO_2	0.35		

MAP 10. 8 mBar, VT 6.1 mL, MV 0.37 L/min

a. What do these results show?
b. What is the most likely explanation?
c. What actions will you take?

29. A 29 week gestation infant weighing 1.15 kg has been placed on synchronised intermittent positive pressure ventilation. He is fighting the ventilator and appears distressed. You are considering either paralysing him or returning him to conventional ventilation. The following arterial blood gas is obtained.

pH	7.20	PIP	20
PaO_2	9.1	PEEP	5
$PaCO_2$	7.1	TI	0.6
HCO_3	20.6	TE	0.6
BE	−8.0	Flow	9.2 L/min
FiO_2	0.55		

MAP 12. 1 mBar, VT 3.1 mL, MV 0.15 L/min

a. What do these results show?
b. What is the most likely explanation?
c. What actions will you take?

30. A 29 week infant is on synchronised intermittent positive pressure ventilation but does not appear to be triggering well. He weighs 1.25 kg. The following blood gas is obtained.

pH	7.48	PIP	18
PaO_2	9.1	PEEP	4
$PaCO_2$	4.1	TI	0.35
HCO_3	23.3	TE	0.35
BE	1.6	Flow	8.1 L/min
FiO_2	0.42		

MAP 10. 6 mBar, VT 5.2 mL, MV 0.46 L/min

a. What do these results show?
b. What is the most likely explanation?
c. What actions will you take?

31. Following on from the case above you have asked a colleague to alter the expiratory time. You return to the baby three hours later and are concerned because your colleague appears to have chosen a longer expiratory time than you would have liked. You take an arterial blood gas, the result of which is shown below.

pH	7.35	PIP	18
PaO_2	7.2	PEEP	4
$PaCO_2$	5.2	TI	0.35
HCO_3	21.6	TE	1.65
BE	−3.2	Flow	8.1 L/min
FiO_2	0.35		

MAP 10. 8 mBar, VT 5.1 mL, MV 0.31 L/min

a. What do these results show?
b. What is the most likely explanation?
c. What actions will you take?

32. A 31 week infant is ventilated on synchronised intermittent mandatory ventilation. The amount of spontaneous breathing is minimal and appears to be less than 10% of the total. The following arterial blood gas is obtained. She weighs 1.6 kg.

pH	7.31	PIP	18
PaO_2	5.5	PEEP	5
$PaCO_2$	7.1	TI	0.35
HCO_3	26.9	TE	0.55
BE	−0.2	Flow	8.8 L/min
FiO_2	0.55		

MAP 10. 1 mBar, VT 9.2 mL, MV 0.69 L/min

a. What do these results show?
b. What is the most likely explanation?
c. What actions will you take?

33. A 27 week infant is one week old and has had RDS. Ventilation is being weaned using synchronised intermittent mandatory ventilation. The following arterial blood gas is obtained. He weighs 1 kg.

pH	7.22	PIP	17
PaO_2	9.1	PEEP	4
$PaCO_2$	8.3	TI	0.3
HCO_3	25.3	TE	1.7
BE	−3.8	Flow	6.4 L/min
FiO_2	0.35		

MAP 5. 8 mBar, VT 4.9 mL, MV 0.15 L/min

  a. What do these results show?
  b. What is the most likely explanation?
  c. What actions will you take?

34. A 3.5 kg term male infant has been ventilated following an asphyxial episode. Ventilation has been easy with excellent tidal volumes and there has been good spontaneous respiratory effort. Ventilation has been so good that he has been extubated into incubator air. Shortly after extubation he has a profound apnoea and bradycardia that does not respond very well to bag and mask ventilation. He is intubated and ventilation is recommenced at the same settings he was effectively ventilated on previously. The following arterial blood gas is obtained.

pH	7.2	PIP	18
PaO_2	6.5	PEEP	5
$PaCO_2$	8.3	TI	0.35
HCO_3	25.3	TE	0.65
BE	−3.8	Flow	10.2 L/min
FiO_2	0.65		

MAP 9. 2 mBar, VT 8.8 mL, MV 0.52 L/min

  a. What do these results show?
  b. What is the most likely explanation?
  c. What actions will you take?

35. A 25 week infant is ventilated for RDS. He has received two doses of surfactant and oxygenation has improved. Carbon dioxide clearance remains poor. The following arterial blood gas is obtained. His weight is 1.05 kg.

pH	7.23	PIP	20
PaO_2	9.1	PEEP	7
$PaCO_2$	8.3	TI	0.35
HCO_3	25.3	TE	0.65
BE	−3.8	Flow	11.6 L/min
FiO_2	0.39		

MAP 10. 5 mBar, VT 2.3 mL, MV 0.13 L/min

  a. What do these results show?
  b. What is the most likely explanation?
  c. What actions will you take?

36. A 29 week infant who weighed 1.3 kg at birth has been ventilated for RDS. He has received three doses of surfactant but his condition has continued to deteriorate. Oxygenation remains poor in 100% oxygen. The following arterial blood gas is obtained.

pH	7.19	PIP	29
PaO_2	6.1	PEEP	5
$PaCO_2$	9.9	TI	0.5
HCO_3	28.1	TE	0.5
BE	−2.4	Flow	10.2 L/min
FiO_2	1.0		

MAP 16. 4 mBar, VT 3.2 mL, MV 0.17 L/min

  a. What do these results show?
  b. What is the most likely explanation?
  c. What actions will you take?

37. Following on from the previous question. Although high-frequency ventilation is available a decision has been made to continue with conventional positive pressure ventilation and to increase the peak pressure and PEEP. After one hour the following arterial blood gas is obtained.

pH	7.14	PIP	34
PaO_2	5.8	PEEP	7
$PaCO_2$	10.1	TI	0.5
HCO_3	24.9	TE	0.5
BE	−6.2	Flow	11.1 L/min
FiO_2	0.95		

MAP 18. 4 mBar, VT 3.1 mL, MV 0.16 L/min

  a. What do these results show?
  b. What is the most likely explanation?
  c. What actions will you take?

38. High-frequency ventilation has been commenced. A blood gas is taken 30 minutes later.

pH	7.16	ΔP	30
PaO_2	6.1	TI:TE	1:2
$PaCO_2$	10.4	Flow	25 L/min
HCO_3	24.6		
BE	−3.6		
FiO_2	1.0		

MAP 18 mBar, VT_{HF} 1.2 mL

  a. What do these results show?
  b. What is the most likely explanation?
  c. What actions will you take?

39. Continuing from the previous case. Two further changes are made in the mean airway pressure and following the second manoeuvre oxygenation starts to improve. A chest X-ray has been performed that has shown good lung expansion. Oxygen saturation has improved and inspired oxygen concentration has been reduced significantly. The following arterial blood gas is obtained two hours after the second change in pressure.

pH	7.15	ΔP	30
PaO_2	8.9	TI:TE	1:2
$PaCO_2$	10.2	Flow	25 L/min
HCO_3	26.3		
BE	−4.9		
FiO_2	0.45		

MAP 22 mBar, VT_{HF} 1.2 mL

a. What do these results show?
b. What is the most likely explanation?
c. What actions will you take?

40. The pressure swing has been adjusted and the baby has been left for 30 minutes. The following arterial blood gas is obtained.

pH	7.38	ΔP	42
PaO_2	10.6	TI:TE	1:2
$PaCO_2$	4.5	Flow	25 L/min
HCO_3	20.1		
BE	−3.6		
FiO_2	0.25		

MAP 22 mBar, VT_{HF} 2.5 mL

a. What do these results show?
b. What is the most likely explanation?
c. What actions will you take?

41. Continuing from above. No changes are made to ventilation and the infant is left while problems are dealt with elsewhere on the neonatal unit. Oxygen saturations start to deteriorate and inspired oxygen is increased. The mean airway pressure is increased further without benefit so is increased once more. Oxygenation continues to deteriorate. The following arterial blood gas is obtained eight hours after the previous one.

pH	7.22	ΔP	42
PaO_2	5.6	TI:TE	1:2
$PaCO_2$	9.8	Flow	25 L/min
HCO_3	29.9		
BE	−0.21		
FiO_2	0.85		

MAP 26 mBar, VT_{HF} 1.4 mL

a. What do these results show?
b. What is the most likely explanation?
c. What actions will you take?

42. A 27 week infant has been ventilated since birth for RDS. Condition has deteriorated over the first two days and ventilation requirements have steadily

increased. The following arterial blood gas is obtained. Her birth weight was 950 g.

pH	7.38	PIP	30
PaO_2	9.1	PEEP	4
$PaCO_2$	3.5	TI	0.4
HCO_3	15.7	TE	0.4
BE	−7.1	Flow	8.9 L/min
FiO_2	0.45		

MAP 16.1 mBar, VT 2.1 mL, MV 0.14 L/min

a. What do these results show?
b. What is the most likely explanation?
c. What actions will you take?

43. A 28 week infant has been ventilated since birth and is now 5 days old. His birth weight was 1.1 kg. The following arterial blood gas is obtained.

pH	7.36	PIP	24
PaO_2	12.2	PEEP	4
$PaCO_2$	5.9	TI	0.5
HCO_3	25.4	TE	0.5
BE	−0.16	Flow	8.1 L/min
FiO_2	0.7		

MAP 12.9 mBar, VT 5.2 mL, MV 0.29 L/min

a. What do these results show?
b. What is the most likely explanation?
c. What actions will you take?

44. A 25 week baby has been ventilated for three weeks for quite severe respiratory distress syndrome. There have been significant problems with oxygenation. The lungs show chronic inflammatory changes on X-ray. The following arterial blood gas is obtained. Most recent weight was 920 g.

pH	7.35	PIP	22
PaO_2	7.2	PEEP	4
$PaCO_2$	9.6	TI	0.4
HCO_3	39.6	TE	0.6
BE	10.9	Flow	9.9 L/min
FiO_2	0.5		

MAP 11.1 mBar, VT 4.2 mL, MV 0.2 L/min

a. What do these results show?
b. What is the most likely explanation?
c. What actions will you take?

45. A 29 week gestation infant has been ventilated for five days. Peak pressure was 26 and maximum inspired oxygen was 70%. There has been steady improvement over the last 24 hours. The following arterial blood gas is obtained. Birth weight was 1.25 kg.

pH	7.32	PIP	14
PaO$_2$	8.2	PEEP	4
PaCO$_2$	7.1	TI	0.4
HCO$_3$	26.1	TE	0.4
BE	0.8	Flow	6.9 L/min
FiO$_2$	0.35		

MAP 9. 0 mBar, VT 5.2 mL, MV 0.39 L/min

a. What do these results show?
b. What is the most likely explanation?
c. What actions will you take?

46. A term infant is found pale and shocked at 3 hours of age on the postnatal wards after birth to a mother with prolonged rupture of membranes. The baby is admitted to the neonatal unit, ventilation is commenced and an arterial line inserted. The following arterial blood gas is obtained. The baby weighs 3.2 kg.

pH	7.01	PIP	28
PaO$_2$	1.3	PEEP	4
PaCO$_2$	6.6	TI	0.6
HCO$_3$	12.1	TE	0.6
BE	−19.6	Flow	14.2 L/min
FiO$_2$	1.0		

MAP 16. 0 mBar, VT 22.0 mL, MV 1.1 L/min

a. What do these results show?
b. What is the most likely explanation?
c. What actions will you take?

47. Continuing with the infant above. Penicillin and gentamicin have been commenced. Peak inspiratory pressures have been increased and an attempt had been made to reverse the ratios (make the inspiratory time longer than the expiratory time). Tolazoline has been given but has only served to drop the blood pressure which now requires boluses of volume and an inotrope infusion to restore it. The following arterial blood gas is obtained.

pH	7.07	PIP	44
PaO$_2$	1.4	PEEP	6
PaCO$_2$	6.3	TI	0.7
HCO$_3$	14.02	TE	0.4
BE	−16.6	Flow	14.1 L/min
FiO$_2$	1.0		

MAP 28. 8 mBar, VT 19.4 mL, MV 1.09 L/min

a. What do these results show?
b. What is the oxygenation index?
c. What is the most likely explanation?
d. What actions will you take?

48. A 25 week infant was ventilated for 4 weeks after birth. She is now nine weeks old and is fully enterally fed. She has occasional bradycardias but is otherwise stable. She is on low flow oxygen through nasal prongs at a rate of 0.3 L/min. She has routine blood tests taken on alternate weeks. On this occasion a capillary blood gas is performed.

pH	7.32	HCO_3	36.4
PO_2	8.6	BE	7.61
PCO_2	9.4	Oxygen	0.3 L/min

a. What do these results show?
b. What is the most likely explanation?
c. What actions will you take?

49. The same infant as in the preceding question was due to be discharged when she developed a viral pneumonia. Her oxygen requirements rose such that she developed serious apnoeas and intubation and ventilation were required. A radial arterial line was inserted. She has been ventilated for 48 hours and the following arterial blood gas is obtained. The last weight was 2.3 kg.

pH	7.47	PIP	24
PaO_2	7.4	PEEP	6
$PaCO_2$	5.2	TI	0.4
HCO_3	28.9	TE	0.8
BE	5.7	Flow	11.4 L/min
FiO_2	0.65		

MAP 11. 8 mBar, VT 13.8 mL, MV 0.72 L/min

a. What do these results show?
b. What is the most likely explanation?
c. What actions will you take?

50. A baby born at 33 weeks gestation had no problems at birth and an uneventful postnatal course. He is about to be discharged at 37 weeks when he starts to vomit profusely after every feed. A capillary blood gas is obtained.

pH	7.52
PcO_2	12.9
$PcCO_2$	6.3
HCO_3	39.5
BE	15.0
FiO_2	0.21

a. What do these results show?
b. What is the most likely explanation?
c. What actions will you take?

ANSWERS

1. **a.** The gas appears to show hypoxia.
   b. There is no information as to what sort of sample this is. If it is a fresh arterial sample the result definitely shows hypoxia. If it is a capillary sample the result cannot be interpreted.

2. **a.** The gas appears to show hypoxia but a capillary sample was used.
   b. Some other indication of oxygenation is essential – pulse oximetry or transcutaneous oxygen measurement would be appropriate. The PaO_2

is underestimated on a capillary sample but the extent to which it differs from an arterial sample cannot be accurately predicted as it will be affected greatly by peripheral capillary perfusion. It is therefore conceivable that a low capillary PO_2 could represent hypoxia, normoxia or hyperoxia and some other means must be used to establish what the result actually means.

3. **a.** The capillary gas sample appears to show a mixture of hypoxia, respiratory acidosis and metabolic acidosis.

   b. Although there is some information in the history to suggest that the infant could have suffered an asphyxial episode – difficult delivery and decelerations on CTG – the description of the infant does not suggest this, nor does it suggest a baby with a significant hypoxia or acidosis. A normal infant who is not ventilated will attempt to respond to the abnormalities in the blood gas if they are genuine. Hypoxia will result in increased respiratory rate and effort, and grunting is likely in an attempt to decrease end-expiratory atelectasis. A respiratory acidosis will normally result in hyperventilation to reduce the carbon dioxide and the normal response to a metabolic acidosis is also hyperventilation. Although a seriously asphyxiated infant may not mount an appropriate response, this does not seem to be the case here as the infant is reported to be responding appropriately to handling. The 'normality' of the infant would suggest that the result is due to a capillary gas sample taken when there is poor peripheral perfusion. This is very common shortly after birth and it is important that such results are interpreted with great caution.

4. **a.** An apparent hypoxia. However, the PO_2 of 3.5 does not seem to be compatible with a saturation of 100% on pulse oximetry.

   b. The most likely explanation is that the umbilical arterial line has been inserted into the umbilical vein by mistake and mixed venous PO_2 is being measured.

   c. A chest and abdominal X-ray should be obtained as quickly as possible to check on the position of the catheter. Until this has been established it would be prudent to reduce the inspired oxygen to obtain a SaO_2 in the mid 80s to low 90s.

5. **a.** The blood gas result shows evidence of a metabolic acidosis. Bicarbonate, base deficit and pH are low; CO_2 is normal.

   b. In any case of a metabolic acidosis it is crucially important that the cause of the acidosis is established. It is not enough to simply establish that an acidosis is present and treat it by giving base. This may temporarily correct the acidosis but leaves the cause untreated. Many conditions may lead to a metabolic acidosis – sepsis, heart failure, haemorrhage, hypovolaemia and hypotension to name but a few – and in many of these cases it is obviously essential that the cause is addressed as a matter of urgency.

   c. In this case the most likely (but not necessarily the correct) cause of the acidosis is hypovolaemia due to acute blood loss. An urgent cross-match should be performed and the haemoglobin monitored closely until blood is available. The haemoglobin is not particularly low but may well not have reached the lowest point yet while fluid shifts from extravascular to intravascular compartments. If the haemoglobin drops further while you are waiting for the cross-matched blood it may be prudent to give emergency O Rh −ve, CMV −ve blood.

6. **a.** Moderate hypoxia in 32% oxygen and mild respiratory acidosis.
   b. The hypoxia can probably be treated by simply increasing the inspired oxygen concentration. The baby must be closely monitored. The respiratory acidosis is not sufficiently severe to warrant CPAP or ventilation but the baby is becoming symptomatic – soft end-expiratory grunt – and may well continue to deteriorate.
   c. A chest X-ray would be very appropriate at this point in time, and if not performed already blood should be sent for inflammatory markers (FBC and CRP) and blood cultures taken. If the X-ray appearances were compatible with respiratory distress syndrome some practitioners would consider briefly intubating the infant so that surfactant could be administered. There is no consensus on this practice and no clinical trial evidence base to justify it.

7. **a.** It is normal.
   b. Although the blood gas is normal the infant is symptomatic. In a term infant developing respiratory symptoms shortly after birth infection is the most worrying possibility and initial investigations should explore this possibility. Blood should be taken for FBC and CRP, blood cultures should be sent and a chest X-ray taken.
   c. Antibiotics should be started. The choice of antibiotic would be determined by local policy which should in turn be determined by any known local resistant organisms.

8. **a.** Significant hypoxia despite a relatively high inspired oxygen concentration. There is a combined respiratory and metabolic acidosis. The carbon dioxide is mildly elevated but the bicarbonate is lower than would be expected in the face of this elevation. The base deficit is moderately high.
   b. Some form of ventilatory support is required. Most practitioners would start either CPAP or positive pressure ventilation at this point. Surfactant could be considered as discussed in the answer to question **6**.

9. **a.** Significant hypoxia despite a relatively high inspired oxygen concentration. pH is satisfactory and there is no evidence of either respiratory or metabolic acidosis. However, the infant is becoming symptomatic. Respiratory rate is quite high and there are frequent bradycardias.
   b. The two issues to be treated are the hypoxia and the symptoms.
   c. Although the inspired oxygen concentration could be increased and this would address the hypoxia it is already quite high and it would be more appropriate to consider some other intervention. It is also unlikely that increasing the inspired oxygen would have a significant impact on either tachypnoea or the bradycardias. Some form of ventilatory assistance would be appropriate and in this instance CPAP would be the most likely option to be considered first. Surfactant could also be considered as discussed in the answer to question **6** above.

10. **a.** Antibiotics must be commenced immediately.

   b. The infant has a marked metabolic acidosis. Ventilation appears satisfactory. There is a strong possibility of infection and although there are other reasons for a metabolic acidosis which may be considered in due course this can be done after antibiotics are commenced. Initiation of treatment for possible infection is much more important than attempting to treat the acidosis.

   c. A septic screen should be performed, of which the most important elements will be full blood count including differential and platelet count, C-reactive protein and blood cultures. A lumbar puncture may be considered but will be decided by local policy, speed with which it can be performed and the opinion as to whether the procedure would be tolerated. It is essential that antibiotics are given as quickly as possible and the delay from added investigations may be regarded as unacceptable.

   d. The infant is 32 weeks old, mother may be colonised with Group B streptococcus and membranes were ruptured for 60 hours. Two major risk factors for infection mean that the infant should have been screened and started on antibiotics as soon as practically possible – three make this even more important. Mother should have received antibiotics before delivery but this would not have altered the need to screen and treat a premature baby with this history. In this case four hours have elapsed and the chance of established infection is very high. Many babies with Group B streptococcal sepsis die within a few hours of birth – any delay is therefore unacceptable.

11. **a.** The gas shows a mixed respiratory and metabolic acidosis and hypoxia.

   b. CPAP on the current settings does not appear adequate for this infant. There is evidence that the infant is having to work, as shown by the recession, but this may not be the sole reason for the metabolic acidosis.

   c. Management will vary between different individuals. There is no doubt that additional management of some form is needed. There are some practitioners who would advocate intubation, administration of surfactant and extubation back onto CPAP. Others would regard it as more appropriate to intubate, administer surfactant and then proceed with positive pressure ventilation. The metabolic acidosis must not be ignored and it is appropriate to look for additional causes and treat as appropriate.

12. **a.** There is a respiratory alkalosis and probable hyperoxia.

   b. The infant has been over-ventilated. The tidal volume is significantly greater than would be expected for this baby's birth weight.

   c. Since intubation the baby has been given surfactant and there has been a significant improvement in the clinical condition. It would probably be most appropriate to return this baby to CPAP. If this is deemed unacceptable, at the very least the inspiratory pressure should be reduced.

   d. There have been two significant errors. Ventilation is being commenced after surfactant has been given and there has been a significant interval before the blood gases have been checked. Secondly, oxygen saturation has been allowed to run in excess of 95% without seeing if inspired oxygen concentration can be reduced further and without checking on the arterial oxygen concentration.

13. **a.** This baby has a metabolic acidosis. Carbon dioxide clearance is satisfactory, as is oxygenation.
    b. It is possible that hypotension is contributing to the metabolic acidosis. Poor tissue perfusion will result in inadequate tissue oxygenation with resultant anaerobic metabolism. However, the obvious course is not necessarily the correct course and it is important to be aware of the other possible reasons for a metabolic acidosis.
    c. The cause of the acidosis must be addressed. In this case it would be appropriate to follow whatever the local policy is for the management of hypertension, be it fluid bolus or commencing inotropic support. This alone may be adequate but if it is not then administration of base may be required.

14. **a.** There is a mixed respiratory and metabolic acidosis. Carbon dioxide is elevated; bicarbonate is relatively low with a significant base deficit.
    b. The infant is under-ventilated. Tidal volume is low. In addition oxygenation is poor at a relatively high inspired oxygen. There is also a metabolic component to the acidosis and there is no obvious reason for this.
    c. An increase in peak inspiratory pressure would probably be the best approach to dealing with both respiratory acidosis and the relative hypoxaemia. If the infant has not received surfactant for some period and a chest X-ray is consistent with respiratory distress syndrome further surfactant should be administered. The reason for the metabolic acidosis is not apparent and therefore should be sought. In the interim it would be appropriate to treat the metabolic acidosis with base.

15. **a.** These results are not easy to explain on first view. The infant has a high CO_2 but bicarbonate does not seem high enough to account for this nor is the pH as acidotic as might be expected. The infant is hypoxic despite high inspired oxygen. Tidal volume is low.
    b. There is a very rapid deterioration and the blood gases were obtained shortly after the deterioration had started. The equilibration of carbon dioxide in the bloodstream and tissues is not instantaneous and there may be a brief delay before the final result of the changes is seen. It is very likely that this gas will deteriorate significantly in the very near future as equilibration happens.
    c. The causes of a sudden deterioration should be sought. The most likely candidates are pneumothorax, a displaced or blocked endotracheal tube or a mechanical failure. It is not appropriate to make changes to the ventilation until the cause of the deterioration is established.

16. **a.** There is a severe respiratory acidosis. The tidal volume is very low and there is severe hypoxia.
    b. The blood gases are now fully equilibrated and the full severity of the deterioration is apparent.
    c. The cause of the deterioration must be addressed. In this case cold light illumination shows a large tension pneumothorax on the right side.

A chest drain is inserted with an immediate improvement in oxygenation and a rapid return to a normal tidal volume.

17. a. There is now a respiratory alkalosis. CO_2 is low and tidal volume is higher than predicted. The arterial oxygen concentration is high.
   b. Following drainage of the pneumothorax the infant has been hyperventilated.
   c. Peak pressures should be returned to values similar to those required before the pneumothorax developed. The inspired option should be reduced.
   d. The ventilator settings were increased at the time of the deterioration. The main problem however was a loss of lung volume due to a pneumothorax. Once this was appropriately managed lung movement was restored but the ventilator settings were not changed. Attention was not paid to the change in tidal volume and the interval before the next arterial blood gas was too long.

18. a. There is a respiratory alkalosis but at the same time this infant remains relatively hypoxic at reasonably high inspired oxygen.
   b. There is some improvement of lung disease allowing better carbon dioxide clearance but still not allowing optimal oxygenation.
   c. If the rate is reduced by increasing expiratory time more time will be spent in inspiration, which would result in a slight increase in mean airway pressure and could improve oxygenation. It might be reasonable to reduce the peak pressure to see whether there was a degree of over-distension but this seems less likely in view of the excellent carbon dioxide clearance.

19. a. There is a respiratory acidosis and poor oxygenation.
   b. The mean airway pressure is much lower than would be expected on the settings. The tidal volume is also surprisingly low. A careful look at the ventilator settings shows a flow rate that is unlikely to be high enough for adequate ventilation in a baby of this size. It is quite likely to be so low that the ventilator will not attain the desired peak pressure.
   c. Flow rate should be increased until adequate ventilation is attained. This should be apparent if any form of pressure wave monitoring is available. If not, blood gases and oxygenation should be closely monitored to make sure that the desired effect is achieved. It is not uncommon to find that flow rates are initially inadequate for larger babies. Options that are much more likely to be used on very small babies are lower flow rates. Flow remains a setting that many people do not adjust on a regular basis and the ventilator may be set up without having considered whether or not the flow is adequate for the baby who is about to be ventilated.

20. a. There is a mixed respiratory and metabolic acidosis. Oxygenation is suboptimal in relatively high inspired oxygen.
   b. This baby appears to be under-ventilated and is trying to make it obvious. The fact that the baby is trying to make respiratory movements suggest that the current ventilation is inadequate and the increased respiratory work may be contributing to the metabolic acidosis. The ventilator rate that has been set is quite low (43 breaths per minute) and the

inspiratory time is sufficiently long to make it likely that the baby will be breathing again before inspiration is over. The slow rate means that carbon dioxide clearance is inadequate. The relatively small number of inspirations means that mean airway pressure is also quite low.

   c. In this situation the first thing to do is to adjust the ventilation to a rate where the majority of breaths appear to be synchronised with the infant's own respiratory rate. In those who use synchronised ventilation, this baby would be an ideal candidate to commence synchronised intermittent positive pressure ventilation. The evidence base for any benefit with this modality is poor and there are practitioners who do not use this technique. Whether or not synchronised ventilation is used the principal aim will be to achieve a respiratory rate that is similar to the spontaneous rate of the baby, thereby reducing the work of breathing and hopefully markedly increasing the efficiency of mechanical ventilation.

21. a. There is a respiratory acidosis with poor oxygenation.

   b. Ventilator pressures appear inadequate and the X-ray changes imply that lung inflation is suboptimal. The fact that both carbon dioxide clearance and oxygenation are affected suggests that better lung inflation may be helpful.

   c. Peak inspiratory pressure could be increased and this would improve both mean airway pressure and tidal volume providing there was better lung recruitment. An increase in the positive end expiratory pressure might help recruit more atelectatic lung. The latter move may reduce the pressure differential that determines tidal volume but it had also secured a greater volume of lung for ventilation and may still improve tidal volume.

22. a. There is a respiratory acidosis with poor oxygenation.

   b. Ventilation pressures are fairly high but mean airway pressure, tidal volume and minute volume are all low. The expiratory time is quite long and respiratory rate is quite slow. The X-ray suggests that the lungs are affected by respiratory distress syndrome.

   c. As a first move it would be wise to reduce the expiratory time, which should have an effect upon both mean airway pressure and minute volume. Surfactant should be administered and a repeat X-ray would be advisable to assess the degree of lung recruitment. Further actions would be determined by the response to this first change.

23. a. The blood gas is almost normal. Oxygen is higher than is desirable.

   b. These results show a dramatic change. There has been a substantial change in both mean airway pressure and tidal volume. The increase in rate means that there has been a very substantial increase in the minute volume. Carbon dioxide has fallen and oxygenation has improved.

   c. These figures might be regarded as reassuring (which to some extent they are) and the dramatic and rapid improvement suggests these figures may continue to change in the relatively near future. The lungs of a more mature baby may respond dramatically to surfactant with a considerable increase in compliance. It is very possible that this improvement will continue and more carbon dioxide may be removed, leading to a respiratory alkalosis. It is almost certainly appropriate to start to reduce pressures at this point but whether or not this is done it is essential that very close monitoring is continued.

24. **a.** There is a metabolic alkalosis and borderline hyperoxia.
    b. Although pressures have been reduced slightly the rate remains high and there is continued excess clearance of carbon dioxide. The changes that were made last time were inadequate and too long has been left since the last change in ventilation before a blood gas is being performed.
    c. The rate should be normalised to somewhere in the region of 60 as a good baseline to start from. Although it is generally a bad idea to alter more than one setting at the time in this case it might be advisable to also reduce the peak pressure. It is very important that closer monitoring is performed until adequate ventilation is achieved at the lowest possible ventilator settings.

25. **a.** There is a respiratory acidosis. Oxygenation is adequate.
    b. The ventilator rate is relatively slow at 46 breaths per minute. Oxygenation is adequate, as is tidal volume, but minute volume is low.
    c. The most logical change will be to reduce the expiratory time to give a faster ventilator rate.

26. **a.** The pH is normal but the arterial oxygen concentration is high despite a reduction in inspired oxygen concentration.
    b. The reduction in expiratory time meant that more time was spent in inspiration with subsequent rise in the mean airway pressure.
    c. Some change should be made which will lead to a reduction in the mean airway pressure. The most logical one in this situation would be to reduce the peak inspiratory pressure.

27. **a.** The acid–base balance is satisfactory but the infant remains hypoxic despite being on 85% oxygen.
    b. There are two major problems with his ventilation. Both inspiratory and expiratory times are short and the background rate is 75 breaths per minute. The second problem is that flow rate in the circuit is low. The mean airway pressure that is currently being achieved is 7.7 where a quick calculation would suggest that it should be above 10. It is likely that the ventilator is unable to attain the peak pressure and ventilation is thus inefficient.
    c. The first, and probably most logical, step would be to increase the flow in the ventilator circuit so that the peak pressure could be obtained relatively rapidly in inspiration and then sustained throughout the rest of the inspiratory period.

28. **a.** This gas shows a combination of a metabolic acidosis and a respiratory alkalosis.
    b. Improvement of the flow has allowed much more effective ventilation and the carbon dioxide has been reduced to very low levels. This has not produced a marked alkalosis however because there appears to be a superimposed metabolic acidosis which has kept the pH within the

acceptable range. The very large base deficit and low bicarbonate show that there is an additional problem. If there were not, one would anticipate a much higher pH and bicarbonate and a much smaller base deficit.

c. An alteration of the ventilation either by reduction of peak inspiratory pressure or by slowing the rate using an increase in expiratory time will allow the carbon dioxide to increase but this is only a small part of the problem. There is a significant metabolic acidosis that has developed over a relatively short period of time and the cause of this must be established. The appropriate treatment will be determined by the cause of the acidosis.

29. a. There is a combination of respiratory and metabolic acidosis. The bicarbonate is lower than would be anticipated for an uncomplicated respiratory acidosis. Oxygenation is adequate.

b. This infant has been placed on synchronised ventilation but the inspiratory time chosen is almost certainly too long to allow effective synchronisation. If the ventilator is set up with a long inspiratory time there is a good chance that the infant will attempt to breathe out during the inspiratory phase and may well be trying to breathe in again either during the same inspiratory cycle or during expiration. The fact that the baby is 'fighting' the ventilator should inform you that the ventilator settings are unsuitable.

c. Reduce the inspiratory time to somewhere around 0.35 seconds. Observe the effect this has on ventilation and on the baby's spontaneous breathing.

30. a. This infant has a respiratory alkalosis.

b. The ventilator settings will not allow effective synchronisation and the background respiratory rate (85 breaths per minute) is leading to hyperventilation. Depending on the model of ventilator in use there may be a short latent period after inspiration is finished during which a further inspiration cannot be initiated. Once this is over the remainder of the inspiratory time is the window during which another breath must be taken for synchronisation to occur. At an expiratory time of 0.35 seconds, even without a latent period, there will be very little time for a breath to be taken if true synchronisation is to occur.

c. Increase the expiratory time significantly to see if true synchronisation will happen and, if it does, what the baby's spontaneous background respiratory rate is.

31. a. The gas is normal.

b. Although there is a long expiratory time a quick calculation using the tidal volume and minute volume will show you that the baby is breathing at a rate of approximately 60 breaths per minute. Although the back-up rate is set at 30 the actual ventilator rate will be determined by the baby's spontaneous respiration which in this case appears to be adequate as it has resulted in a normalisation of the previously abnormal blood gas. The mean airway pressure is also significantly higher than you would expect if the baby was breathing at the back-up rate.

c. No action is needed.

32. a. There is a mild respiratory acidosis and moderate hypoxia.

  b. Ventilation is inadequate and the current settings on synchronised intermittent mandatory ventilation are not supporting adequate gas exchange.
  The choice of this particular modality can be questioned in this instance.
  With SIMV the baby is expected to take unsupported breaths during the
  expiratory period. In this case the expiratory time is so short that it is
  unlikely that effective spontaneous breathing will be allowed. Whatever
  modality is being used it would appear that ventilation is inadequate.

  c. The respiratory acidosis and moderate hypoxia could be addressed by
  an increase in peak inspiratory pressure. A change to either conventional
  ventilation or synchronised intermittent positive pressure ventilation
  could allow an optimisation of ventilation.

33. a. There is a respiratory acidosis.

  b. As this infant is on synchronised intermittent mandatory ventilation with
  a relatively long expiratory time there is the potential for him to be taking a large number of unsupported breaths. The back-up rate would be
  30 breaths per minute and with the measured tidal volume of 4.9 mL
  and minute volume of 0.15 L/min it would appear that there is no spontaneous ventilation. If this is the case it will explain the carbon dioxide
  retention.

  c. The first thing is to check whether or not the infant is breathing spontaneously. If not, it would be reasonable to search for any reason why.
  Is the infant sedated or even paralysed? (This may sound stupid but it
  has been known.) Would the infant benefit from a respiratory stimulant
  such as caffeine? Although these issues should be addressed it is important to note that ventilation remains inadequate and a respiratory acidosis
  will persist unless action is taken. The first most logical step would be
  to increase the respiratory rate to eliminate more carbon dioxide. The
  expiratory window could be reduced to permit more supported breaths
  or the infant could be changed to positive pressure or synchronised positive pressure ventilation.

34. a. There is a respiratory acidosis and oxygenation is poor.

  b. This infant was ventilating well prior to his extubation on exactly the
  same ventilator settings. Following intubation he is no longer able to do
  so. Although a degree of atelectasis may happen following extubation this
  would have to be quite severe and does not seem the most likely explanation in view of how well the infant was previously. Tidal volumes prior
  to extubation were good but are now poor with both tidal volume and
  minute volume approximately half of what one would anticipate if the
  lungs were inflating normally (tidal volume 4–6 mL/kg; weight 3.5 kg
  therefore normal tidal volume in the region of 17 mL; respiratory rate
  60 therefore predicted minute volume 1.05 L). It is conceivable that a
  mucus plug has been dislodged during extubation (not an uncommon
  phenomenon) and has occluded a main bronchus.

  c. If the poor ventilation continues a chest X-ray is indicated and selective bronchial intubation and suction may be warranted. The exact
  reason for the deterioration of ventilation is difficult to establish without

some X-ray evidence. If there is no evidence of bronchial occlusion it may just be that there was atelectasis following extubation and a period of ventilation at a higher peak pressure may be needed to recruit lung again.

35. a. The gas shows a respiratory acidosis. Oxygenation is satisfactory.

    b. Tidal volume and minute volume are low. The positive end expiratory pressure is relatively high and this may explain why tidal volumes are low. The high PEEP is helping maintain a high mean airway pressure and therefore oxygenation is satisfactory.

    c. The PEEP should be reduced while watching the tidal volume. No other changes should be made until the effect of this manoeuvre becomes apparent.

36. a. There is a respiratory acidosis and poor oxygenation.

    b. Ventilation is obviously unsatisfactory. The mean airway pressure is quite high but is still insufficient to maintain oxygenation or good carbon dioxide clearance. The tidal volume is low and suggests that lung inflation is poor.

    c. Action at this point will depend upon what ventilation modality is in use. Many practitioners would regard this baby as suitable for commencing high-frequency ventilation. Others do not believe there is a role for this modality as no benefit has been established over conventional ventilation. If high frequency is not to be used then conventional ventilation must be adjusted to attempt to secure better tidal volumes. An increase in peak inspiratory pressure is indicated and it is possible that increasing the level of PEEP may help to recruit atelectatic lung.

37. a. The respiratory acidosis is slightly worse and there is borderline improvement in the oxygenation. Mean airway pressure has increased but there has been no net change in the tidal volume.

    b. It is likely that the lung remains atelectatic and high pressures have not resulted in further lung recruitment.

    c. It would be possible to increase peak inspiratory pressures further and possibly also inspiratory time and/or PEEP. At these pressures anyone using high-frequency oscillation would almost certainly have opted for this alternative.

38. a. There has been no significant improvement. The respiratory acidosis persists and there is still poor oxygenation.

    b. It is likely that the MAP is not high enough to recruit the atelectatic lung. Without recruitment oscillation will be ineffective and gas exchange will remain poor. It is recommended that when oscillation has commenced with a poorly aerated lung the MAP used should be at least $2\,cmH_2O$ higher than the MAP on conventional ventilation before switching to oscillation.

    c. Poor lung recruitment could be confirmed with an X-ray but in a situation where gas exchange remains poor and an appropriate MAP has not been selected in the first place a further change in MAP should be made first.

39. **a.** Oxygenation is much improved but carbon dioxide clearance has not been affected and the respiratory acidosis persists.

  b. As oxygenation has improved this would imply that lung filling is now adequate. The fact that carbon dioxide clearance remains poor suggests that the magnitude of the oscillation around the MAP is inadequate. Rule of thumb guidelines suggest that the tidal volume in high frequency (VT_{HF}) should be approximately 2 mL/kg initially and changes can be made thereafter to determine the optimal tidal volume for the individual baby. This baby has a VT_{HF} of 1.2 mL and body weight of 1.3 kg. The tidal volume is therefore obviously insufficient.

  c. The magnitude of the pressure swing should be increased using whatever control is available on the ventilator in question. If it is possible to measure the VT_{HF} then the pressure swing should be adjusted until it is approximately 2 mL/kg.

40. **a.** The gas has normalised.

  b. Appropriate mean airway pressure and pressure swing have been selected.

  c. Oxygenation is now very good with high saturations in 25% oxygen. Carbon dioxide clearance has improved dramatically and has normalised within 30 minutes of making the change in pressure settings. Although it might be tempting to leave the baby at this point very close observation is necessary. It is very conceivable that lung recruitment will continue, with the possibility of hyper-expansion and it is also possible that carbon dioxide clearance will continue and the baby may rapidly become hypocarbic. It could be prudent to reduce the mean airway pressure and it will certainly be necessary to repeat a blood gas fairly soon.

41. **a.** Again there is poor oxygenation and a respiratory acidosis.

  b. Although the assumption has been made that there is a loss of lung volume responsible for the poor ventilation – hence the increase in mean airway pressure – an alternative explanation is that the lungs had become hyper-inflated. They will therefore be less compliant and air entry will be impaired. If pressures continue to be increased the situation will only worsen and, furthermore, significant lung damage may ensue.

  c. An urgent chest X-ray should be performed to assess the degree of lung filling. If this is not immediately available it may be prudent to try and reduce the mean airway pressure to see the effect it has on oxygenation. Ideally radiological examination should be performed first so that any changes are made on the basis of information rather than speculation.

42. **a.** There is a metabolic acidosis and a respiratory alkalosis.

  b. This combination is often missed as the normal pH reassures the operator that everything is acceptable. In this case the carbon dioxide is very low and were there not a metabolic acidosis the pH would probably be in the region of 7.5. However something is responsible for a metabolic acidosis that has moved the pH back towards the normal range.

  c. There are two separate elements to management here. Firstly, the cause of the metabolic acidosis must be sought and appropriate management initiated. Secondly, the ventilation must be adjusted so that the carbon dioxide returns towards the normal range. The easiest initial move would be to increase expiratory time, thereby reducing the respiratory rate.

43. a. Arterial oxygen concentration is too high; otherwise the blood gas is acceptable.

    b. Ventilation is satisfactory but the inspired oxygen concentration has not been turned down rapidly enough.

    c. The inspired oxygen should be decreased immediately. The blood gas is very good and there is room to start weaning this infant. A reduction in the peak inspiratory pressure could be considered. It would also be reasonable to reduce the inspiratory time while increasing the expiratory time and keeping respiratory rate the same.

44. a. There is a compensated respiratory acidosis. The pH is normal but the carbon dioxide is high. This is associated with a high bicarbonate and a base excess of >10 mmol/L.

    b. This infant is likely to have developed chronic lung disease. The combination of ventilation for 3 weeks and inflammatory changes on X-ray are highly suggestive.

    c. It would be appropriate to try to reduce the peak respiratory pressure and wean ventilation. Babies with chronic lung disease may appear stuck on a ventilator because they have a high carbon dioxide and there are concerns that reducing ventilation will allow this to rise further. This is possibile but it is still important that attempts are made to reduce the pressures further to try to reduce the inflammation.

45. a. The blood gas is satisfactory.

    b. Ventilation is currently appropriate.

    c. At pressures of 14/4 extubation should be considered. Whether this is directly into incubator oxygen or onto CPAP will depend upon the policy of the individual unit. Although lower pressures are less damaging to the lungs than higher pressures, it is still not advisable to leave an infant with an endotracheal tube in place and with positive pressure ventilation. The ventilator rate is still high (75) and it would also be reasonable to slow this down to make sure the baby is capable of spontaneous respiration.

46. a. There is severe hypoxaemia and a mixed metabolic and respiratory acidosis.

    b. The most likely diagnosis here is persistent pulmonary hypertension of the newborn. Tidal volumes are good and thus there is unlikely to be a problem with pulmonary atelectasis. The history of a term baby found collapsed when there is a history of prolonged rupture of membranes is highly suggestive of PPHN secondary to sepsis.

    c. A chest X-ray is essential and an echocardiogram would be very helpful. Blood must be sent for a septic screen but this infant is too sick for a lumbar puncture. First-line antibiotics which will cover both Group B *Streptococcus* and *E. coli* must be started immediately. The management of the respiratory condition will be determined by what modalities are available in the hospital. At the very least the peak inspiratory pressures must be increased to see whether oxygenation can be improved. Pulmonary vasodilators should be considered and it is important that systemic blood pressure is maintained.

47. **a.** Profound hyperoxia remains and there is a severe metabolic acidosis and a degree of respiratory acidosis.

   b. The oxygenation index is extremely high at 270 [OI = MAP × FiO$_2$ (%)/PaO$_2$ (mmHg)].

   c. Current manoeuvres have not worked. There is, presumably, severe pulmonary hypertension with very little blood perfusing the lungs.

   d. This infant urgently needs either nitric oxide or ECMO. Because of the severity of this infant's condition ideally he should be transferred to an ECMO centre, receiving nitric oxide en route. Should further attempts be made to stabilise him rather than transfer it is unlikely he will survive. There is evidence to suggest that delaying referral for ECMO while other modalities are tried is associated with a reduced success rate for ECMO and longer runs when on ECMO.

48. **a.** This baby has compensated respiratory acidosis.

   b. As this baby requires continuing oxygen it is very likely that she has chronic lung disease of prematurity and a persistently elevated carbon dioxide. As she is nine weeks old this is now compensated as the renal threshold for bicarbonate increases and plasma bicarbonate rises. The combination of an elevated carbon dioxide, a normal or near normal pH and elevated bicarbonate and base excess are the key features of a compensated respiratory acidosis.

   c. No action is indicated. This is the normal body reaction to a persistently elevated carbon dioxide and any attempts to normalise it will lead to destabilisation of the acid–base balance. As this infant has chronic lung disease the only thing that should be ensured is that oxygenation is adequate and appropriate. Insufficient oxygen can, over a long period of time, lead to right ventricular hypertrophy and pulmonary hypertension. There is good evidence that maintaining adequate oxygenation can prevent this from happening in the majority of cases.

49. **a.** There is a respiratory alkalosis in combination with a compensated respiratory acidosis.

   b. This baby has been ventilated in an attempt to normalise the carbon dioxide. 'Normal' for this infant is likely to be significantly higher than it would be for an infant who did not have chronic lung disease. As the compensation has led to a normalisation of the pH a further reduction of the carbon dioxide will drive the pH to the alkaline side of normal. The tidal volume for this infant is at the upper end of the normal range which is surprising in a baby with chronic lung disease where lung volumes are typically reduced.

   c. Ventilatory support should be reduced to allow the carbon dioxide to return to what is the 'normal range' for this infant. This is likely to be higher than one would expect in an unaffected infant. A carbon dioxide at which the pH is either normal or slightly on the acidotic side of normal should be the aim.

50. a. There is a metabolic alkalosis.
  b. This infant is vomiting stomach acid which means there is a surplus of alkali in the body, hence the metabolic alkalosis.
  c. An intravenous infusion must be established and the reason for the vomiting determined. Blood samples should be sent for haematology and biochemistry. A septic screen should be performed and antibiotics commenced. Manual examination of the abdomen is indicated and with a plain abdominal film and/or ultrasound. In this baby's case examination revealed a palpable mass at the pylorus.

Chapter 7

X-rays

High quality X-ray images and their accurate and reliable interpretation are of central importance in neonatal care. Many of the abnormalities and appearances that are seen are only encountered in the immediate postnatal period and expertise in the interpretation of X-rays of other age groups of the population does not necessarily bring with it expertise in the interpretation of neonatal images. Although some appearances are common – respiratory distress syndrome and chronic lung disease for example – others such as certain skeletal dysplasias may be extremely rare and a supra-regional specialist opinion may be needed. All those who work with newborn babies should be competent at interpretation of neonatal images as the response to problems detected may need to be very fast.

The questions in this chapter cover a variety of appearances. In all questions interpretation of the X-ray will be needed. In many the probable diagnosis and a management plan will also be expected.

QUESTIONS

1. A term baby is noted to be grunting shortly after birth. The baby is tachypnoeic and there is marked recession. The following chest X-ray has been obtained.

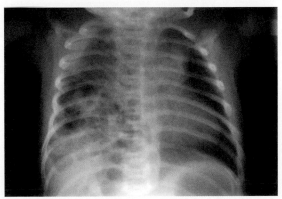

Figure 7.1

   a. Describe the abnormalities on the X-ray.
   b. What is the diagnosis?
   c. What is the management of the baby?

2. A 28 week baby is 10 days old. Abdominal distension has been noted and the following X-ray is obtained.

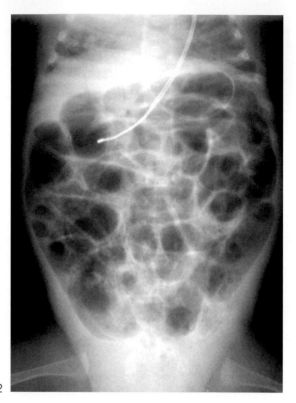

Figure 7.2

    a. Describe the abnormalities on the X-ray.

    b. What is the diagnosis?

3. The same baby as in question **2** is reviewed a few hours later. His abdomen has become more distended and discoloured. The following abdominal X-ray is obtained.

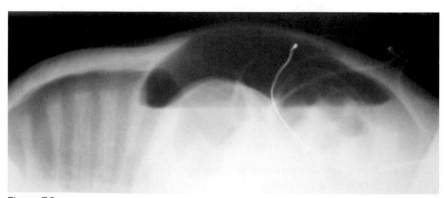

Figure 7.3

a. Describe the abnormalities on the X-ray.
b. What is the diagnosis?
c. What is the management of this baby?

4. A 37 week gestation baby is noted to have frequent small vomits. At 24 hours of age he is noted to be tachypnoeic and he is admitted to the neonatal unit. A chest X-ray is obtained.

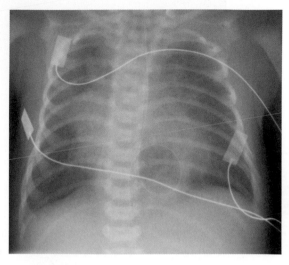

Figure 7.4

a. Describe the abnormalities on the X-ray.
b. What are the diagnoses?
c. What is the management of the baby?

5. A 36 week baby is admitted to the neonatal unit after a choking episode. The following chest X-ray is obtained.

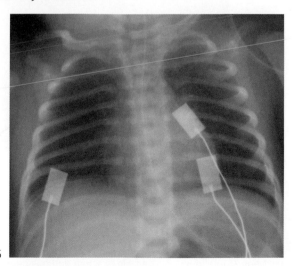

Figure 7.5

a. Describe the abnormalities on the X-ray.
b. What is the diagnosis?
c. What is the management of the baby?

6. A 27 week infant is ventilated for RDS. Ventilatory requirements have increased over the last hour. A chest X-ray is obtained.

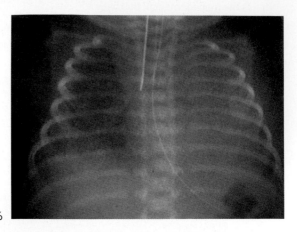

Figure 7.6

    a. Describe the abnormalities on the X-ray.
    b. What is the management of the baby?

7. A term baby is noted to have a degree of frontal bossing, as does his mother. A chest X-ray is performed.

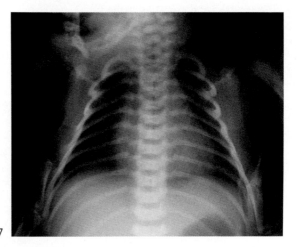

Figure 7.7

    a. Describe the abnormalities on the X-ray.
    b. What is the diagnosis?
    c. What is the inheritance of this condition?

8. A 29 week gestation baby has been on CPAP for moderate respiratory distress and has been stable in 35% oxygen. He is active and has been noted to have quite marked intercostal recession on occasion. He suddenly deteriorates with persistent recession and an increase in oxygen requirements to 95%. A chest X-ray is taken.

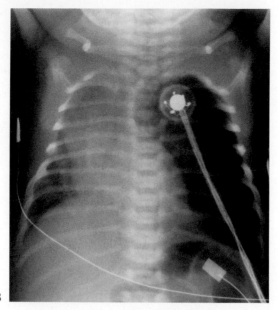

Figure 7.8

   a. Describe the abnormalities on the X-ray.

   b. What is the management of the baby?

9. A 27 week gestation infant is ventilated for respiratory distress. Ventilation requirements have been moderately high and two doses of surfactant have been given. Oxygen requirements have steadily risen from 55% to 95%. In response to a profound bradycardia and desaturation he receives ventilation down his endotracheal tube using a resuscitation bag. He deteriorates further and a chest X-ray is obtained.

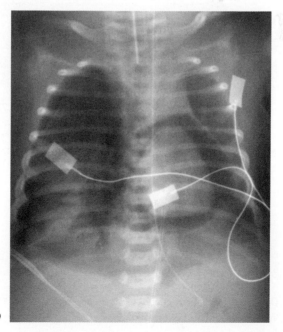

Figure 7.9

a. Describe the abnormalities on the X-ray.
b. What is the management of the baby?

10. A 31 week gestation infant is admitted to the intensive care unit. Mother booked late and there has been minimal antenatal care. The baby needs resuscitation at delivery and is transferred to the unit ventilated. Ventilation proves very difficult and a chest X-ray is obtained.

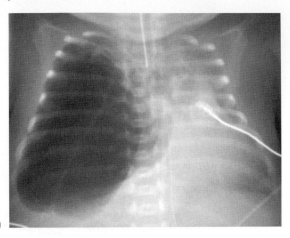

Figure 7.10

a. Describe the abnormalities on the X-ray.
b. What is the differential diagnosis?
c. What is the management of the baby?

11. A 32 week gestation infant is stable at birth but a problem is noted at admission and a chest X-ray obtained.

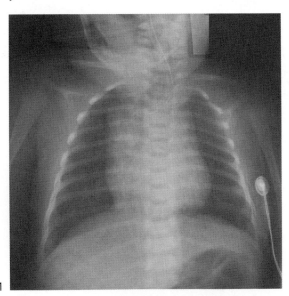

Figure 7.11

a. Describe the abnormalities on the X-ray.
b. What is the management of the baby?

12. A term baby is thought to have an absent Moro reflex and limited movement of the arm. An X-ray is taken. In view of these changes a chest X-ray is then performed.

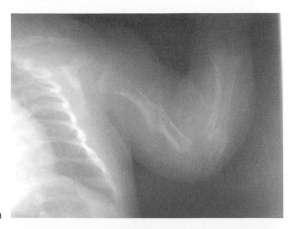

Figure 7.12a

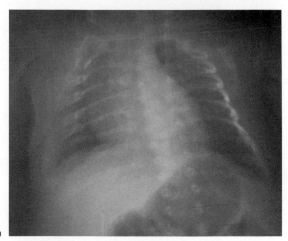

Figure 7.12b

    a. Describe the abnormalities on the arm X-ray.
    b. Describe the abnormalities on the chest X-ray.
    c. What is the most likely diagnosis?
    d. What management would you consider?

13. A 27 week gestation infant is now 4 weeks old. She needs 0.4 L/min supplementary oxygen but this has recently risen to 0.8 L/min. A chest X-ray is performed.
    a. Describe the abnormalities on the X-ray.
    b. What management has this baby had in the past that is clearly evident on the X-ray?
    c. What management will you initiate in response to the abnormality on this chest X-ray?

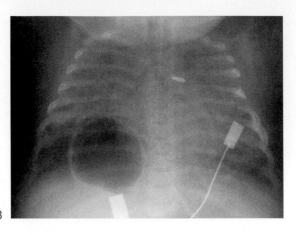

Figure 7.13

14. Antenatal ultrasounds have suggested a growth retarded fetus. At birth, the baby has obvious limb abnormalities and requires ventilation. Limb and chest X-rays are performed.

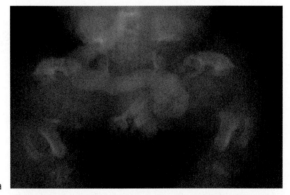

Figure 7.14a

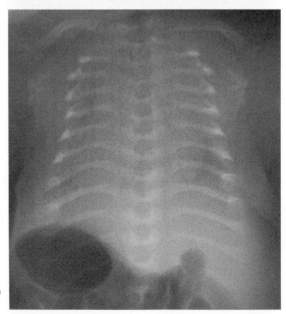

Figure 7.14b

a. Describe the abnormalities on the limb X-ray.
b. Describe the abnormalities on the chest X-ray.
c. What is the most likely diagnosis?
d. What is the prognosis?

15. A baby is born at term and is noted to be cyanosed at rest. There is moderate recession. There is bilateral lower limb oedema. Femoral pulses are weak. The anterior fontanelle is bulging and a loud bruit can be heard when listening over it. A chest X-ray is performed.

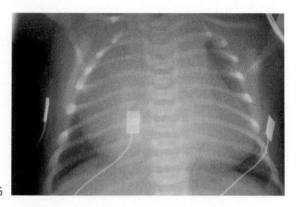

Figure 7.15

a. What abnormalities are there?
b. What possible explanation do you have?
c. What initial further investigations would you consider?

16. A baby is born at 26 weeks and requires ventilation from birth. Surfactant was given on delivery suite. Ventilation has steadily increased and the baby is in 95% oxygen at pressures of 28/6 at 24 hours of age. Blood gases are poor. A chest X-ray is performed.

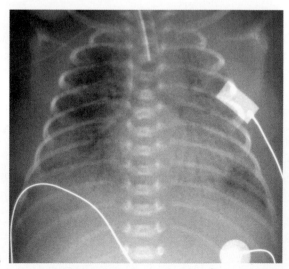

Figure 7.16

a. What abnormalities are there?
b. What is the most likely diagnosis?
c. What treatment would you consider?

17. A term infant is born following a severe asphyxial insult. There is thick meconium present and the oro-pharynx and trachea are suctioned under direct vision and meconium is removed. Ventilation is required and requirements steadily increase. At 8 hours of age the pressures are 32/4 and 100% oxygen is required. The blood gas shows a pH of 7.01, PO_2 of 3.4 and PCO_2 of 7.2.

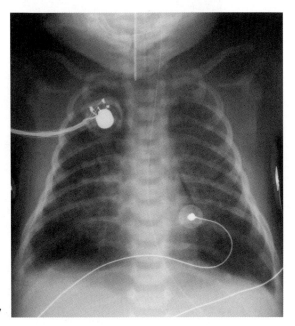

Figure 7.17

a. What does the X-ray show?
b. What is the diagnosis and what complication may be present?
c. What action could be taken?

18. A 36 week gestation infant has mild respiratory distress at birth. He requires 30% oxygen and there is mild recession. As symptoms persist an X-ray is performed at 6 hours of age.
a. What does the X-ray show?
b. If this is the only problem with the baby, what is the most likely diagnosis?
c. If the baby is asymptomatic, what should you do?
d. If the baby is symptomatic, what would you consider?
e. What other investigations would be warranted?

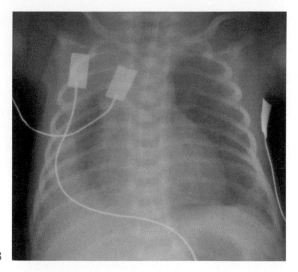

Figure 7.18

19. A term infant is born by elective caesarean section because of previous caesarean sections. Shortly after birth the baby is noted to be mildly dusky and grunting and there is mild recession. A septic screen is performed and a chest X-ray obtained. Antibiotics are started.

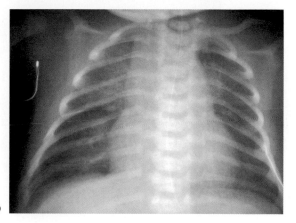

Figure 7.19

    a. What abnormality is seen on this X-ray?
    b. What is the most likely diagnosis?
    c. What management steps do you need to take?
    d. What is the prognosis for the baby?

20. A preterm infant has chronic lung disease. Her condition worsens and following investigations a surgical procedure is performed. The following day a chest X-ray is performed.
    a. Describe the X-ray.
    b. What surgical procedure was performed?
    c. What treatment may be indicated?

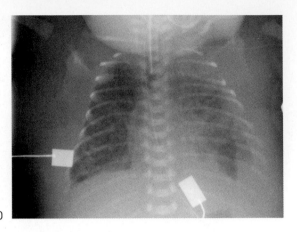

Figure 7.20

21. A 26 week infant is in 0.5 L/min of supplementary oxygen at 36 weeks corrected age. He has mild recession and capillary gases show a fully compensated respiratory acidosis. A chest X-ray is taken as part of a work-up for chronic lung disease.

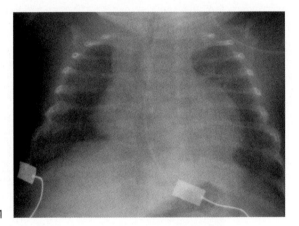

Figure 7.21

    a. Describe the X-ray.
    b. What is the likely diagnosis?

22. A baby born at 24 weeks gestation is 2 weeks old. He has been stable on low ventilation pressures but has not tolerated CPAP. Attempts have been made to start nasogastric feeds on several occasions but he does not appear to tolerate them as there are reasonable volume gastric aspirates on most occasions. Over the last 48 hours the aspirates have become increasingly bilious and an abdominal X-ray is taken.

    a. Describe the X-ray abnormalities.
    b. What is the diagnosis?
    c. What is this diagnosis commonly associated with?
    d. What is your immediate management plan?
    e. What is the likely outcome for this baby?

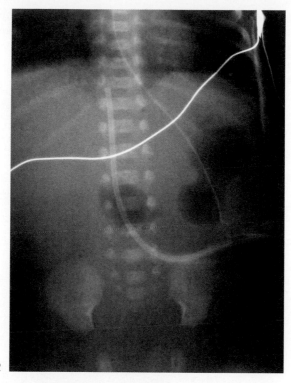

Figure 7.22

23. A 26 week infant has been ventilated for RDS. He was weaned onto CPAP after 16 days and was initially stable. Six days after starting CPAP his oxygen

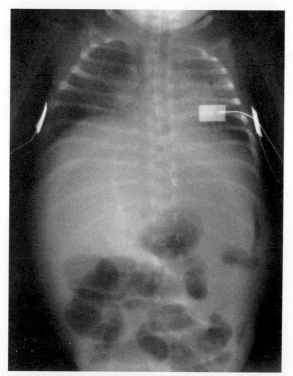

Figure 7.23

requirements started to rise (from 35% to 65%) and he was commenced on a course of dexamethasone; 36 hours after starting dexamethasone he deteriorates substantially. An X-ray is taken.

   a. What abnormalities are seen on this X-ray?
   b. What is the diagnosis?
   c. What is your management plan?

24. A term baby becomes cyanosed 6 hours after birth. Increasing the inspired oxygen concentration only partially treats this. On examination the chest is clear and there are no abnormal sounds. A chest X-ray is obtained.

   a. Describe the chest X-ray.
   b. What is your diagnosis?
   c. What will you do next?

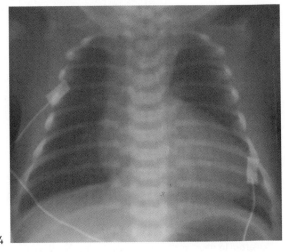

Figure 7.24

25. A 28 week gestation infant has been born. A chest and abdominal X-ray is taken at 4 hours of age.

   a. Describe the X-ray.
   b. What is your diagnosis?
   c. What will you do next?

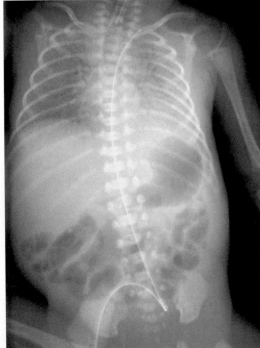

Figure 7.25

26. A term infant is born to a mother who is known to have insulin dependent diabetes. He is grunting from birth and oxygen saturations are poor. A chest X-ray is obtained.

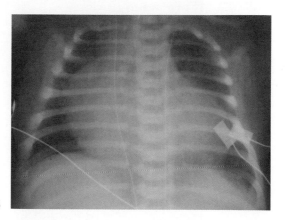

Figure 7.26

    a. Describe the X-ray.
    b. What is your diagnosis?
    c. What will you do next?

27. A 32 week gestation infant has been born. There has been a 10-week history of oligohydramnios. The baby has required ventilation from birth. Blood gases are poor at high ventilation pressures. A chest X-ray is taken at 3 hours of age.

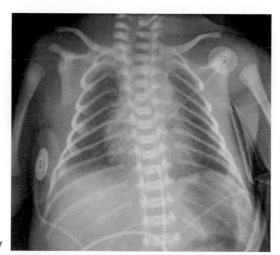

Figure 7.27

    a. Describe the X-ray.
    b. What is your diagnosis?

28. A term baby has not fed well since birth. Bilious vomiting has been noted, as has mild abdominal distension. At 48 hours the distension becomes much worse and an abdominal X-ray is taken.

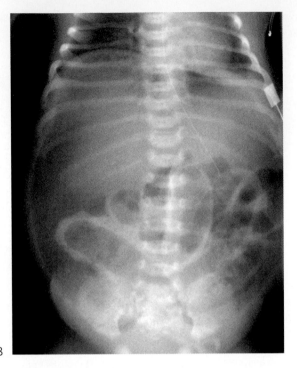

Figure 7.28

    a. What does the X-ray show?

    b. What do you think has happened?

    c. What will you do next?

29. A 27 week gestation infant has had a central venous line inserted. A chest X-ray is taken to confirm line position.

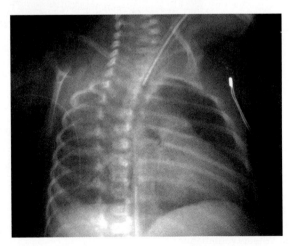

Figure 7.29

    a. What does the X-ray show?

    b. Is the line position acceptable?

    c. What will you do next?

30. A 28 week gestation infant has been ventilated for 12 days. He is now 6 weeks old and requires 0.6 L/min of oxygen. A chest X-ray is taken.

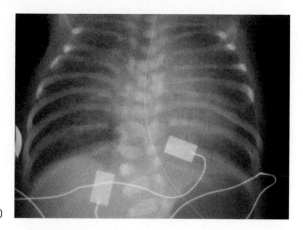

Figure 7.30

    a. What does the X-ray show?
    b. What action will you take?

31. A 25 week gestation infant has been ventilated since birth and is now 9 days old. A chest X-ray is taken.

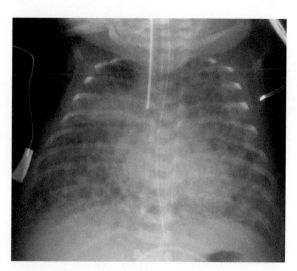

Figure 7.31

    a. What does the X-ray show?
    b. What is responsible for these changes?

32. A 26 week gestation infant has received one dose of surfactant in the delivery room and a further dose 12 hours later. A chest X-ray is taken at 24 hours of age.

a. What does the X-ray show?

b. What do you think has happened?

c. What will you do next?

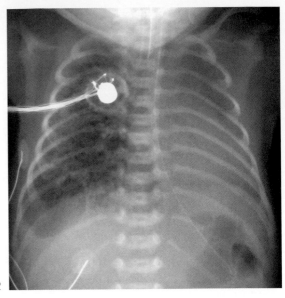

Figure 7.32

33. A baby is born at 36 weeks to a mother with insulin dependent diabetes. He does not tolerate feeds and abdominal distension is noted. A chest and abdominal X-ray is taken at 36 hours of age.

    a. What does the X-ray show?

    b. What do you think has happened?

    c. What will you do next?

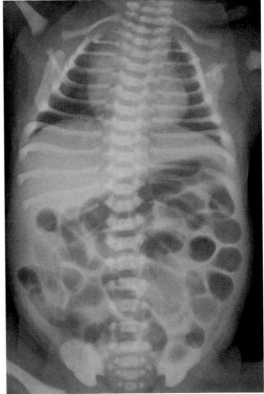

Figure 7.33

34. A term infant shows minimal respiratory effort and requires ventilation. A chest X-ray is taken. On talking to the parents you notice that the mother shows little expression in her facial movements.

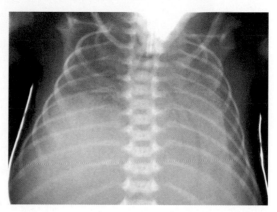

Figure 7.34

    a. Describe the X-ray?
    b. What do you think may be the explanation for these appearances?
    c. What will you do?

35. A 25 week gestation infant has been ventilated since birth. Three doses of surfactant have been given with little effect. A chest X-ray is taken at 48 hours of age.

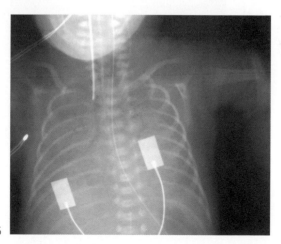

Figure 7.35

    a. What does the X-ray show?

36. A 28 week gestation infant has developed moderate RDS and is stable on CPAP. Abdominal distension is noted and an abdominal X-ray is requested. By mistake a chest X-ray is taken instead.

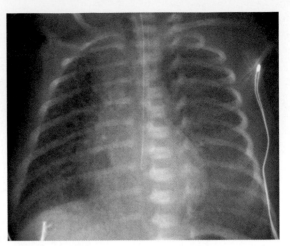

Figure 7.36

    a. What does the X-ray show?
    b. What action will you take?

37. A 24 week infant requires ventilation from birth and is now 4 weeks old. He is known to have duodenal atresia but the surgeons do not want to operate until he is a lot bigger. He has been to theatre for a surgical procedure. A chest X-ray is taken to check that the procedure has been performed correctly. The appearance of the right lung is as it has been since birth.

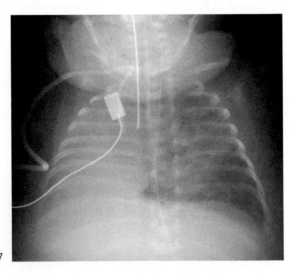

Figure 7.37

    a. What does the X-ray show?
    b. What was the surgical procedure?
    c. What is the explanation for the appearances of the right lung?

38. A 28 week gestation infant has been born and has needed relatively little ventilatory support. Feeds are introduced on day 3 and increased slowly. On day 5 he deteriorates and there is obvious abdominal distension. An X-ray is obtained.

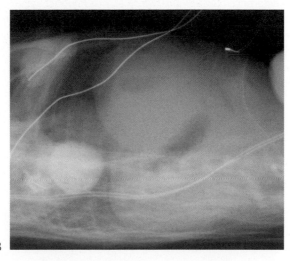

Figure 7.38

    a. What does the X-ray show?
    b. What do you think has happened?
    c. What will you do next?

39. A term infant is born in poor condition following an ante-partum haemorrhage. The infant takes a few deep gasps and then stops breathing. Heart rate is 57 bpm.

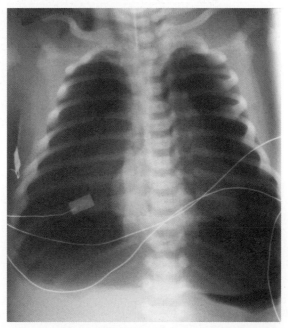

Figure 7.39

Bag and mask ventilation is commenced. There is poor chest movement and there is little response to ventilation. Transillumination is performed and there is no difference between the two sides. An endotracheal tube is inserted and ventilation does not improve. A butterfly needle is inserted into the right chest. A few bubbles are seen but this then stops. An X-ray is taken.

   a. What does the X-ray show?
   b. How do you explain the clinical story?
   c. What will you do next?

40. A 36 week gestation infant has been born and is in poor condition. She is very growth retarded and there is a widespread petechial rash. An X-ray is taken at 6 hours of age.

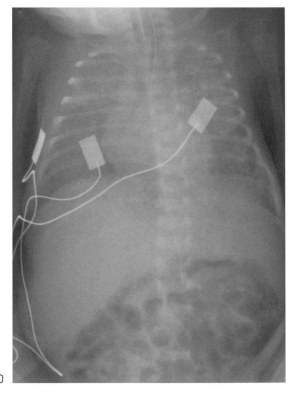

Figure 7.40

   a. What does the X-ray show?
   b. How might these appearances link with the clinical history?
   c. What treatment would you consider?

41. A 26 week gestation infant is 4 days old. A central venous line has been inserted into the left long saphenous vein and shortly afterwards abdominal distension is noted. An X-ray is performed.

   a. List three major abnormalities in the intestines.
   b. How is the position of the central line relevant?
   c. What are the underlying diagnoses?

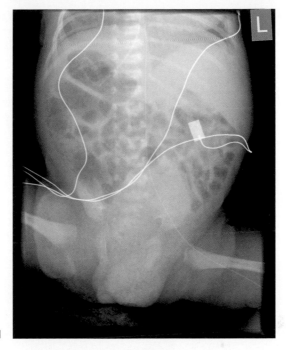

Figure 7.41

42. A 26 week gestation infant has had severe RDS and has not responded well to surfactant. Because of deteriorating gases at high peak pressures high frequency oscillation is commenced. He initially improves and his inspired oxygen falls from 100% to 45%. After 24 hours he starts to deteriorate again and inspired oxygen increases to 90%. A chest X-ray is taken at 4 hours of age.

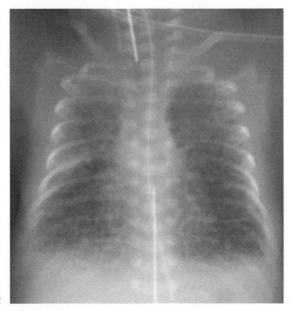

Figure 7.42

    a. What does the X-ray show?
    b. What action will you take?

43. A 27 week gestation infant has had moderate RDS and ventilation is weaning fairly rapidly. Extubation to CPAP is being considered when she deteriorates and abdominal distension is seen. NEC is suspected and a chest and abdominal X-ray is requested.

  a. What does the X-ray show?

  b. What is the reason for her deterioration?

  c. What action will you take?

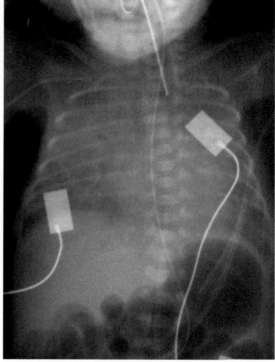

Figure 7.43

44. A 26 week infant is born in poor condition and needs high pressure ventilation from the outset. The baby has caused considerable concern to the fetal medicine

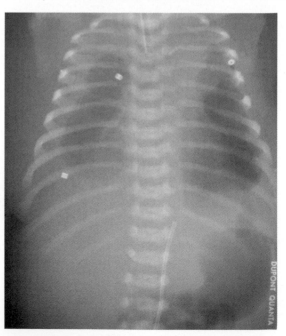

Figure 7.44

specialists and an intra-uterine procedure has been performed. A chest and abdominal X-ray is obtained shortly after birth.

    a. What does the X-ray show?

    b. What intra-uterine procedure was performed?

    c. What do you think the underlying diagnosis is?

45. A 28 week gestation infant has mild RDS. There was significant growth retardation and Dopplers showed reversed end-diastolic flow. The abdomen looks moderately distended and stage 1 NEC is suspected. A decision has been taken not to feed for at least for 10 days. A chest X-ray is obtained.

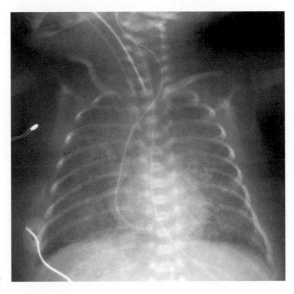

Figure 7.45

    a. What does the X-ray show?

    b. What action will you take?

46. In the same infant as in question **45** the procedure is repeated. A further chest X-ray is taken.

    a. What does the X-ray show?

    b. What will you do next?

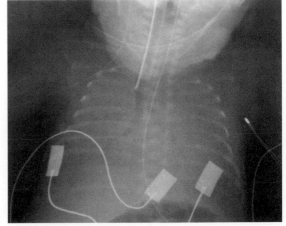

Figure 7.46

47. A 26 week gestation infant has required ventilation from birth. A chest and abdominal X-ray is taken at 4 hours of age.

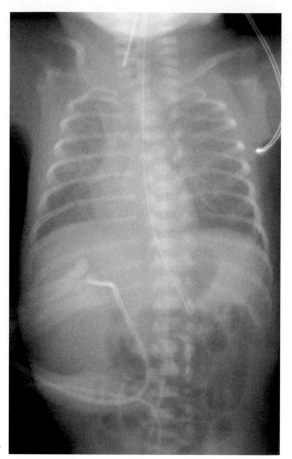

Figure 7.47

    a. What does the X-ray show?

    b. What action will you take?

48. A 25 week gestation infant has required ventilation from birth and has needed high pressures. She is now 2 weeks old and there has been a sudden deterioration. The cause is not obvious on examination and a chest and abdominal X-ray is requested.

    a. What does the X-ray show?

    b. Why was this not detected on examination?

    c. What action will you take?

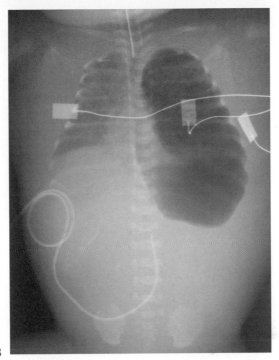

Figure 7.48

49. A 26 week infant has been unwell since birth. At 6 days of age abdominal distension is noted. Three abdominal X-rays are obtained at 24-hour intervals.

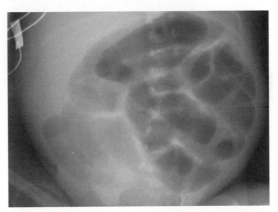

Figure 7.49a

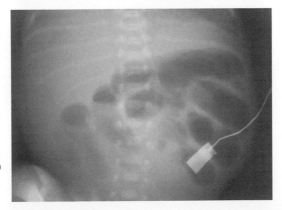

Figure 7.49b

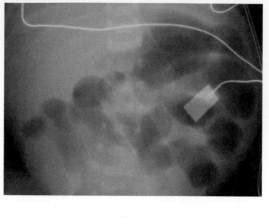

Figure 7.49c

a. What do the X-rays show?
b. What is the diagnosis?
c. What actions should be taken?

50. A 29 week gestation infant deteriorates rapidly after birth and requires ventilation. A chest and abdominal X-ray is taken at 24 hours of age.

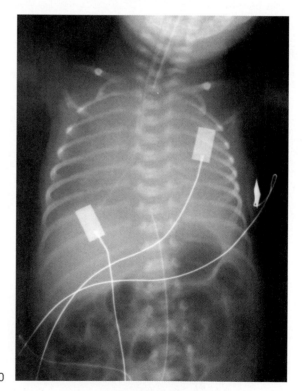

Figure 7.50

a. What does the X-ray show?
b. What is the explanation?
c. What will you do next?

1. a. i. The heart is displaced to the left of the chest.
  ii. There are bowel loops visible in the chest cavity on the right.
  b. Right-sided diaphragmatic hernia. These are much less common than left-sided diaphragmatic hernias. The baby is not ventilated (no endotracheal tube visible on CXR) and this therefore suggests that this defect was not recognised antenatally. The optimal management for these babies is intubation and ventilation immediately after birth avoiding lung inflation using a mask.
  c. This baby should be ventilated to prevent the bowel from distending any more with swallowed air. A paediatric surgical opinion should be sought.

2. a. i. There is a nasogastric tube in situ.
  ii. The bowel loops are dilated.
  iii. The bowel wall is thickened.
  iv. There is no air in the rectum.
  v. There is widespread intramural gas.
  b. The diagnosis is necrotising enterocolitis. There are staging criteria for NEC described by Bell. The features described in the above X-ray are consistent with Bell stage 2 NEC.[1]

3. a. The lateral abdominal X-ray shows free air. There are loops of bowel extending into the gas filled area.
  b. The baby has a perforation. This would increase the stage of NEC to Bell stage 3.
  c. The baby should be reviewed by a paediatric surgeon. If ventilation is compromised a drain should be inserted through the abdominal wall to release the pressure from build up of free gas in the abdomen. There have been recent studies to compare drain insertion with laparotomy for NEC. These have not demonstrated superiority of one technique over the other, but have confirmed the poor outlook of babies requiring surgery for perforated NEC.[2,3]

4. a. i. There is a large patch of opacification in the mid zone on the right side of the chest. There is some patchy shadowing elsewhere.
  ii. There is a nasogastric tube in place.
  iii. The nasogastric tube is coiled in a pouch in the thorax, behind the heart.
  b. This baby has a sliding para-oesophageal (hiatus) hernia. The prevalence in newborns is unknown but it is thought to be relatively uncommon. It can be discovered on a routine X-ray but usually presents with features of gastro-oesophageal reflux. In this case the changes in the lung would be compatible with aspiration in association with reflux.
  c. No interventions are needed if the child is asymptomatic. However, in this case it would be appropriate to commence antibiotics and consider anti-reflux treatment if vomiting remains problematic.

5. a. With the exception of chest leads and a nasogastric tube there are no abnormalities on this X-ray. It is normal.
   b. Normal.
   c. The chest X-ray does not reveal anything that needs treatment.

6. a. i. The endotracheal tube is down the right main bronchus.
   ii. The left lung is inadequately aerated.
   iii. There is a nasogastric tube in situ.
   b. The endotracheal tube should be withdrawn and the correct position confirmed with a repeat chest X-ray.

7. a. The clavicles are absent.
   b. Cleidocranial dysostosis. In this condition, the clavicle is either hypoplastic or absent and the ribs are short. The anterior fontanelle often closes late and there may be delayed eruption of teeth. There can be bossing of the forehead.
   c. Autosomal dominant. It results from a mutation in the CBFA1 gene, which controls a key transcription factor in osteoblast differentiation.

8. a. i. Large tension pneumothorax on the left.
   ii. Mediastinal shift to the right with tracheal deviation.
   iii. Transcutaneous oxygen electrode on left upper chest.
   iv. Surprisingly the infant is not intubated.
   b. i. Immediate drainage of the pneumothorax.
   ii. Intubation and ventilation is very likely to be needed.

9. a. i. Intubated infant.
   ii. Right pneumothorax.
   iii. Pneumopericardium.
   iv. Umbilical arterial catheter.
   v. Bilateral hyperinflation of the chest.
   vi. There is abnormal shadowing at the right base which is difficult to assess without other X-rays. This turned out to be a cystic adenomatoid malformation.
   b. The pneumothorax should be drained. The decision to drain the pneumopericardium will be dictated by the clinical condition of the infant, specifically with respect to cardiac function.

10. a. i. Intubated infant.
   ii. High UAC.
   iii. Large cystic mass in right lung with a septum running across the middle.
   b. These appearance would be consistent with a large cystic adenomatoid malformation (which was the case in this infant) or lobar emphysema. The latter is unlikely as this condition usually develops after birth as opposed to presenting with problems at birth. There is debate about the use of the word 'congenital' as some authorities maintain that the lobar emphysema develops as a result of airway problems that develop postnatally.
   c. The management of these conditions is extremely difficult. Close co-operation with paediatric surgeons is essential. Direct puncture has a high chance of leading to formation of a broncho-pleural fistula. The infant may be too sick to tolerate thoracotomy, yet respiratory compromise may become so severe that intervention is necessary.

11. a. There is a large bore (Replogle) nasogastric tube, partially coiled in the upper oesophagus. There is a shadow of air in the upper oesophagus but none lower down, suggesting an oesophageal atresia. There is evidence of gas in the gastrointestinal tract, suggesting a tracheo-oesophageal fistula.

   b. Management is complex and requires close collaboration with paediatric surgeons. If the infant is mature and clinically stable, surgery should be considered in the relatively near future. If the infant is very sick or immature, then a decision may be made to defer surgery until a more stable state is achieved, or the baby has grown.

12. a.   **i.** The X-ray shows a fracture of the left humerus.

       ii. There is marked osteopenia of all bones, especially marked in the bones of the forearm.

   b.   **i.** Marked rotation of the film.

       ii. There is thinning of the ribs with what are almost certainly fractures with callous formation.

     iii. Osteopenia of all bones.

   c. Osteogenesis imperfecta.

   d. Pamidronate infusions have been used to improve bone density and reduce the risk of further fractures. Such management should only be undertaken in specialist centres as general experience of this management is extremely limited.

13. a.   **i.** Clip in left upper chest.

       ii. Abnormal separation of left 4th and 5th ribs.

     iii. Widespread patchy opacification of both lungs.

     iv. Large bulla in right lung base.

       v. Nasogastric tube in situ.

   b. The PDA has been clipped.

   c. None. This infant is not intubated and ventilated and unless there are signs of severe respiratory distress, no action is needed. The infant has what appears to be quite severe chronic lung disease and would not benefit from re-ventilation. Although the bulla looks fairly large on X-ray, it is only occupying a relatively small proportion of the intra-thoracic space. The majority resolve spontaneously over time, as was the case with this infant.

14. a.   **i.** Short long bones (compare to size of cord clamp).

       ii. Marked bowing of bones, particularly noticeable in femurs.

   b. The chest is very narrow with abnormal ribs that are short and thin with splayed ends. The vertebral bodies are flattened with wide intervertebral spaces.

   c. The appearance is that of a congenital skeletal dysplasia. In this case the most likely diagnosis is thanatophoric dysplasia as indicated by the extremely short limbs with classic 'telephone receiver' shaped femurs.

   d. Thanatophoric dysplasia is invariably fatal, usually shortly after birth.

15. a. The heart is grossly enlarged in all dimensions.

   b. The enlarged heart does not in itself point to a specific diagnosis and conditions such as a cardiomyopathy, structural heart defect, storage disorder, maternal diabetes and heart failure are all possibilities. In this case the combination of a large heart, peripheral oedema and a bruit over the bulging anterior fontanelle should raise the possibility of an intracranial arteriovenous malformation resulting in high output cardiac failure (as was the case in this baby).

   c. **i.** Echocardiogram.

      ii. Cranial ultrasound, CT scan or MRI.

      iii. Four limb BP and oxygen saturations.

      iv. Check maternal history and antenatal ultrasounds.

16. a. **i.** There is widespread opacification throughout both lung fields.

      ii. There are clear air bronchograms on both sides.

      iii. The heart border is not clearly defined.

      iv. The costophrenic and cardiophrenic angles are not clearly visualised.

      v. There is an endotracheal tube.

      vi. There is a central venous line entering by the left arm and with a tip at the junction of the SVC and right atrium.

   b. Respiratory distress syndrome is the most likely diagnosis.

   c. Surfactant should be given if the dose has not been repeated since birth. Ventilatory requirements are high and some centres would consider high frequency oscillatory ventilation at this point. If this is not available ventilation will probably need to be adjusted to improve the blood gases.

17. a. **i.** There is patchy opacification that is most marked in the perihilar region.

      ii. There are basal bullae, most apparent on the right.

      iii. The lungs are relatively hyperexpanded, 11 posterior rib ends are showing.

      iv. There is a transcutaneous oxygen electrode, chest leads and a nasogastric tube.

      v. There is an endotracheal tube.

   b. The history and chest X-ray appearances are typical of meconium aspiration syndrome. It is very possible that a significant degree of persistent pulmonary hypertension is contributing to the clinical picture.

   c. There is evidence that both high frequency ventilation and nitric oxide may be useful in this condition, and are particularly useful in combination. In severe cases extracorporeal membrane oxygenation may be life saving and referral should be made early. There is some evidence from animal studies and limited human data to support the use of surfactant, either by bolus administration of by surfactant lavage.

18. a. **i.** There is a nasogastric tube in situ.

      ii. There is loss of the costophrenic angle on the right and increased shadowing in the lower peripheral right chest.

   b. Right pleural effusion. Pleural effusions can occur for many reasons. If diagnosed antenatally, they are associated with chromosomal or congenital abnormalities. Congenital viral infections can also cause effusions. Isolated effusions can be a chylothorax or idiopathic.

   c. If asymptomatic and there are no other concerns it is appropriate to simply observe the infant. Idiopathic effusions may resolve while a chylothorax may increase once feeding is commenced. Careful observation and repeat X-rays are essential.

d. If there is respiratory distress the infant may need respiratory support and draining of the effusion.

e. This would depend upon how unwell the baby was and whether fluid had been drained. In an asymptomatic baby baseline haematology and biochemistry may be indicated and little else. If unwell, viral titres may be indicated, as may chromosome analysis. If pleural fluid is drained, the fluid should be sent for cytology, biochemical and microbiological analysis. A high lymphocyte count indicates a chylothorax.

19. a. There is fluid in the horizontal fissure and some peri-hilar streaking.
b. The most likely diagnosis is transient tachypnoea of the newborn. However due to the difficulty in accurately diagnosing infection it is common to consider this as a possible differential diagnosis.
c. Close observation and respiratory support such as CPAP may be needed for a short while. Affected infants rarely require more than 40% oxygen or respiratory support for more than three days. Antibiotics should be given until infection has been excluded.
d. The prognosis is good. Most infants recover over 24 hours. There is debate regarding whether infants with TTN are more prone to wheezing in childhood.[4]

20. a.　i. There is an endotracheal tube in situ.
　　ii. There is a nasogastric tube in situ.
　　iii. Both lungs show inflammatory and cystic change consistent with bronchopulmonary dysplasia.
　　iv. The lungs appear hyperinflated – note the bulging pleura on the right.
　　v. There is loss of the left costophrenic angle and obvious outlining of the lungs on the left side with fluid.
　　vi. There is abnormal separation of the upper ribs on the left.
　　vii. There is a long line in situ in the left subclavian vein. The position of the tip seems satisfactory.
　　viii. There is marked oedema visible most obviously outside the chest.
b. The separation of the ribs on the left side of the chest is highly suggestive of a ductal ligation in the recent past. The chylothorax which is present is a well recognised complication of the procedure.
c. This infant has bronchopulmonary dysplasia and is still ventilated. The treatment options available at this stage would be a short course of diuretics or steroids. Diuretics can improve oxygenation and lung compliance, but it is prudent to give a short course to assess for response before embarking on long-term diuretic use due to the high incidence of side effects.

21. a.　i. Generalised patchy opacification throughout the lung fields.
　　ii. Small volume lungs.
　　iii. Tracheal deviation to the right.
　　iv. Rib fractures on the right with callus formation.

b. The chest appearances are consistent with chronic lung disease and in this case the tracheal deviation is likely to be due to fibrotic changes in the right upper chest. The baby is likely to have been in hospital for some weeks and osteopenia of prematurity has developed. The rib fractures are probably a result of the osteopenia. In this particular case it is of interest to note that alkaline phosphatase and plasma calcium and phosphate had been within the normal ranges throughout the majority of the admission.

22. a. There is a 'double bubble' with a dilated stomach and duodenum.
   b. Duodenal atresia.
   c. Additional problems may be Down syndrome, cardiac abnormalities and malrotation.
   d. A large-bore nasogastric tube must be inserted and left on free drainage; electrolyte and blood gas anomalies must be corrected.
   e. Isolated duodenal atresia can be successfully corrected by surgery although experience at such early gestation is very limited. Other anomalies such as cardiac defects (which are much commoner with duodenal atresia) will affect the prognosis.

23. a. **i.** There is a naso–jejunal tube in situ.
   ii. There is a very large translucency covering much of the abdomen. This 'football sign' indicates free air in the peritoneal cavity.
   iii. There is a white line running to the right of and almost parallel to the vertebral column. This is the falciform ligament and it only becomes visible when there is free intraperitoneal gas.
   iv. The lung fields are patchy throughout. They are extremely low volume yet appear hyperinflated with marked upward slanting of the ribs. It is difficult to interpret how many of these changes are due to intrinsic lung disease and how much to compression from abdominal distension.
   b. There is obvious chronic lung disease and definite gastrointestinal perforation. The latter is quite possibly related to the administration of steroids.
   c. Management will depend upon the severity of illness. If his condition has become unstable and gases have deteriorated, ventilation will be required. If the abdominal distension compromises ventilation an abdominal drain may well be required. Surgical review and consideration for a laparotomy will be needed early in the process.

24. a. **i.** The heart shape is ovoid (egg-shaped).
   ii. The upper mediastinum is narrow.
   iii. The lung fields appear normal.
   b. Transposition of the great arteries.
   c. The diagnosis should be confirmed by echocardiography. A prostaglandin infusion should be started and the case should be discussed with the nearest paediatric cardiac centre as soon as possible.

25. a. **i.** Both lung fields show a diffuse granular appearance.
   ii. There are bilateral air bronchograms.
   iii. The end of the endotracheal tube is high.
   iv. The tip of the UAC appears to be somewhere close to the right subclavian artery.

b. Respiratory distress with incorrectly placed UAC and ET tube.

c. **i.** The UAC will need to be withdrawn into a more appropriate position.

   ii. The endotracheal tube will need to be inserted further.

   iii. A nasogastric tube should be inserted and the intestines decompressed.

   iv. Surfactant administration should be considered.

26. a. **i.** The heart is much larger than normal.

   ii. The lung fields appear well aerated.

   iii. Pleura bulging on both sides.

   iv. UAC on the left – very high (probably – this cannot be confirmed to be the UAC until the abdomen is X-rayed and the caudal loop is seen).

   v. UVC on the right, very high (position confirmation needed as above).

b. A diabetic cardiomyopathy is the most likely diagnosis. Although septal hypertrophy is the best described association, biventricular hypertrophy may develop with significant and serious reduction in stroke volume.

c. **i.** Reposition the lines.

   ii. Echocardiography.

   iii. Seek expert advice if haemodynamically unstable.

27. a. **i.** The chest is small.

   ii. The ribs are thin and slope downwards steeply.

   iii. There is a UVC about 1 cm above the diaphragm.

   iv. The UAC tip is at T9.

   v. The endotracheal tube tip is very high and is only just visible on the X-ray.

b. Pulmonary hypoplasia secondary to oligohydramnios.

28. a. **i.** There is free gas in the peritoneal cavity.

   ii. There are dilated loops of bowel, several of which appear to have very irregularly thickened walls.

   iii. The right diaphragm appears thickened.

   iv. There is no gas in the rectum.

b. There is intestinal perforation which has probably been present some time to result in the degree of bowel wall thickening that is apparent. The presence of irritant material is also probably responsible for thickening of the diaphragm. It is not clear why the bowel has perforated but the absence of rectal gas may be suggestive of an obstruction. In this baby's case there was colonic atresia.

c. The free gas will need drain insertion, unless a laparotomy is performed immediately. Surgical review is essential and the baby should be stabilised as dictated by clinical condition.

29. a. **i.** The film is extremely rotated and it is difficult to accurately place anything in the picture.

   ii. There is a line to the right of the vertebral column that could be a UAC, but this cannot be stated with any certainty.

   iii. There is an endotracheal tube which is slightly high.

   iv. There is a central venous line coming in from the right arm. It is very likely to be actually ending lateral to the chest.

b. The line position is almost certainly unsatisfactory.

c. The line should be removed. A further non-rotated film could be obtained but the position of the line is likely to be more lateral if this is done.

30. a.
  i. The lungs show diffuse patchy opacities consistent with chronic lung disease.
  ii. The lungs are relatively small volume and hyperinflated, with upward sloping ribs.
  iii. There are vertebral abnormalities.

b. No action is indicated although it is assumed that a detailed examination has already been performed to exclude any other anomalies that may be associated with the vertebral abnormalities.

31. a.
  i. The lungs are hyperinflated.
  ii. There is a nasogastric feeding tube in place.
  iii. There is what is probably a UAC, with the tip at around T8.
  iv. There is an endotracheal tube.
  v. There is widespread patchy shadowing which appears consistent with cystic changes throughout both lung fields.

b. These apparently cystic changes are compatible with chronic lung disease. Although the diagnosis of CLD (or BPD) is dependent on a prolonged oxygen requirement changes may be present well before then and can be seen histologically in infants who have died only a few days after birth. The distribution and pattern of the changes is different from that expected with pulmonary interstitial emphysema, which also gives widespread cystic changes.

32. a.
  i. There is an endotracheal tube.
  ii. There is a nasogastric tube.
  iii. There is opacification of the left lung, consistent with RDS.
  iv. The right lung has cystic change throughout, consistent with pulmonary interstitial emphysema.
  v. There is a large bulla at the base of the right lung.

b. The presence of pulmonary interstitial emphysema in the right lung and what appears to be quite severe RDS in the other lung suggests that the endotracheal tube may have been in the right main bronchus at the time of the first surfactant administration. As one lung is now well expanded and the other solid, any further surfactant is likely to also go into the right lung.

c. Ventilatory management of this baby will be difficult. The left lung needs aeration and thus recruitment of alveoli. The ideal way to do this is to use higher ventilatory pressures to both recruit and retain alveolar expansion. Unfortunately the right lung is showing signs of cystic change and over-distension with a bulla in the right base, and high pressures will result in further damage. High frequency may be useful and anecdotally it has been suggested that paralysing the baby and ventilating with the PIE side down may minimise damage to the PIE side and facilitate inflation of the atelectatic side.

33. a. **i.** There is a nasogastric tube.
      ii. There are loops of dilated bowel but no evidence of inflammatory changes, thus making NEC unlikely.
      iii. There is no air in the rectum.

b. Either structural or functional bowel obstruction is likely. There is nothing on the X-ray that allows differentiation between possible causes. Maternal diabetes is associated with a small left colon in the newborn baby. This results in a functional obstruction that usually resolves with time (as it did with this infant).

c. A contrast study is probably indicated. Further investigations will depend on the result of this. The baby should not be fed, intravenous fluids should be given and a nasogastric tube should be left on free drainage.

34. a. **i.** There is extremely poor lung inflation.
      ii. The diaphragms are very high.
      iii. The ribs are thin, particularly on the posterior aspect.

b. Myotonic dystrophy.

c. The baby will need ventilating. There is normally some improvement over time, although it may be a long time before breathing is strong enough to allow extubation.

35. a. **i.** There is an endotracheal tube in place.
      ii. There is a line with a tip at approximately T11. It is not clear what this line is.
      iii. There is an endotracheal tube at an appropriate position.
      iv. There is what appears to be a central venous line with the tip below the sternal end of the left clavicle.
      v. Both lungs are very poorly aerated.
      vi. There is a fracture of the left arm. The bones do not appear particularly osteopenic and this is presumably traumatic in origin.

36. a. **i.** There is a nasogastric tube with the end in the mid-thoracic oesophagus.
      ii. The lungs have diffuse patchy opacification consistent with chronic lung disease.

b. The nasogastric tube needs to be repositioned and as much gas removed from the intestines as possible.

37. a. **i.** There is an endotracheal tube and nasogastric tube.
      ii. There is a fine-bore central venous catheter with the tip in the thoracic inlet.
      iii. There is a large-bore central venous catheter on the right with the tip at the junction of the SVC and right atrium.
      iv. The right lung is opaque with no areas of aeration.

b. Surgical placement of a central venous catheter. The large-bore catheter is a Broviac line.

c. There is aplasia/hypoplasia of the right lung. The fact that the lung has always had this appearance and the infant is now 4 weeks old is strongly against collapse or consolidation as the cause of this appearance.

38. a. i. There is free gas above the liver in this lateral X-ray.
  b. Gastrointestinal perforation.
  c. Surgical referral. A drain may need to be inserted pending laparotomy.

39. a. i. There are bilateral pneumothoraces.
  ii. There is an endotracheal tube in position.
  b. Pneumothoraces may have been present at birth, following the gasping respirations or following initial ventilation. Bilateral pneumothoraces may be difficult to diagnose because all signs are equal on both sides. Although a needle drain may allow re-inflation the lung will expand onto the needle which can easily become blocked.
  c. Immediate insertion of bilateral chest drains.

40. a. i. There is an endotracheal tube, the tip of which is too high.
  ii. There is a nasogastric tube.
  iii. There is patchy opacification of both lungs.
  iv. There is enlargement of both liver and spleen.
  b. The combination of growth retardation, a petechial rash and hepato-splenomegaly is highly suggestive of a congenital infection. Cytomegalovirus is the most likely candidate. A pneumonitis may develop with CMV infection although it is rarely present at birth and most commonly associated with perinatally acquired infection.
  c. i. Blood needs to be sent for CMV testing.
  ii. Further investigations should look for other evidence of CMV damage – an echocardiogram to look for congenital heart defects and cerebral ultrasound, CT or MRI to look for intracranial calcification and evidence of lissencephaly or polymicrogyria that may occur with early infection.
  iii. If the diagnosis is confirmed, treatment with anti–CMV chemotherapy should be considered. There is some encouraging information on the use of ganciclovir.

41. a. i. There is dilated bowel with thickened walls, mainly on the right side of the abdomen.
  ii. There are areas of bowel with intramural gas.
  iii. The gut distribution is opposite to that expected. The stomach (see NGT position) is on the right, liver on the left.
  b. The central line is passing to the left of the spine.
  c. The appearances suggest necrotising enterocolitis in a baby with situs inversus. The appearances are typical of NEC. The distribution of the abdominal contents and the left sided position of the inferior can only be explained by situs inversus. The very small amount of heart visible appears to be on the left but further investigation would be needed to exclude dextrocardia.

42. a. i. There is an endotracheal tube with a high tip.
  ii. There is a central line which is probably an umbilical arterial line with the tip at T8.
  iii. There is patchy opacification throughout both lungs.

    iv. The lungs are hyperinflated with 11 posterior rib ends showing and with flat diaphragms.

    v. The heart appears moderately compressed.

  b. Mean airway pressure should be reduced or ventilation should be changed to a different modality.

43. a.   **i.** There is a central venous catheter entering from the right arm.

    ii. There is patchy shadowing of both lungs.

    iii. There is a nasogastric tube, the end of which cannot be seen.

    iv. There is gaseous distension of the stomach and intestines.

    v. The endotracheal tube is not in the trachea – it is almost certainly in the oesophagus.

  b. Ventilation of the gastrointestinal tract.

  c. Remove the ET tube and either re-intubate or try CPAP. Gas should be sucked out of the gastrointestinal tract if possible and the nasogastric tube should then be put on free drainage.

44. a.   **i.** There is an endotracheal tube in the correct position.

    ii. There is a central line which is probably an umbilical arterial catheter with the tip at T11–12.

    iii. The lungs are very small volume.

    iv. There are pleural effusions, more marked on the right than the left.

    v. There are two echodensities over the right lung field and one over the left. Each has the appearance of a small cylinder.

  b. In-utero drainage of pleural effusions using drains with pigtails on both ends. The echodense bodies are markers – one on each end of the drains.

  c. Pleural effusions of this severity are uncommon. In the absence of other signs of hydrops, pulmonary lymphangiectasia is a definite possibility.

45. a.   **i.** There is an endotracheal tube that is high.

    ii. There is a nasogastric tube in position.

    iii. The lungs show patchy shadowing in both fields.

    iv. There is a central venous line which appears to have been inserted through a scalp or neck vein. The end is resting within the right atrium.

  b. The central venous line needs to be withdrawn to lie outside the heart.

46. a.   **i.** There is an endotracheal tube.

    ii. There is a nasogastric tube.

    iii. There is a central venous line which appears to have been inserted through a vein in the right arm. It has passed in a cephalad direction. The tip is not visible but probably lies in either the neck or the head.

  b. The line needs to be withdrawn until the tip lies in the region of the thoracic inlet.

47. a.   **i.** There is an endotracheal tube that is very high.

    ii. There is a nasogastric tube with the tip in the stomach.

    iii. There is an umbilical arterial line with the tip at T5.

    iv. There is an umbilical venous catheter which deviates to the right and appears to lie within the liver.

  b. Umbilical venous and arterial lines and the endotracheal tube need to be repositioned.

48. a.   **i.**   There is an endotracheal tube that is slightly high.

   ii.   There is a central venous line with the tip at the thoracic inlet.

   iii.   There is an umbilical venous line with a very low tip.

   iv.   There is a large amount of oedema, very obvious on the sides of the chest.

   v.   The lungs show dense shadowing and there may be some parenchymal cysts compatible with pulmonary interstitial emphysema.

   vi.   There is a left tension pneumothorax with mediastinal shift to the right.

b.   Although a pneumothorax of this size should be easily detected by transillumination the oedema around the chest will have resulted in a diffuse brightness that may well have concealed the pneumothorax.

c.   A chest drain must be inserted immediately.

49. a.   There are fixed loops of dilated bowel that do not change from one X-ray to another.

b.   This unchanging appearance is highly suggestive of dead bowel. NEC is the most likely underlying cause.

c.   Surgical referral is needed. A laparotomy will be required at some point and an abdominal drain may be required as an interim measure.

50. a.   **i.**   There is an endotracheal tube that is high.

   ii.   There is a central venous line entering from the right arm that is slightly too long.

   iii.   There is what is probably an umbilical arterial line, with the tip at T8/9.

   iv.   The lung fields are poorly aerated.

   v.   There is a nasogastric tube which is passing down into the right lung.

   vi.   There is gas in the stomach.

b.   There is a tracheo-oesophageal fistula or cleft. Although it is possible to pass a nasogastric tube into the trachea it should not be possible to do so when an endotracheal tube is in place as is the case here. The nasogastric tube is gaining access to the trachea through a fistula or cleft lower down.

c.   The nasogastric tube needs to be removed. The endotracheal tube should be inserted further to see if it can block a fistula, otherwise ventilation will be very difficult. A surgical opinion should be sought.

REFERENCES

1. Bell MJ, Ternberg JL, Fagin RD et al. Neonatal necrotizing enterocolitis. Therapeutic decisions based upon clinical staging. Ann Surg 1978;187:1–7

2. Blakely ML, Tyson JE, Lally KP. Laparotomy versus peritoneal drainage for necrotizing enterocolitis or isolated intestinal perforation in extremely low birth weight infants: outcomes through 18 months adjusted age. Pediatrics 2006;117:e680–e687

3. Moss RL, Dimmitt RA, Barnhart DC et al. Laparotomy versus peritoneal drainage for necrotizing enterocolitis and perforation. N Engl J Med 2006;354:2225–34

4. Shohat M, Levy G. Transient tachypnoea of the newborn and asthma. Arch Dis Child 1989;64:277–79

Chapter 8

Scans

In recent years, advanced scanning techniques have become an integral part of neonatal practice. Before delivery, high quality antenatal ultrasound imaging may identify a range of abnormalities. In many cases, antenatal detection may allow a postnatal action plan to be put in place prior to the delivery thereby ensuring that delivery is in the best place with the most appropriate personnel in attendance. Regular cranial ultrasound scans are regarded by many as an essential part of the routine management of the preterm infant, with most neonatal units now screening all infants under 32 weeks gestation. This safe, movable and repeatable investigation gives immediate images that can be interpreted at the cot side. The prognostic value of abnormal scans is an area over which there is still considerable debate and this will be addressed in the questions.

More recently, the availability of high quality magnetic resonance imaging (MRI) has increased, and the detail possible with this technique may be invaluable in the assessment of infants with congenital neurological abnormalities or those who have suffered an episode of perinatal asphyxia.

This chapter contains ultrasound, CT and MRI scans along with relevant clinical histories. As with X-rays, interpretation is required as well as proposed management in some. In others you will be asked to comment upon the possible long-term significance of the abnormality that has been detected. There are many textbooks available for reference.[1–4]

QUESTIONS

1. A term baby presents in heart failure shortly after birth. The fontanelle is noted to be bulging outward and a bruit is audible over the fontanelle. A further investigation is performed.

   a. What type of scan is this?

   b. What does it show?

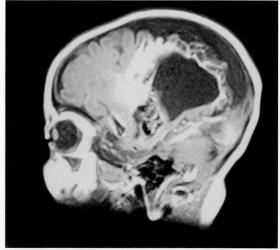

Figure 8.1

2. The same infant had the following chest X-ray taken.
  a. Describe the chest X-ray.
  b. What is the diagnosis from the chest X-ray?
  c. How is this image linked with the MRI scan?

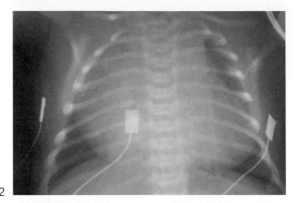

Figure 8.2

3. A term baby is born following a difficult vaginal delivery. No resuscitation is required and he is returned to his mother. Paediatricians are asked to review him at 18 hours of age as it is thought that he may have made some abnormal movements. He appears well on examination and an MRI scan is performed.

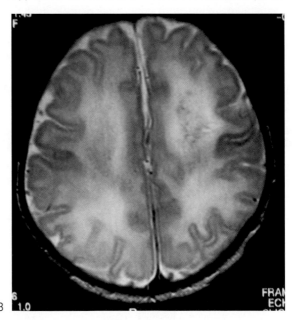

Figure 8.3

  a. Describe the scan.
  b. What is this likely to be due to?
  c. What clinical signs would this infant demonstrate, if any?
  d. What is the most likely underlying cause?
  e. What one other investigation would you consider to give more information about prognosis?

4. A preterm baby, born at 28 weeks' gestation has a follow-up scan carried out at 34 weeks corrected gestational age.

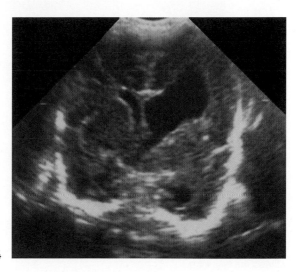

Figure 8.4

   a. What type of scan is this?
   b. What does it show?
   c. Why has this happened?
   d. What is the outlook for this baby?

5. This scan was carried out on a 25 week gestation infant, who is now 72 hours old. He had a very stormy first two days, requiring maximal inotropic support and high ventilatory pressures. He is now requiring no blood pressure support and is on minimal ventilation.

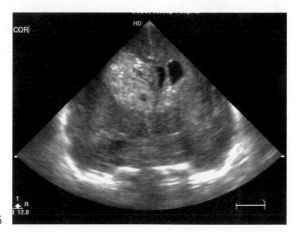

Figure 8.5

   a. Describe the scan.
   b. What has happened?
   c. What is the outlook for this baby?

6. A 27 week gestation baby has a routine head scan performed at 2 days of age.

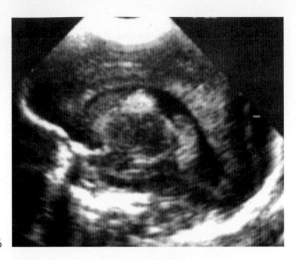

Figure 8.6

    a. Describe the scan.

    b. Will this affect the baby's long-term outcome?

7. A routine head scan is performed in a 29 week gestation infant. Parents want to know what it shows and whether it means that their baby is going to be normal or not.

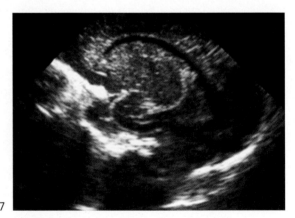

Figure 8.7

    a. Describe the scan.

    b. What is the likely outcome for this baby?

8. A baby is known to have a congenital abnormality of the head antenatally. This scan is carried out after birth.

    a. Describe the scan.

    b. What is the diagnosis?

    c. What are the associations?

    d. What is the long-term outlook for this condition?

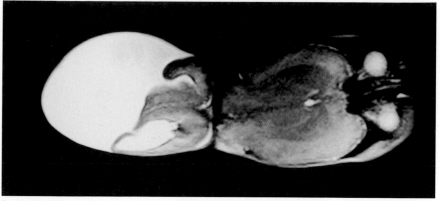

Figure 8.8

9. This scan was carried out on day 7 in an ex-26 week gestation infant.

    a. Describe the scan.

    b. What is the most likely cause?

    c. What is your management?

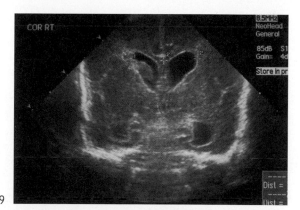

Figure 8.9

10. A 25 week gestation infant has a scan performed at the age of 10 days.

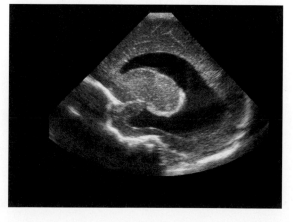

Figure 8.10

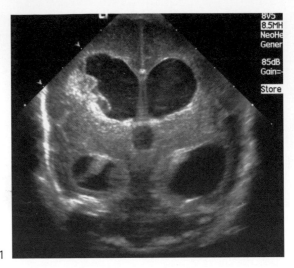

Figure 8.11

   a. What do these images show?

   b. What is your management?

11. This is a routine scan carried out on a baby born at 30 weeks' gestation who requires no ventilatory support and is tolerating full milk feeds by 5 days of life.

   a. Describe the scan.

   b. What is the diagnosis?

   c. What is the outcome for this baby?

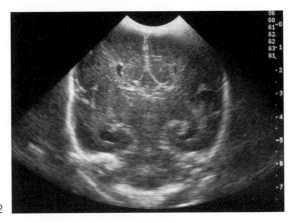

Figure 8.12

12. Examine the scan below.

   a. What type of scan is this?

   b. What does it show?

   c. What would the management of this baby be?

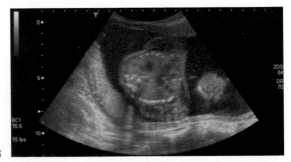

Figure 8.13

13. A 29 week infant has a routine cranial ultrasound scan performed.

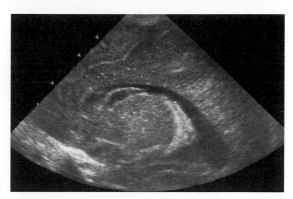

Figure 8.14

    a. Describe the scan.
    b. Why has this happened?
    c. What is the outlook for this baby?

14. A baby is born at term through meconium-stained liquor and requires full resuscitation. She has seizures noted at 1 hour of age and is given a loading dose of phenobarbitone. She is ventilated for the first 12 hours and then copes without respiratory support. She has established feeding by day 7 and is discharged at day 10. An MRI is carried out the day before discharge.

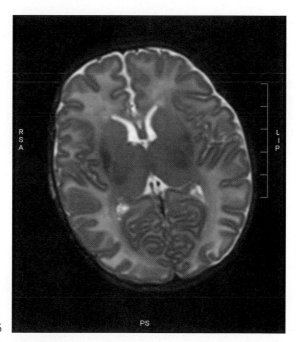

Figure 8.15

    a. What does the MRI show?
    b. Why has this occurred?

15. A baby girl is delivered by caesarean section for failure to progress. She has a large abdomen at birth with masses palpable bilaterally.

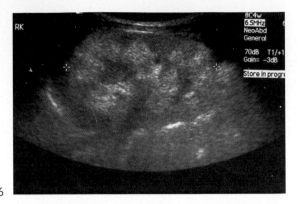

Figure 8.16

    a. Describe the scan.
    b. What is the likely diagnosis?
    c. What problems might the baby have?
    d. What are the known associations?

16. A routine cranial ultrasound scan is carried out on a 31 week gestation infant.

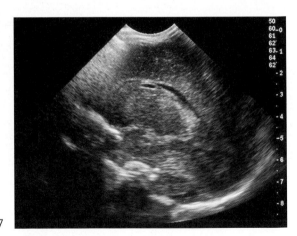

Figure 8.17

    a. Describe the scan.
    b. What is the diagnosis?
    c. What is the outlook for this baby?

17. A baby born at 36 weeks gestation has severe RDS with a history of prolonged rupture of membranes for 5 days. He is treated with antibiotics and is transferred for high frequency oscillation ventilation. He was initially hypotensive requiring maximal inotropic support. A scan is carried out on day 3 after transfer.

a. Describe the scan.

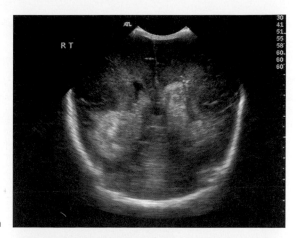

Figure 8.18a

A few days later, a further scan was obtained.

b. Describe the changes.

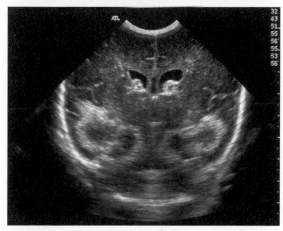

Figure 8.18b

18. Following an abnormal cranial ultrasound scan, further imaging is carried out.

a. Describe the scan.

b. What might this be associated with?

c. What is the long-term outlook for this baby?

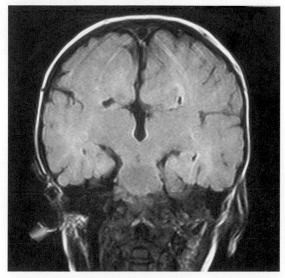

Figure 8.19

19. A woman is scanned antenatally at 30 weeks.

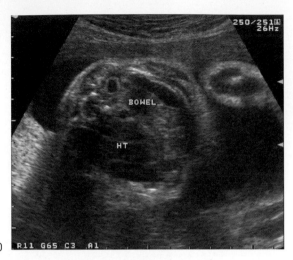

Figure 8.20

a. What does the scan show?
b. What will be your management of the baby at birth?
c. What are the baby's chances of survival?

20. Examine the scan below.

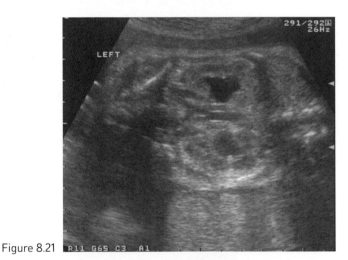

Figure 8.21

a. Describe the antenatal scan of the fetus's renal tract.
b. What would your postnatal management of this infant be if any?

21. A woman is referred for a detailed fetal scan and has been found to have a raised alphafetoprotein.

    a. What is the abnormality on this scan?

    b. What other investigations would you carry out postnatally?

    c. What conditions is this anomaly associated with?

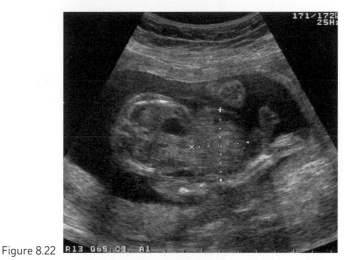

Figure 8.22

22. A term infant is born vaginally following a rapid delivery. At 24 hours of age she is noted to be irritable and feeding is poor. A cranial ultrasound is performed and raises some concerns. Another investigation is performed.

    a. What type of scan is this?

    b. What does it show?

    c. What is the outcome for this baby?

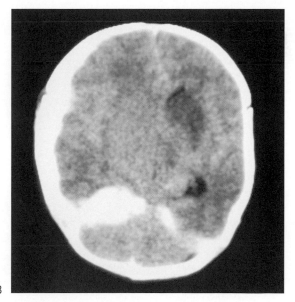

Figure 8.23

23. An infant is noted on postnatal examination to have a large head circumference, with a bulging fontanelle. He is asymptomatic and feeding well by bottle. An MRI scan is performed.

    a. Is this a T1 or T2 weighted MRI?

    b. What does it show?

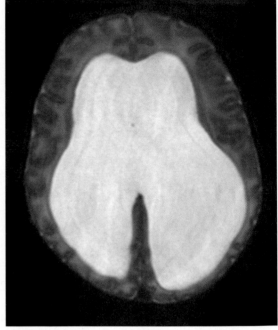

Figure 8.24

24. A CT scan has been performed on a growth retarded baby born at 38 weeks gestation. There is mixed hyperbilirubinaemia and a petechial rash.

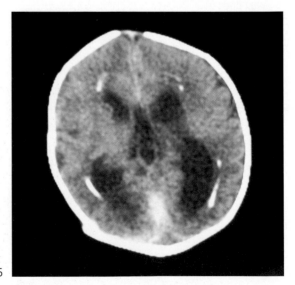

Figure 8.25

    a. What does the scan show?

    b. What is the diagnosis?

    c. What other investigations must be performed?

25. An MRI scan is carried out on a six month old infant.
   a. Describe two abnormalities with this scan.
   b. What is the likely cause?

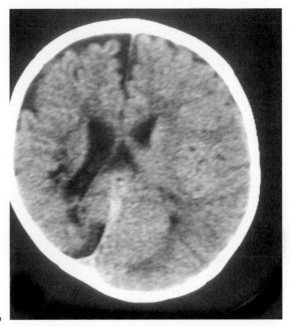

Figure 8.26

26. A term baby is delivered with a growth at the back of the skull. She has an MRI scan as shown below.
   a. Describe the scan.
   b. What is the likely diagnosis?

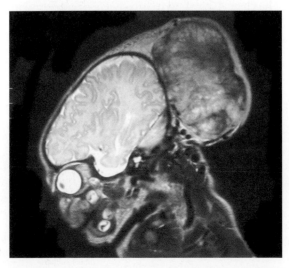

Figure 8.27

27. A cranial ultrasound scan is carried out in a 25 week infant. She has been transferred in for intensive care from a level 2 unit. She seemed to be relatively stable for the first 24 hours after birth but at the age of 26 hours becomes acidotic and pale and required fluid resuscitation and increasing ventilation. A scan is carried out and is shown. Describe the scan.

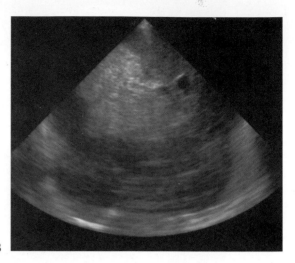

Figure 8.28

ANSWERS

1. a. This is an MRI scan of the brain.

   b. It shows a loss of cortex in the centre of the brain with an area filled with fluid. There is also increased extra-axial fluid around the brain. Blood vessels are tortuous and highlighted on the scan above the area filled with fluid.

2. a. The chest X-ray shows a grossly enlarged heart with very little lung tissue visible.

   b. The chest X-ray would be consistent with cardiac failure or possibly a cardiomyopathy.

   c. The two images are linked. The MRI shows a large AV malformation and the chest X-ray shows cardiac failure. Arteriovenous malformation is a rare cause of neonatal intracranial haemorrhage. The vein of Galen is most commonly involved, but a malformation here rarely presents as an intracranial haemorrhage. Approximately half of all cases present with cardiac manifestations, especially heart failure due to high cardiac output. Other clinical presentations, depending on the site of the AVM, may be seizures, hydrocephalus due to increased venous pressure or obstruction of CSF drainage, or opisthotonus with other brain stem signs in association with malformations originating in the posterior fossa.

3. a. There is an area of abnormally high signal on the left side of the brain (seen on the right side of the picture).

b. It is likely to be due to an infarction of the middle cerebral artery. The left middle cerebral artery is more commonly affected than the right, up to 3 or 4 times so.

c. Infants with focal infarction do not usually have encephalopathy. The most common presentation is seizures, starting unilaterally but then becoming more generalised. Abnormalities in tone can also be present. Abnormal signs in the neonatal period are not predictive of later outcome.[5] The prognosis for neurodevelopmental outcome is variable. Normal outcome has been reported in between one-third and one-half of all affected infants but some may develop signs of a hemiplegia.[5,6]

d. In most cases of arterial infarction, the aetiology is unknown. Where a cause can be defined it is usually due to either thrombus, embolus or ischaemia. Of these, embolic phenomena appear most common and there is an association with twin-to-twin transfusion and congenital heart disease including the presence of a PDA. Other causes that have been reported include maternal cocaine abuse, polycythaemia, and elevated maternal cardiolipin and anti-phospholipid antibodies. Activated protein C deficiency in association with factor V Leiden deficiency is becoming increasingly recognised. Adverse perinatal events are reported in nearly 50% of affected infants.[7]

e. It would be useful to carry out an EEG as this may have prognostic value. If the background activity on the EEG is abnormal, there is likely to be an abnormal motor outcome.[7]

4. a. This is a coronal section on a cranial ultrasound scan.

b. It shows a very large single cavity cyst which is in communication with the left lateral ventricle. The right lateral ventricle appears unaffected. This is a porencephalic cyst.

c. Porencephalic cysts are the end results of a destructive process in the brain, such as intracranial haemorrhage, infection or surgery. The parenchyma is replaced by fluid, hence the cyst formation. Communication with the ventricles, as in this case, may or may not be present.

d. The prognosis depends on the size and whether unilateral or bilateral. Anecdotally every neonatologist knows of one or more infants who had such a lesion and were normal on long-term follow-up. There is no doubt that with extensive infarction, particularly bilaterally, outcome is likely to be poor.[8] However, for infants with unilateral and relatively small lesions a substantial number of infants may be normal at follow-up.[9]

5. a. This is a cranial ultrasound scan, coronal view. It shows midline shift, with complete obliteration of the right lateral ventricle with marked echodensity through much of the hemisphere. The left lateral ventricle can be seen but is displaced and distorted. There is pressure on the right side of the cavum of the septum pellucidum.

b. There has been an intraventricular haemorrhage in the right lateral ventricle with secondary haemorrhage into the parenchyma. It is difficult to say from the scan whether this is solely extensive haemorrhage but it is likely that there is venous infarction occurring as well as this is thought to be the major contributory factor for parenchymal involvement after intraventricular bleeding. Following the bleed on the lateral wall and floor of the ventricle, pressure is exerted on a venous plexus that drains the periventricular cerebral cortex. Ischaemia develops in this region resulting in haemorrhagic infarction.

  c. Outlook is difficult to define in the early period. The long-term outlook will be influenced by the size and position of the lesion, and the degree of cystic degeneration that results. Sources quoting neurodevelopmental outcome have widely differing estimates ranging from an incidence of significant neurological deficit from as low as 20% to in excess of 90%. There are also widely varying estimates of mortality with figures as high as 60% quoted. As the likely final extent of damage is uncertain early on, sequential scans are essential.

6. a. This is a parasagittal view of a cranial ultrasound showing the lateral ventricle. It shows an area of echo density in the floor of the lateral ventricle. The diagnosis is a subependymal haemorrhage or germinal matrix haemorrhage. There is no intraventricular haemorrhage seen. Using a grading system, this is a grade I GMH-IVH.

  b. Previously it was thought that babies with a subependymal haemorrhage would have no long-term complications. However, a recent study looking at infants with grade I and II intraventricular haemorrhages, i.e. germinal matrix bleeds with or without blood in the ventricles with no dilatation or parenchymal involvements, has demonstrated an increased risk of neurodevelopmental problems. When compared with infants with normal cranial ultrasounds, those with grade I–II IVH at 20 months corrected age had a significantly lower mean Mental Development Index (MDI) score than infants with a normal scan (74 ± 16 compared to 79 ± 14, $p = 0.006$). They were more likely to have an MDI < 70 (45% compared to 25%; OR, 2.00; 95% CI, 1.20–3.30; $p = 0.008$), major neurological abnormality (13% compared to 5%; OR, 2.60; 95% CI, 1.06–6.36; $p = 0.036$), and neurodevelopmental impairment (47% v 28%; OR, 1.83; 95% CI, 1.11–3.03; $p = 0.018$) at 20 months corrected age, even when adjusting for confounding factors. Advanced imaging such as MRI may give further information about other injuries that are associated with grade I–II IVH, which could explain these outcomes.[10] It is important to appreciate that this implies an association between these grades of IVH and an abnormal outcome but does not demonstrate causation.

7. a. This is a normal cranial ultrasound scan.

  b. It is likely, but by no means certain, that this baby will do well in the long term. Severe abnormalities on cranial scans are important predictors of cerebral palsy and mental retardation, and a normal head scan commonly implies the absence of major impairment. However, a recent study followed infants with normal head scans and showed that up to 30% of ELBW infants had either cerebral palsy or a low score on the mental development index. Risk factors associated with this high rate of adverse outcome included pneumothorax, prolonged exposure to mechanical ventilation, and educational and economic disadvantage. The authors suggest that improvements in neonatal care to reduce duration of ventilation and avoidance of pneumothoraces might improve neurodevelopmental outcome for ELBW infants.[11] When counselling parents about a normal head scan, it is important to emphasise that all premature babies will need long-term follow-up to assess growth and neurodevelopment.

8. a. This is an MRI scan of an infant's head and neck. There is a large lesion at the back of the skull, with protrusion of cerebral and meningeal tissue into the sac.

b. This infant has an occipital encephalocele, a congenital defect of the skull which has allowed herniation of brain tissue into the sac. A cerebral meningocele only contains meninges and CSF. The lesion shown above clearly contains brain as well, thus is an encephalocele; 75% of encephaloceles are occipital (as in this case), the other 25% are frontal.

c. Encephaloceles are seen in a variety of chromosomal disorders – trisomy 13 and 18 in particular and also with deletions of 13q and 16q. They can be seen in several syndromes such as Meckel–Gruber (polycystic kidneys, polydactyly, cleft lip and palate), Dandy–Walker (hydrocephalus, absence of cerebellar vermis, cranial nerve palsies), Joubert (cerebellar vermian aplasia, ataxia, coloboma, and renal cysts) and others.

d. Severe intellectual and motor deficits are seen with microcephaly. There is also weakness and spasticity. Intellectual impairment is seen more often in posterior encephaloceles. The long-term outlook depends on presence of brain tissue in the sac, development of hydrocephalus, development of the brain (e.g. presence of microcephaly) and the presence of other brain malformations such as microgyria, optic pathway dysgenesis.[3]

9. a. This is a coronal midline view of a cranial ultrasound. It shows bilateral dilatation of the anterior and posterior horns of the lateral ventricles. The third ventricle is not clearly seen. The parenchyma of the brain looks normal.

b. This is most likely due to resolving haemorrhage in the ventricles. There is a blood clot on the wall of the right ventricle.

c. This baby needs regular follow-up scans to look for progressive dilatation of the ventricles. The scans should be carried out weekly, at a minimum, with a shorter time between scans if the dilatation is significant. The optimum way to assess this is to measure the ventricular index. This is the distance between the midline and the lateral border of the lateral ventricle in a coronal view in the plane of the 3rd ventricle. There is a chart of normal ranges.[12] The baby should be assessed clinically with regular head circumference measurements (plotted on growth charts) and assessment of the fontanelle and sutures. Serial assessment with scans is crucial as the clinical signs of hydrocephalus (rapid head growth, full fontanelle) do not appear for days, or even weeks, after the dilatation has started.

10. a. The scan is a sagittal view of a cranial ultrasound scan. It shows a uniformly dilated lateral ventricle. This scan would be consistent with post-haemorrhagic hydrocephalus.

   b. Continued monitoring is essential and if head circumference continues to increase progressively further from the 95th centile the only option that can be considered is the removal of some cerebrospinal fluid. The exact point at which this should be considered is uncertain and there is considerable variation between practitioners as to when they will start drainage. Repeated taps by insertion of a needle cannot be recommended and appears to be associated with a worse long-term prognosis thus leaving the options of insertion of a reservoir or shunt. Treatment with acetazolamide and furosemide has been associated with worse outcome and no benefit has been demonstrated following a DRIFT procedure (drainage, irrigation and fibrinolytic therapy).[13]

11. a. This is a cranial USS showing a coronal section, in the midline. There is mild asymmetry of the lateral ventricles, which are widely separated and of abnormal shape.

   b. This baby has agenesis of the corpus callosum (ACC).

   c. ACC can be an isolated abnormality, which usually means there is no obvious neurological abnormality. Its prevalence is therefore unknown in the general population as it may be asymptomatic. It can be associated with other abnormalities, and this may change the outcome, e.g. Chiari malformation and neuronal migration disorders. With other abnormalities, the prognosis is considered to be poor. Isolated ACC has a much more variable prognosis with some infants having normal neurodevelopment to others having severe neurological handicap. Infants with ACC require careful neurodevelopmental follow-up. Infants with this finding on USS warrant an MRI to look for other abnormalities.

12. a. This is an antenatal scan of a fetus.

   b. It shows a cross section of the fetus and the chest. The rib ends are clearly visible, as is the heart. The most striking abnormalities are the growths on the outer chest wall which can be seen bilaterally. From the ultrasound it is difficult to say what the masses are. Doppler would be useful to see if these are haemangiomas.

   c. Serial antenatal scans would be needed to assess the rate of growth of the masses. Depending on the size, mode of delivery may be affected. Detailed postnatal examination would be necessary plus imaging, initially ultrasound followed by CT or MRI for more detail and involvement of underlying structures.

13. a. This a parasagittal view of a cranial ultrasound. The obvious abnormality is a cystic lesion in the floor of the lateral ventricle, known as a subependymal cyst.

   b. This occurs as a germinal matrix haemorrhage resolves and is replaced by a cavity. The bright white line above the cyst, which can extend around the whole of the ventricle, is due to haemosiderin-laden macrophages. These post-haemorrhagic cystic lesions are most commonly detected at the caudothalamic notch. They are often tear-shaped and measure 2–11 mm in size.[14]

c. Generally, infants with subependymal cysts have no long-term sequelae. However, these have occurred after a germinal haemorrhage and therefore there does appear to be an increased risk of long-term sequelae as discussed in detail in the answers to question **6**.

14. a. There is an equal and symmetrical signal within the posterior limb of the internal capsule (PLIC), and there is asymmetry of signal in the basal ganglia. There is also some mild cortical highlighting.

b. This infant has suffered an episode of perinatal asphyxia. The usual pattern seen on an MRI scan with perinatal asphyxia is loss of the normal signal intensity with the PLIC. Abnormalities within the basal ganglia and thalami, and cortical highlighting are also seen following asphyxial episodes. The prevalence of changes in the basal ganglia and thalami are thought to be due to the high metabolic rate in this region due to myelination.

15. a. This is a renal ultrasound scan. It shows a large hyperechogenic kidney. As a rule of thumb the kidney measurements should be the number of gestation weeks in millimetres. There are areas of different echogenicity, with loss of the normal intrarenal architecture. The kidney contains multiple tiny cysts measuring 1–2 mm each, giving the 'bright' appearance.

b. The likely diagnosis is autosomal recessive polycystic kidney disease (ARPCKD). Multi-cystic dysplastic kidneys have a different appearance with the classical appearance of numerous cysts resembling a bunch of grapes with no normal renal parenchyma seen.

c. Severe early problems for these babies may develop due to pulmonary hypoplasia because of inadequate liquor volume in utero. Antenatal scans can show enlarged hyperechoic kidneys from 14 weeks gestation, along with oligohydramnios and an empty bladder. Infants may require prolonged periods of ventilation which can be difficult. If infants survive the acute neonatal period, then up to 33% will develop end-stage renal failure in childhood, necessitating dialysis and eventual renal replacement.

d. ARPCKD is associated with hepatic duct ectasia, cysts and peripheral fibrosis. A gene locus on 6p21 has now been found.

16. a. This is a sagittal section of a head ultrasound scan. It shows a small cyst at the front of the lateral ventricle.

b. The most likely diagnosis is a connatal cyst. Synonyms for connatal cysts are coarctation of the lateral ventricles and frontal horn cysts. Connatal cysts are located at or just below the superolateral angles of the frontal horns or body of the lateral ventricles and are mainly anterior to the foramina of Monro. They can be hard to differentiate from subependymal cysts that are located below the external angle and posterior to the foramen of Monro. They represent a normal variant due to approximation of the walls of the frontal horns of the lateral ventricles proximal to their external angles. When the ventricular walls are close enough to touch each other, the most external portion of the ventricle acquires a round shape which on ultrasound appears to be a cyst.[15]

c. Connatal cysts have a reported incidence of 0.7% in low birth weight preterm infants and are thought to be benign. These cysts have been reported to resolve in follow-up studies.[16]

17. a. There are large intraventricular haemorrhages in both lateral ventricles. The temporal horns of the ventricles are distended. There is extension of the clot into the frontal horns, especially on the left. There is also an area in the left periventricular region which is suspicious of a venous infarct.

b. The lateral ventricle still contains some blood and there is now dilatation of the frontal horns. There are bilateral parenchymal echodensities lying posteriorly around the temporal horns, consistent with venous infarction. One paper described this pattern of infarction, however only with unilateral lesions and associated with mild to moderate intraventricular haemorrhage. The survivors did not have a uniform type of cerebral palsy but had a lower Bayley Mental Development Index. Some developed temporal lobe epilepsy.[17] The infant in the case above obviously has bilateral large intraventricular haemorrhages associated with bilateral venous infarcts. This is an unusual lesion and data regarding long-term prognosis is sparse.

18. a. This MRI scan shows agenesis of the corpus callosum. The lateral ventricles are abnormal and crescentic in shape. They are shifted laterally resulting in the formation of a large midline interhemispheric subarachnoid space. The abnormal shape is due to deformation by fibres of the cerebral hemisphere that were meant to cross in the corpus callosum, but due to the agenesis, run longitudinally as the bundles of Probst.

b. Agenesis of the corpus callosum can be an isolated finding but can be associated with other structural brain anomalies. It is seen in Aicardi, Apert's, Smith–Lemli–Opitz, Goldenhaar, Fryns', Meckel–Gruber, Zellweger's and Walker–Warburg syndromes. It is also seen with inborn errors of metabolism and in fetal alcohol syndrome. It is therefore important not only to look for other anomalies on the MRI scan, but to look at the infant for anomalies in other systems.

c. Agenesis of the corpus callosum involves a spectrum of abnormalities including abnormalities in the pericallosal nervous tissue. It is thus difficult to give the parents a definitive idea of long-term outlook as the wide range of abnormalities will also imply a wide spectrum of intelligence and of associated neurodevelopmental problems. Normal intelligence is not unusual, but severe compromise may be present, especially if other abnormalities are present.

19. a. The scan shows a congenital diaphragmatic hernia. The heart is visible in the chest and there are loops of bowel present at the same level.

b. An experienced neonatal team should attend the delivery of an infant with a know CDH. Affected babies should be delivered in a tertiary centre where paediatric surgery is accessible. Rapid intubation with gentle ventilation is recommended, with permissive hypercapnia. The lungs are frequently hypoplastic and pneumothoraces are common. It is known that infants with CDH are surfactant deficient and some reports have shown that exogenous surfactant could be beneficial. More recent papers have shown that in term infants the use of surfactant leads to higher ECMO use, more chronic lung disease and lower survival rates.[18] The use of nitric oxide as a pulmonary vasodilator has also been used in the treatment of infants with CDH. It can cause a rapid improvement in oxygenation but the effect is usually transient. It has been not shown to improve survival[19] but there are varying reports on whether it decreases the need for ECMO.[19,20] A Cochrane review in 2001 found no clear data to support use in infants with CDH.[21] There are however cases where a trial of nitric oxide is warranted.

  c. It is extremely difficult to accurately predict the chance of survival in these infants. The first paper to describe survival in a surgical series was in 1946 with 100% survival.[22] Clearly it depends on whether the infant is stable enough to be operated on. There are a group of infants who are difficult to ventilate from birth due to severe pulmonary hypoplasia and die within the first few days without surgery. If infants are operated on, their survival increases up to 75% in some series.[23] Left-sided defects are more common and have a better outcome than right-sided defects. Late presenting defects have a better prognosis due to less lung hypoplasia and pulmonary hypertension.

20. a. The scan shows dilatation of the pelvis (prominent echo-poor component) surrounded by normal renal cortex. This is consistent with hydronephrosis. Both kidneys are visible in this scan, one of top of the other. The upper kidney is the abnormal one. The lower kidney is difficult to assess in this view; however the renal pelvis does appear prominent.

  b. Approximately 1% of fetuses present some dilatation of their urinary tract in utero.[24] The significance of mild antenatally detected hydronephrosis remains controversial. Further investigations are warranted if scans show a progressive enlargement or the anteroposterior diameter is >10 mm, as this is more likely to be associated with pathology. Studies have show that mild dilatation (4–10 mm) progresses to hydronephrosis (>10 mm) in approximately a quarter of cases,[25] and other groups have shown that it can be associated with vesicoureteral reflux.[26] This infant should have a postnatal scan to assess the degree of dilatation, and if the dilatation is progressive, should be commenced on prophylactic antibiotics and a micturating cystogram performed to look for obstruction in the urinary tract.[27]

21. a. This antenatal scan shows an abdominal wall defect. It is an exomphalos because of its covering of omphaloperitoneal membrane, and its relationship to the umbilical cord. The dark area within the fetal abdomen could represent a displaced stomach, or dilated bowel. The mass (with the markers on) is the exomphalos. The mass is within the base of the umbilical cord which can be seen continuing from it on the right of the image.

  b. Exomphalos is a spectrum of anomalies ranging from a small defect with gut herniating into the cord to a large defect (exomphalos major), where bowel and liver are enclosed in the sac. It is frequently associated with other anomalies and echocardiography, karyotyping, and in some cases contrast studies should therefore be performed to assess gut rotation. It can be associated with other midline defects including involvement of diaphragm, heart and bladder.

   c. 30% of cases of exomphalos are associated with chromosomal abnormalities, particularly trisomy 13 and 18, and less so 21,[28] and there is a higher rate of chromosomal abnormalities in smaller defects that do not include the liver.[29] More than half of infants with exomphalos have other malformations, with cardiac defect being the most common.[30] There is also an association with neural tube defects.[31] The most well recognised association is with Beckwith–Wiedemann syndrome (omphalocele, macroglossia and hyperinsulinism).

22. a. This is a CT scan.

   b. The interhemispheric fissure is deviated to the left. There is an area of high attenuation along both leaves of the tentorium cerebelli which is more pronounced on the right. There appears to be a widening of the extra-axial space on the right with a density compatible with the presence of blood. Although a ventricular space can be seen on the left none is visible on the right. This could be due to a degree of swelling of the right side of the brain causing both midline deviation and ventricular compression. These findings are consistent with a subdural haematoma on the right side.

   c. In the most severe forms outlook is poor with neurological abnormalities in approximately half at follow-up. This is presumably due to related cerebral injury. In less severe forms the majority do well.

23. a. It is a T2 scan. Following application of a magnetic field, the time required for a certain percentage of the tissue's nuclei to realign is termed 'Time 1' or T1, which is typically about 1 second. T2 imaging employs a spin echo technique, in which spins are refocused to compensate for local magnetic field inhomogeneities. In practical terms this has a major effect on the appearance of the scans. In T1 weighting white matter appears white and grey matter grey while CSF appears black. In T2 imaging this is reversed with CSF appearing white.

   b. The scan shows severe hydrocephalus with very marked reduction of the cortical mantle. The inter-ventricular septum is absent. Although cranial ultrasound is an ideal way to measure ventricular dilatation, more detailed imaging with MRI is usually carried out prior to shunt insertion. The diagnosis in this case is Dandy–Walker malformation. This is associated with severe hydrocephalus, as seen in this scan.

24. a. This is a CT scan of the brain. The striking abnormalities are ventriculomegaly and the areas of brightness (same as bone) in the periventricular regions due to calcification.

   b. This scan is consistent with congenital cytomegalovirus.

   c. Urine should be sent for CMV detection by PCR, and blood for serology for CMV IgM. This has a sensitivity of approximately 70%.

For further information on CMV see Chapter 10, questions **1** and **2**.

25. a. The two abnormalities seen on the scan are marked asymmetry of the cortex, with one hemisphere being much smaller than the other and with asymmetry of the lateral ventricles.

   b. This is likely to be secondary to a middle cerebral artery infarct in the neonatal period and the scan shows the long-standing deficit.

26. a. There is a large mass at the back of the skull which seems to be separate from the brain contents. The brain looks relatively normal and the mass seems to be full of vessels and covered with skin.

   b. It is difficult to say from the scan what the diagnosis is, but the most likely is an arterio-venous malformation (as was the case here) as no extension of brain tissue into the sac is visible.

27. This is a coronal view of a cranial scan. There is extensive haemorrhage seen on the right with complete obliteration of the right ventricle. There is deviation of the midline with the left ventricle pushed to the far left of the image. This baby has suffered a large intraventricular bleed with parenchymal extension. There are three clinical syndromes described by Volpe.[4] This baby has had a catastrophic deterioration, presenting with pallor, acidosis and a change in ventilation. Other signs can be a fall in blood pressure or feed intolerance. If these changes occur along with a drop in haematocrit, a full fontanelle or seizures, a GMH-IVH is likely to have occurred as in this case. The saltatory syndrome is more common and more gradual in onset. This generally presents with a change in type of movements and seizures can occur. Most GMH-IVH however are asymptomatic – in fact up to 50% have no obvious clinical signs.

REFERENCES

1. Rennie JM. Neonatal cerebral ultrasound. Cambridge University Press, Cambridge, 1997
2. Rutherford M. MRI of the neonatal brain. WB Saunders, Oxford, 2001
3. Levene MI, Chervenak FA, Whittle M (eds). Fetal and neonatal neurology and neurosurgery, 3rd edn. Churchill Livingstone, Edinburgh, 2001
4. Volpe JJ. Neurology of the newborn. WB Saunders, Oxford, 2001
5. Sreenan C, Bhargava R, Robertson CM. Cerebral infarction in the term newborn: clinical presentation and long-term outcome. J Pediatr 2000;137(3):351–55
6. Estan J, Hope P. Unilateral neonatal cerebral infarction in full term infants. Arch Dis Child Fetal Neonatal Ed 1997;76(2):F88–F93
7. Mercuri E, Rutherford M, Cowan F et al. Early prognostic indicators of outcome in infants with neonatal cerebral infarction: a clinical, electroencephalogram, and magnetic resonance imaging study. Pediatrics 1999;103(1):39–46
8. Guzzetta F, Shackelford GD, Volpe S et al. Periventricular intraparenchymal echodensities in the premature newborn: critical determinants of neurologic outcome. Pediatrics 1986;78:995–1006
9. de Vries LS, Roelants-van Rijn AM, Rademaker KJ et al. Unilateral parenchymal haemorrhagic infarction in the preterm infant. Eur J Paediatr Neurol 2001;5:139–49
10. Patra K, Wilson-Costello D, Taylor HG et al. Grades I–II intraventricular hemorrhage in extremely low birth weight infants: effects on neurodevelopment. J Pediatr 2006;149(2):169–73
11. Laptook AR, O'Shea TM, Shankaran S, Bhaskar B. NICHD Neonatal network. Adverse neurodevelopmental outcomes among extremely low birth weight infants with a normal head ultrasound: prevalence and antecedents. Pediatrics 2005;115(3):673–80
12. Levene MI. Measurement of the growth of the lateral ventricles in preterm infants with real-time ultrasound. Arch Dis Child 1981;56(12):900–904

13. Whitelaw A, Evans D, Carter M et al. Randomised clinical trial of prevention of hydrocephalus after intraventricular hemorrhage in preterm infants: brain-washing versus tapping fluid. Pediatrics 2007;119:e1071–e1078

14. Larcos G, Gruenewald SM, Lui K. Neonatal sub-ependymal cysts detected by sonography: prevalence, sonographic findings, and clinical significance. Am J Roentgenol 1994;162:953–56

15. Rosenfeld DL, Schonfeld SM, Underberg-Davis S. Coarctation of the lateral ventricles: an alternative explanation for subependymal pseudocysts. Pediatr Radiol 1997;27:895–97

16. Pal BR, Preston PR, Morgan ME et al. Frontal horn thin walled cysts in preterm neonates are benign. Arch Dis Child Fetal Neonatal Ed 2001;85:F187–F193

17. Govaert P, Smets K, Matthys E et al. Neonatal focal temporal lobe or atrial wall haemorrhagic infarction. Arch Dis Child Fetal Neonatal Ed 1999;81(3):F211–F216

18. Van Meurs K. Congenital Diaphragmatic Hernia Study Group. Is surfactant therapy beneficial in the treatment of the term newborn infant with congenital diaphragmatic hernia? J Pediatr 2004;145(3):312–16

19. Neonatal Inhaled Nitric Oxide Study Group (NINOS). Inhaled nitric oxide and hypoxic respiratory failure in infants with congenital diaphragmatic hernia. Pediatrics 1997;99(6):838–45

20. Neonatal Inhaled Nitric Oxide Study Group (NINOS). Inhaled nitric oxide in term and near-term infants: neurodevelopmental follow-up of the neonatal inhaled nitric oxide study group. J Pediatr 2000;136(5):611–17

21. Finer NN, Barrington KJ. Nitric oxide for respiratory failure in infants born at or near term. Cochrane Database Syst Rev 2001;(2):CD000399

22. Gross RE. Congenital hernia of the diaphragm. Am J Dis Child 1946;71:580–92

23. Boloker J, Bateman DA, Wung JT et al. Congenital diaphragmatic hernia in 120 infants treated consecutively with permissive hypercapnea/spontaneous respiration/elective repair. J Pediatr Surg 2002;37(3):357–66

24. Cachat F, Ramseyer P, Meyrat BJ et al. Antenatally detected hydronephrosis: practical approach for the pediatrician. Rev Med Suisse 2005;1(7):505–6, 509–12

25. Persutte WH, Koyle M, Lenke RR et al. Mild pyelectasis ascertained with prenatal ultrasonography is pediatrically significant. Ultrasound Obstet Gynecol 1997;10(1):12–18

26. Gloor JM, Ramsey PS, Ogburn PL et al. The association of isolated mild fetal hydronephrosis with postnatal vesicoureteral reflux. J Matern Fetal Neonatal Med 2002;12(3):196–200

27. John U, Kähler C, Schulz S et al. The impact of fetal renal pelvic diameter on postnatal outcome. Prenat Diagn 2004;24(8):591–95

28. Reddy VN, Aughton DJ, DeWitte DB et al. Down syndrome and omphalocele: an under recognized association. Pediatrics 1994;93(3):514–15

29. Benacerraf BR, Saltzman DH, Estroff JA et al. Abnormal karyotype of fetuses with omphalocele: prediction based on omphalocele contents. Obstet Gynecol 1990;75:317–19

30. Hughes MD, Nyberg DA, Mack LA et al. Fetal omphalocele: prenatal US detection of concurrent anomalies and other predictors of outcome. Radiology 1989;173:371–76

31. Calzolari E, Bianchi F, Dolk H et al. Omphalocele and gastroschisis in Europe: a survey of 3 million births 1980–1990. EUROCAT Working Group. Am J Med Genet 1995;28(58):187–94

Chapter 9

Feeds and growth

Feeding and adequate growth are vital to both the preterm and term infant. After birth, the infant undergoes many changes, not only in gut structure but also in gut function and metabolism. Premature infants are slow to establish effective peristalsis and suck and swallow reflexes may be some weeks or even months before becoming strong enough to allow full oral feeding. An infant who has required prolonged ventilation may become orally defensive and in the worst cases may not tolerate any oral feeding and require long-term nasogastric tube feeding. In addition the preterm gastrointestinal tract appears to be particularly vulnerable to ischaemic damage, and necrotising enterocolitis may occur in up to 8% of neonatal admissions.[1] It is not surprising that studies have documented a degree of postnatal growth failure in the majority of infants born prematurely. For those born extremely prematurely growth failure may be prolonged and severe and final stature may be affected.

It is now clear that nutrition and growth, both as a fetus and in the early weeks of postnatal life, may have major implications on long-term health. The concept of programming suggests that cardiovascular and cerebrovascular disease as well as insulin resistance and diabetes may have an early origin in some individuals and there is a small amount of evidence to suggest that premature infants may be more vulnerable to this early programming than are other, more mature infants. Infants who are born small for gestational age are at risk of developing later risk factors for cardiovascular disease, such as high blood pressure. Promotion of postnatal growth was thought to ameliorate these effects, but there is now evidence in human infants and other animals born prematurely that promotion of growth by increased postnatal nutrition increases later cardiovascular risk. It would therefore seem crucial that while preterm and small for gestation age infants should be fed appropriately, they should not be 'over fed' in the neonatal period.[2]

Once enteral feeding has been established, the most common problem seen on a day-to-day basis is gastro-oesophageal reflux. A recent paper documented that 25% of all extremely low birth weight (<1 kg) infants are discharged home from the neonatal unit on treatment for reflux.[3] The diagnosis and management of reflux remains a subject of considerable debate with a relative lack of strong consistent evidence.

This chapter aims to cover the common problems described above as well as other topics such as nutritional supplementation.

QUESTION 1

i) A baby is reviewed in clinic and his mother describes episodes of vomiting post feeds and says that he seems uncomfortable. She has tried positioning the baby after feeds but feels this has not made any difference. A friend has said that her baby has gastro-oesophageal reflux and she has been extensively reviewing this subject on the internet. She would like you to discuss the pros and cons of the following investigations for GOR.

    a. pH probe
    b. Oesophageal manometry
    c. Oesophageal impedance
    d. Fluoroscopy
    e. Endoscopy
    f. Chiropractice
    g. Empiric therapy.

ii) Mother elects to have empiric treatment. Which of the following treatments would you suggest?

    a. Cisapride
    b. Gaviscon
    c. Gripe water
    d. Antacids
    e. Thickeners
    f. Hydrolysed formula milk
    g. Erythromycin
    h. Ranitidine
    i. Metoclopramide
    j. Omeprazole
    k. Domperidone
    l. Buscopan (hyoscine butylbromide)
    m. Coleif
    n. Infacol.

QUESTION 2

Match the following milks and ingredients/uses

Infatrini	Milk protein, soy and lactose free
Nutramigen	Gluten free
Neocate	Gluten, sucrose and lactose free
Infasoy	Disaccharide/whole protein intolerance with medium-chain triglycerides
Peptijunior	Lactose intolerance, galactosaemia

QUESTION 3

Which of the following statements about iron and its supplementation are correct?

i) Maternal iron deficiency affects 30–50% of pregnancies

ii) Maternal iron deficiency anaemia is associated with an increased risk of preterm delivery

iii) Maternal smoking can cause perinatal iron deficiency

iv) Maternal diabetes can cause perinatal iron deficiency

v) Iron supplementation prevents early anaemia

vi) Can lead to an increased risk of infection

vii) Should be given at the same time as calcium and phosphorus supplements

viii) Can be started safely at about 4–6 weeks of life

ix) Is only needed in infants fed formula milk

x) Supplements should be started immediately after birth

xi) Iron deficiency can lead to problems with neurodevelopment which are reversed once treatment is started.

QUESTION 4

Which of the following are risk factors for NEC?

i) Early feeds

ii) Indomethacin

iii) Blood transfusion

iv) Fortified feeds

v) Thickened feeds

vi) H2 receptor antagonists.

QUESTION 5

Which of the following statements concerning feeds and feed supplements are correct?

i) All preterm formula fed infants should receive folic acid

ii) Infants with haemolytic anaemia should always receive folate supplementation

iii) Human milk contains sufficient vitamin A for the preterm infant

iv) Vitamin A supplementation is associated with a reduction in the incidence of chronic lung disease

v) All preterm infants should receive a minimum of 1000 IU vitamin D a day to prevent rickets

vi) Vitamin supplementation should be increased in hepatic failure

vii) Rickets can be prevented by adequate vitamin D supplementation

viii) Increasing calcium intake is usually helpful when there is evidence of poor bone mineralisation

ix) Nucleotide supplementation of formula milk may enhance growth in preterm infants

x) Human milk does not contain nucleotides

xi) Beta-carotene supplementation is of proven benefit in preterm babies

xii) Vitamin E supplementation is essential in infants receiving human milk

xiii) Vitamin E supplementation is useful in the prevention of haemolytic anaemia, ROP, BPD and IVH

xiv) Vitamin C levels in preterm infants are normally satisfactory and supplementation is not recommended

xv) The vitamin content of breast milk is affected by maternal diet.

QUESTION 6

You have admitted a baby to the neonatal unit who is 30 weeks gestation. The baby requires no respiratory support and her blood glucose is stable. The mother wants to breast feed and the practice on your unit is to give bolus feeds.

The mother wants to know why the baby cannot be fed continuously as she has heard about necrotising enterocolitis and is worried her baby may develop it if the baby is fed by bolus feeds. What do you tell her?

QUESTION 7

You review a 4-month-old baby in clinic who you have been treating for reflux with thickened feeds and erythromycin. The mother has been researching on the internet and thinks her child may actually be allergic to cows' milk but then talks about protein intolerance.

i) Is this a plausible explanation for the symptoms?

ii) How do you explain the difference between CMA and CMPI?

iii) What is the prognosis for both conditions?

The mother wants her baby tested for cows' milk allergy.

iv) What investigations do you carry out?

She wants to try soy milk as alternative milk. She has heard that it is good for the regurgitation and crying that her baby suffers with.

v) What do you tell her?

vi) Do you alter your treatment of the baby? If so, what do you do?

QUESTION 8

Which of the following are true?

i) Long-chain polyunsaturated fatty acids improve retinal sensitivity in preterm infants

ii) LCPUFA enriched formula milk can decrease the incidence of bronchopulmonary dysplasia

iii) LCPUFA enriched formula milk leads to a decrease in the incidence of sepsis

iv) A protein intake of above 3 g/kg/day is needed to support the same rate of growth as in utero for a preterm baby

v) Amino acids in total parenteral nutrition should be started on day 3 after renal function has improved to prevent elevation in blood urea nitrogen (BUN)

vi) The addition of glutamine improves feeding tolerance in ELBW infants

vii) The addition of glutamine may decrease the incidence of infection in ELBW infants.

ANSWER 1

i) a. pH probe study. This is a simple bedside test that gives reproducible data. Oesophagitis may be predictable and comparative data may be produced. However acid reflux only will be detected and there is evidence that up to 90% of GOR is due to milk or gas and is not acid. Normal values have only been established for term infants and cannot be applied to preterm infants. Furthermore the upper limit of acceptable reflux index (12%) is substantially higher than that regarded as acceptable in adults or older children (6%). Studies have shown poor correlation between pH probe reflux and symptoms. Infants should not be receiving antacids, H2 antagonists or proton pump inhibitors.

  b. Oesophageal manometry. Allows assessment of motility and an understanding of the pathophysiology of GOR and of sphincter function. This tends to be used only in specialist centres as both operation and evaluation of results are complex. There is no role for this method in normal practice.

  c. Oesophageal impedance. Allows detection of acid and non–acid events with an immediate result (in comparison to the delay with pH probe). Normal values are not available in either preterm or term infants and analysis is time consuming. As with pH probes there is poor correlation between episodes of reflux and symptoms. The predictive value for different treatments is not established.

  d. Fluoroscopy. Allows visualisation of sucking and swallowing activity, structural anatomy and brief episodes of reflux. Studies are of short duration and episodes of reflux may be seen in normal and asymptomatic infants. It should not be used to evaluate the severity of reflux but has a role in the exclusion of other problems that may mimic reflux.

  e. Endoscopy. Permits visualisation of areas of oesophagitis and biopsy if necessary. Requires considerable expertise particularly if biopsy is considered and especially in a preterm baby. An infant will require heavy sedation or anaesthesia.

  f. Chiropractice. This has been recommended by several groups although evidence is lacking to support this therapy in this condition.

  g. Empiric treatment. The commonest means of assessment. Not associated with the risk of other investigations but does carry a risk as does use of any medication. Effect is difficult to evaluate as a large placebo effect is associated with use of any medication in a condition associated with parental anxiety. Appropriate doses and associated risks are not clearly defined.

  ii) There is a lack of evidence of efficacy and safety for all medications and none can be recommended routinely in the absence of evidence to suggest that

GOR is the cause of symptoms. As several studies have failed to demonstrate such an association an argument could be made that none of these agents are appropriate. There are, however, specific considerations with some of these agents.

a. Cisapride. Prokinetic agent without central anti-dopamine effects which directly stimulate the myenteric plexus. In infants born under 36 weeks gestation, cisapride should not be used for up to 3 months, due to the risk of Q–T interval prolongation in this age group.

b. Gaviscon. A compound alginate preparation that forms a raft that floats on the surface of the stomach contents to reduce reflux. Contains sodium and magnesium alginate. Half sachet = 1 dose = 1mmol Na.

c. Gripe water. A variety of products are marketed as 'gripe water' and all contain different ingredients – ginger, fennel, essential oils, peppermint, chamomile, caraway, aloe, lemon balm and activated charcoal just to name a few. All claim to bring immediate relief and many claim to be recommended by health care professionals. Supportive evidence is missing.

d. Antacids. Should not be used due to complications such as constipation (calcium- and aluminium-containing antacids), diarrhoea (magnesium-containing antacids), and metabolic bone disease (aluminium-containing antacids which bind to phosphate).

e. Thickeners. The number of reflux episodes may be decreased in term infants by adding a thickener to the milk to increase viscosity. In preterm babies or babies who are sick, thickened milk may lead to difficulties with sucking or swallowing. In these cases, simply increasing the concentration of the feed slightly may lead to less gastric distension, which in turn would decrease the likelihood of reflux, while maintaining calorie intake.

f. Hydrolysed formula. There is evidence that cows' milk allergy can be indistinguishable from gastro-oesophageal reflux. Therefore, a trial of a hydrolysed formula (partially hydrolysed feed also known as semi-elemental, e.g. Nutramigen) may be beneficial in a baby who is showing symptoms of reflux and irritability. Improvement is usually seen within 1 week of changing the milk.

g. Erythromycin. This is used for its pro-kinetic effects but has no effect on oesophageal motility or on the lower oesophageal sphincter. May improve gastro-duodenal contractility in babies older than 33 weeks. Randomised controlled trials have not confirmed efficacy. It has been associated with an increased incidence of hypertrophic pyloric stenosis.

h. Ranitidine. An H2 receptor antagonist that limits the interaction of histamine released from mast cells. There is a dose-dependent response in both preterm and term babies. If pH monitoring shows increased acid exposure leading to oesophagitis, then it would be reasonable to try ranitidine. However, use of ranitidine to treat airway symptoms, irritability or feeding intolerance lacks supportive data. Cimetidine should not be used in babies as it interacts with cytochrome P450 and reduces oxidative drug metabolism in the liver.

i. Metoclopramide. Dopamine antagonist with prokinetic effect upon the gut. It also enhances the strength of the oesophageal sphincter action. Lack of proven benefit and well recognised extra-pyramidal side effects including oculo-gyric crises mean use is not recommended.

j. Omeprazole. Proton-pump inhibitor with superior acid reducing effect when compared with the H2 receptor antagonists. Also metabolised by the cytochrome P450 pathway and there is a genetically determined defect in the pathway that impairs metabolism in some individuals. This may affect both efficacy of treatment and potential toxicity. Problems with reducing gastric acid production include promotion of bacterial overgrowth, increased risk of hypertrophic pyloric stenosis due to increased serum gastrin, and altered digestion due to decreased activity of acid-dependent lipases.

k. Domperidone. Also a dopamine antagonist, principally active in the gastrointestinal tract and prokinetic in the upper gut. It is less likely to cause extra-pyramidal side effects as it does not cross the blood–brain barrier. Efficacy not established.

l. Buscopan. Antimuscarinic that is primarily used for smooth muscle spasm in the gut. Should not be used in children or neonates as the risk of side effects is high.

m. Colief. Lactase – this theoretically reduces symptoms when lactose intolerance contributes to colic. Anecdotally may be highly effective in selected infants. No convincing experimental data.

n. Infacol. Simeticone (activated dimeticone) – which is a foaming agent and works in a similar way to Gaviscon, although evidence for benefit is uncertain.

ANSWER 2

Infatrini – gluten free

Nutramigen – gluten, sucrose and lactose free

Neocate – milk protein, soy and lactose free

Infasoy – lactose intolerance, galactosaemia

Peptijunior – disaccharide/whole protein intolerance with medium-chain triglycerides.

ANSWER 3

i) Yes[4] – it is the commonest cause of perinatal iron deficiency worldwide.

ii) Yes – iron deficiency anaemia, when detected early in pregnancy, is associated with a more than two-fold increase for the risk of preterm delivery.[4]

iii) Yes – maternal smoking can cause perinatal iron deficiency. Smoking leads to increased carbon monoxide and decreased utero-placental blood flow. This in turn leads to erythropoiesis which depletes the iron stores.[5]

iv) Yes – poorly controlled maternal diabetes can cause perinatal iron deficiency by increased fetal metabolic rate and oxygen consumption. The relative hypoxia again causes increased erythropoiesis and the additional iron required cannot be met by increasing maternal–fetal transport.[6]

v) No – does prevent late anaemia. Use of erythropoietin and iron can result in a better response to iron

vi) Yes – iron supplements have a high osmolality if given undiluted and if mixed with breast milk can cause disruption of anti-infective properties. Parenteral iron is more likely to do so.

vii) No – insoluble compounds may be formed which would decrease bioavailability.

viii) Yes – most preterm babies have received multiple blood transfusions while in the neonatal unit, and have thus received intravenous iron. They are likely to have extremely high ferritin levels and thus iron supplements can be delayed.

ix) No – human milk has inadequate supplies of iron and preterm infants fed human milk are more likely to suffer from iron deficiency.

x) No – it is generally recommended that iron supplements should not be given in the first 4 weeks after birth when enteral feeds have only just begun as it may be associated with an increased risk of gastrointestinal disturbance.

xi) No – iron deficiency between 6 months and 2 years can lead to long-term neurodevelopmental problems that are not reversed despite adequate treatment.[7] Iron is needed for neurotransmission, myelination and brain growth. Areas such as the hippocampus and striatum are particularly vulnerable to iron deficiency. Studies have shown both short- and long-term effects due to perinatal iron deficiency.[8]

ANSWER 4

i) Several studies have shown that it is safe to use small feeding volumes early in life, even in selected circumstances, such as feeding during the use of indomethacin to treat symptomatic patent ductus arteriosus. Prolonging small feeding volumes, sometimes called trophic feeding, has been shown to be associated with a marginally significant reduction in necrotising enterocolitis in very low birth weight infants. Cochrane Review concluded that, comparing trophic feeds with no enteral nutrient intake, there was no significant difference in necrotising enterocolitis, infants required more days to reach full enteral feeding and tended to have a longer hospital stay.[9–11]

ii) Patent ductus arteriosus is a risk factor for the development of necrotising enterocolitis. The use of indomethacin to treat patent ductus arteriosus in preterm infants may either decrease the incidence of necrotising enterocolitis by stabilising or closing the ductus arteriosus or increase its incidence by a direct constricting effect on mesenteric blood vessels. Although some small studies have suggested that indomethacin does increase the risk of NEC, recent papers have concluded that PDA is an independent risk factor for the development of necrotising enterocolitis in very low birth weight infants and therapy with indomethacin did not have a significant effect on the risk for necrotising enterocolitis.[12,13]

iii) While anecdotal reports suggest that NEC has developed quickly after a blood transfusion, this information is not reflected in published studies. However, neonatal exchange transfusion and intrauterine transfusion have been shown to be associated with an increased incidence of NEC. Blood transfusions may unmask latent NEC, and apnoeas and desaturations could potentially be an early symptom of NEC. It may be that the anaemia for which a blood transfusion is requested is an independent risk factor for NEC, or an early manifestation of NEC still developing, which then becomes recognised several hours later (during or after the transfusion). Some units omit feeds for the duration of a blood transfusion. There are several reports of blood transfusion causing acute haemolysis in babies with established NEC and red cell T antigen activation although the use of low anti-T titre plasma products has not been shown to reduce mortality and the current neonatal transfusion guidelines remain non-committal about the importance of T activation.

iv) Fortified feeds – many neonatal units are routinely using milk fortifier to enhance the nutrition and growth of preterm infants. It is thought that breast milk fortifier may increase the incidence of NEC stage I–III.[14]

Berseth et al[15] compared two human milk fortifiers, one with iron and one with without, showing that there was no difference in the incidence of sepsis and NEC. This refutes the premise that the inclusion of iron in fortifiers increases the incidence of sepsis and NEC.

v) Thickened feeds – although descriptive case reports have linked some feeding interventions such as thickened feedings to NEC, there is no evidence to establish a causal relation. There are however several anecdotal reports of infants being fed with thickened feeds and later developing NEC. The theory is that thickened feeds may have led to NEC as a result of bowel obstruction with subsequent bacterial overgrowth or following direct mucosal injury by calorifie dense milk.[16,17]

vi) A recent case-control study of NEC of Bell stage II or greater showed a higher incidence if treated with ranitidine. This may support the hypothesis that gastric pH level may be a factor in the pathogenesis of NEC.[18]

ANSWER 5

i) Although this remains common practice and is recommended in certain textbooks, the composition of current formula milk is sufficient for adequate supplementation. Human breast milk contains approximately twice the minimum folate supplementation in formula milk.

ii) Although this practice has been recommended, this is based upon old studies when folate levels in milk were almost certainly inadequate. Evidence to suggest that this practice should be continued is conflicting and the composition of current formula milk and breast milk is sufficient for adequate supplementation.

iii) Human milk does not supply enough vitamin A for the preterm infant and this situation is compounded by the fact that most preterm infants are born with low stores. Supplementation is recommended but the exact dose is uncertain.

iv) Systematic review has suggested that vitamin A supplementation may lead to a reduction in both supplementary oxygen requirements and death. Treatment regimes have involved intramuscular injection and the treatment has not gained widespread acceptance. Some studies have not shown evidence of benefit.

v) There is good evidence that supplementation of 400 IU vitamin D a day is adequate and higher doses are not required.

vi) Infants with liver failure should be on higher vitamin supplementations including vitamin K.

vii) Radiological rickets may be found in infants with normal vitamin D levels. Hypophosphataemia is now recognised as a more important contributory factor than vitamin D.

viii) Calcium supplementation may be beneficial if intake is poor, but is unlikely to be effective if intake is already adequate. High calcium intake may decrease fat absorption and can lead to calcium soap intestinal bolus obstruction.

ix) There is evidence that babies can utilise preformed nucleotides in supplemented formula milks and that utilisation increases at times of deficiency. Studies in term infants have shown improved growth and reduced gastrointestinal disturbance but this benefit has not been shown in preterm infants.

x) Breast milk contains at least 15 different nucleotides which represent a significant proportion of the non-protein nitrogen. It is for this reason that supplementation of formula feeds has been suggested.

xi) Beta-carotene supplementation of milk is now common. This is almost certainly because of an absence of carotenoids in formula milk which are present in human milk. Beta-carotene is only one of these. Although supplementation is now common, there is no clear information as to what it is supposed to do and currently no evidence of benefit from randomised controlled trials exists.

xii) Human milk contains adequate levels of vitamin E and there is no evidence that supplementation is of additional benefit.

xiii) Vitamin E supplementation may be useful in the prevention of haemolytic anaemia in preterm infants but there is no consistent advice on this. Although it has been suggested and given to prevent ROP, BPD and IVH, there is no evidence of benefit from randomised trials and supplementation with high doses has risks of potential toxicity. A Cochrane Review in 2003 concluded that vitamin E supplementation in preterm infants reduced the risk of IVH but increased the risk of sepsis including NEC. The evidence does not support the routine use of vitamin E supplementation by intravenous route at high doses.[19]

xiv) Vitamin C levels are usually low and supplementation is recommended. Standard multivitamin preparations contain vitamins A, B, C and D.

xv) Levels of water-soluble vitamins in breast milk are influence by dietary changes and breast feeding mothers should be encouraged to eat fruit and vegetables. Routine supplementation with proprietary vitamin preparations is not normally necessary for the mother.

ANSWER 6

Most premature infants are unable to suck effectively or co-ordinate sucking, swallowing and breathing. She must initially be fed by a nasogastric tube to give milk feeds. Milk can be given by tube either intermittently, typically over 10–20 minutes every hour, progressing up to every two or three hours, or continuously, using an infusion pump. Although theoretical benefits and risks of each method have been proposed, the effects on clinical outcomes are not certain. A Cochrane Review in 2003 summarised the differences in outcomes which were feeding tolerance, days to reach full enteral feeding, growth, length of stay and incidence of necrotising enterocolitis (NEC).[20]

It concluded that infants fed by continuous tube feeding took longer to reach full enteral feeds, but there was a slight trend towards earlier discharge. There was however no difference in weight gain or growth including length, head circumference and skin fold thickness. To reassure this mother, there was no difference in the incidence of NEC.

ANSWER 7

i) This is a plausible explanation. It is thought that up to half the cases of gastro-oesophageal reflux in infants under a year of age may be associated with cows' milk allergy. It is also thought that the reflux may be induced by the allergy.[21] The association has been well described by several groups, one quoting it in up to 42% of infants who previously had received a diagnosis of reflux.[22] The symptoms and age of presentation are similar in both conditions. One group treated a group of infants with reflux who had not responded to pharmacological treatment with a cows' milk free diet – 20% improved.[23] The overlapping symptoms include crying, irritability, vomiting, failure to thrive, apnoeas, ALTEs and colic. A recent paper has said that umbilical erythema can be a sign of food intolerance and a useful diagnostic tool for CMPI.[24]

ii) Many people use the terms cows' milk allergy (CMA) and cows' milk protein intolerance (CMPI) interchangeably. CMA is an immunologically mediated reaction to cows' milk proteins that can involve the gut, skin, respiratory tract, or cause systemic anaphylaxis. Prevalence is about 1–3%, being most common in infants. CMPI, however, should refer to a non-immunological reaction to cows' milk. The most common cause is lactase deficiency, which is mostly acquired during late childhood or adulthood. It has marked racial variation with lowest incidence in northern Europeans.

iii) The prognosis for true cows' milk allergy is worse than for CMPI. It can cause severe morbidity and even fatality if not recognised and treated. Dietary elimination is associated with good prognosis. CMPI, commonly due to a lactase deficiency, is generally a benign condition, with symptoms limited to the gastrointestinal tract.[25]

iv) There are no definitive investigations for cows' milk protein intolerance or allergy because in general the immunological basis of the involved mechanisms is commonly undetermined. Some tests, however, may reinforce clinical suspicions.

Cavataio et al found that IgG anti-beta-lactoglobulin assay was the most useful test for making a diagnosis of both gastro-oesophageal reflux and cows' milk allergy. The test was positive in 27/30 subjects with GER and CMA and in 4/42 patients with GER only.[26] Generally a diagnosis is made if there is resolution of symptoms with elimination.

v) Concerns have recently been raised regarding potential risks with soy protein. Most recent advice is to use soy protein formulae only in certain cases. They should not be used in preterm infants or infants with food allergy before the age of 6 months. Soy protein formulae can be used for feeding term infants, but they have no nutritional advantage over cows' milk protein formulae and contain high concentrations of phytate, aluminium and phytoestrogens (isoflavones), which may have side effects. There is no evidence supporting the use of soy protein formulae for the prevention or management of infantile colic, regurgitation, or prolonged crying.[27,28]

vi) As this baby is not responding to your usual treatment of reflux, it may well be worth trying a cows' milk free diet due to the overlap of symptoms in these conditions. The baby should be started on an extensively hydrolysed formula milk of which there are many on the market, such as Peptijunior, Nutramigen, Neocate or Progestamil. A 6–8-week course should be tried as a minimum for resolution of symptoms. These milks can also be thickened if regurgitation symptoms persist.

ANSWER 8

i) True – LCPUFA are concentrated at synapses within the retina and there is improved retinal sensitivity and visual acuity with LCPUFA added to formula milk.

ii) False – although one study did show that infants fed with an enriched formula had longer duration of ventilation,[29] there has been no difference shown in the rates of BPD in this group of babies compared to controls.[30]

iii) False – many trials have reported no difference in sepsis in babies fed with LCPUFA enriched formula milk.[29]

iv) True – the most commonly applied standard is that of intra-uterine growth. The protein accretion rate between 24 and 32 weeks' gestation is approximately 2 g/kg/day, and the estimated rate of obligate protein loss is 1.1–1.5 g/kg/day.

v) False – generally TPN and amino acid solutions are started later in the most sick and preterm infants who are in greatest need of nutrition. Concerns usually raised are problems with acid–base balance and an increase in BUN and ammonia levels. However, studies have shown that there is no difference in plasma levels of cholesterol, triglycerides, bicarbonate, blood urea nitrogen, creatinine and pH in infants with early TPN compared to late (after 48 hours).[31] In early life BUN reflects fluid status rather than amino acid intake.

vi) False – glutamine is one of the most abundant amino acids in plasma and in breast milk, but is unstable in aqueous solutions, hence generally not included in amino acid solutions. Glutamine depletion has negative effects on the functional integrity of the gut and leads to immunosuppression. Glutamine-enriched enteral nutrition does not improve feeding tolerance in VLBW infants.[32]

vii) True – studies in adults have shown that glutamine-supplemented amino acid solution decreased the incidence of infections. One study has suggested that the use of glutamine-enriched enteral nutrition in VLBW infants should be seriously considered.[32]

REFERENCES

1. Kosloske AM. Epidemiology of necrotising enterocolitis. Acta Paediatr Suppl 1994;396:2–7
2. Singhal A, Cole TJ, Fewtrell M et al. Promotion of faster weight gain in infants born small for gestational age: is there an adverse effect on later blood pressure? Circulation 2007;115(2):213–20
3. Malcolm W, Gantz M, Das A et al. Anti-reflux medications at NICU discharge for extremely low birthweight infants [abstract]. Presented at Annual Meeting of the Pediatric Academic Societies, San Francisco, April 2006
4. Scholl TO. Iron status during pregnancy: setting the stage for mother and infant. Am J Clin Nutr 2005;81(5):1218S–1222S
5. Sweet DG, Savage G, Tubman TR et al. Study of maternal influences on fetal iron status at term using cord blood transferrin receptors. Arch Dis Child Fetal Neonatal Ed 2001;84(1):F40–F43
6. Petry CD, Eaton MA, Wobken JD et al. Iron deficiency of liver, heart, and brain in newborn infants of diabetic mothers. J Pediatr 1992;121(1):109–14
7. Lozoff B, Georgieff MK. Iron deficiency and brain development. Semin Pediatr Neurol 2006;13(3):158–65
8. Armony-Sivan R, Eidelman AI, Lanir A et al. Iron status and neurobehavioral development of premature infants. J Perinatol 2004;24(12):757–62
9. Tyson JE, Kennedy KA. Trophic feedings for parenterally fed infants. Cochrane Database Syst Rev 2005;20(3)
10. Berseth CL, Bisquera JA, Paje VU. Prolonging small feeding volumes early in life decreases the incidence of necrotizing enterocolitis in very low birth weight infants. Pediatrics 2003;111:529–34
11. Berseth CL. Feeding strategies and necrotizing enterocolitis. Curr Opin Pediatr 2005;17(2):170–73
12. Dollberg S, Lusky A, Reichman B. Patent ductus arteriosus, indomethacin and necrotizing enterocolitis in very low birth weight infants: a population-based study. J Ped Gastroenterol Nutr 2005;40(2):184–88
13. O'Donovan D, Baetiong A, Adams K et al. Necrotizing enterocolitis and gastrointestinal complications after indomethacin therapy and surgical ligation in premature infants with patent ductus arteriosus. J Perinatol 2003;23.286–90
14. Hallstrom M, Koivisto AM, Janas M et al. Frequency of and risk factors for necrotizing enterocolitis in infants born before 33 weeks of gestation. Acta Paediatr 2003;92(1):111–13
15. Berseth CL, Van Aerde JE, Gross S et al. Growth, efficacy, and safety of feeding an iron-fortified human milk fortifier. Pediatrics 2004;114(6):e699–e706
16. Clarke P, Robinson MJ. Thickening milk feeds may cause necrotising enterocolitis. Arch Dis Child 2004;89:F280
17. Berseth CL. Feeding strategies and necrotizing enterocolitis. Curr Opin Pediatr 2005;17(2):170–73
18. Guillet R, Stoll BJ, Cotton CM et al. Association of H_2-blocker therapy and higher incidence of necrotizing enterocolitis in very low birth weight infants. Pediatrics 2006;117(2):e137–e142
19. Brion LP, Bell EF, Raghuveer TS. Vitamin E supplementation for prevention of morbidity and mortality in preterm infants. Cochrane Database Syst Rev 2003;(4)
20. Premji S, Chessell L. Continuous nasogastric milk feeding versus intermittent bolus milk feeding for premature infants less than 1500 grams. Cochrane Database Syst Rev 2003;(1)
21. Salvatore S, Vandenplas Y. Gastroesophageal reflux and cow milk allergy: is there a link? Pediatrics 2002;110(5):972–84
22. Iacono G, Carroccio A, Cavataio F et al. Gastroesophageal reflux and cow's milk allergy in infants: a prospective study. J Allergy Clin Immunol 1996;97(3):822–27
23. McLain BI, Cameron DJ, Barnes GL. Is cow's milk protein intolerance a cause of gastro-oesophageal reflux in infancy? J Paediatr Child Health 1994;30(4):316–18

24. Iacono G, Di Prima L, D'Amico D. The 'red umbilicus': a diagnostic sign of cow's milk protein intolerance. J Pediatr Gastroenterol Nutr 2006;42(5):531–34

25. Bahna SL. Cow's milk allergy versus cow milk intolerance. Ann Allergy Asthma Immunol 2002;89(6 Suppl 1):56–60

26. Cavataio F, Iacono G, Montalto G et al. Gastroesophageal reflux associated with cow's milk allergy in infants: which diagnostic examinations are useful? Am J Gastroenterol 1996;91(6):1215–20

27. ESPGHAN Committee on Nutrition. Agostoni C, Axelsson I, Goulet O et al. Soy protein infant formulae and follow-on formulae: a commentary by the ESPGHAN Committee on Nutrition. J Pediatr Gastroenterol Nutr 2006;42(4):352–61

28. Turck D. Soy protein for infant feeding: what do we know? Curr Opin Clin Nutr Metab Care 2007;10(3):360–65

29. Fewtrell MS, Abbott RA, Kennedy K. Randomized, double-blind trial of long-chain polyunsaturated fatty acid supplementation with fish oil and borage oil in preterm infants. J Pediatr 2004;144(4):471–79

30. Fewtrell MS, Morley R, Abbott RA et al. Double-blind, randomized trial of long-chain polyunsaturated fatty acid supplementation in formula fed to preterm infants. Pediatrics 2002;110(1 Pt 1): 73–82

31. Ibrahim HM, Jeroudi MA, Baier RJ et al. Aggressive early total parental nutrition in low-birth-weight infants. J Perinatol 2004;24(8):482–86

32. van den Berg A, van Elburg RM, Westerbeek EA et al. Glutamine-enriched enteral nutrition in very-low-birth-weight infants and effects on feeding tolerance and infectious morbidity: a randomized controlled trial. Am J Clin Nutr 2005;81:1397–404

Chapter 10

Infection

Infection remains an extremely important cause of both morbidity and mortality in the neonatal population. The fetus is extremely vulnerable to congenital infection while the newborn baby is susceptible to early and late onset sepsis. Nosocomial infection can affect a significant number of infants, particularly those who are sickest and most dependent.

Congenital infections with organisms that may have little effect on an adult or older child can have a devastating effect on the fetus and infant, resulting in profound long-term damage. The commonest cause of congenital infection is cytomegalovirus affecting 0.5–3% of live births worldwide. In very low birth weight infants who need prolonged intensive care, rates of culture-proven infection of up to 30% have been quoted, with mortality rates that are equally high. Neonatal units are busy and as they become busier both time and staffing constraints lead to an increase in nosocomial infections.

Questions in this chapter will cover different aspects of congenital infections, the presentation of sepsis, prevention of infection and other common situations such as contact with chickenpox on the neonatal unit.

QUESTION 1

Which of the following statements about cytomegalovirus (CMV) are correct (answer true or false)?

i) CMV is an RNA virus

ii) It is the most common intra-uterine infection

iii) Congenital CMV can be caused by maternal primary infection or reactivation and both are of the same severity

iv) The incidence of primary CMV infection acquired during pregnancy is 5–10%

v) Primary CMV infection is associated with a 40% risk of congenital CMV infection

vi) At least 50% of infected infants will show clinical signs at birth

vii) There is a 20% mortality associated with symptomatic congenital CMV

viii) Infants can become infected by breast feeding if the mother is seropositive.

QUESTION 2

You are called to counsel a mother who is 31 weeks gestation. The baby was noted to be small on scans. Karyotyping from the amniotic fluid is normal and the fluid is positive for CMV by PCR. The fetus is noted to have unilateral ventriculomegaly.

   i) What other abnormalities should be looked for on the antenatal scans?

   ii) Which of the following symptoms could be present in the newborn period? Choose six correct answers.

      a. Seizures
      b. Hepatosplenomegaly
      c. Thrombocytopenia
      d. Unconjugated hyperbilirubinaemia
      e. Chorioretinitis
      f. Cataracts
      g. Defective enamelisation
      h. Inguinal hernia.

   iii) What is the likely prognosis if the baby shows symptoms at birth?

   iv) If the baby is asymptomatic at birth, what is the likely prognosis?

   v) Which is the preferred method for testing for congenital CMV? Choose one answer.

      a. Detection of pp65 antigen in white blood cells
      b. Virus isolation from placenta
      c. PCR assay of urine
      d. Serology testing for IgG and IgM
      e. Histology of skin biopsy.

   vi) What action would you take after birth to confirm the diagnosis of congenital CMV and over what time scale?

The baby's investigations support the diagnosis of congenital CMV. On examination, the baby has a large liver and spleen, thrombocytopenia and imaging reveals intracranial calcification.

   vii) What treatment options are available?

QUESTION 3

Regarding parvovirus B19, which of the following statements are correct?

   i) It is a large double stranded DNA virus

   ii) It is a small single stranded DNA virus

   iii) It replicates in rapidly dividing cells

   iv) Approximately 25% of adults show evidence of a previous infection

   v) A rash and arthralgia occur in the second phase of the illness. At this point, the child is still infectious

   vi) The more severe the infection in a pregnant woman, the more severe the fetal infection

vii) If parvovirus B19 infection occurs during pregnancy, the majority of fetuses will be affected

viii) The outcome of the fetus depends on the point at which the infection occurred in pregnancy.

QUESTION 4

The following features are typically associated with which intrauterine infection – hydrocephalus, epilepsy, cerebral calcification and chorioretinitis. Choose the best answer.

i) Congenital CMV

ii) Congenital toxoplasmosis

iii) Congenital Epstein Barr virus

iv) Congenital varicella

v) Congenital rubella

vi) Congenital herpes

vii) Congenital TB.

QUESTION 5

Which of the following statements are true of toxoplasmosis?

i) The risk of congenital infection remains constant throughout pregnancy

ii) The risk of congenital infection is up to 90% in the third trimester

iii) Congenital infection is more severe if maternal infection is acquired in the third trimester

iv) In the UK, about 60% of women are sero-positive

v) Congenital infection occurs in 1 in 100 exposed babies

vi) Increasing gestational age at seroconversion is associated with an increased risk of mother-to-child transmission

vii) CSF will show a lymphocytosis

viii) Toxoplasmosis cannot be treated

ix) If diagnosed antenatally in the first trimester the mother can be treated with pyrimethamine and sulfadiazine to decrease the risk of fetal infection

x) If there are no eye signs within the first year of birth, the infant is unlikely to develop ocular problems.

QUESTION 6

You are called to the postnatal ward to review a baby who is 8 hours old.

The midwife reports that the baby is not feeding well. His mother says he tried to feed after birth but now is not interested. On examination, the infant looks pale, and feels slightly floppy. He is mottled with cool peripheries and has a heart rate of 160 bpm and mild recession. He has normal heart sounds, and both femoral pulses can be felt.

i) What is your first management step?

ii) What questions if any do you ask the mother?

iii) List five investigations you should carry out.

iv) What other investigations may be useful?

v) What is your next step in managing this baby?

The results of the initial investigations are obtained and shown below:

Hb	14.7 g/dL
WBC	21.4×10^9/L
Neut	1.7×10^9/L
Platelets	104×10^9/L
CRP	94 mg/L

Urine SPA sample – no cells, no organisms seen

Chest X-ray shows a diffuse, fine, reticulogranular pattern, much like that seen in RDS.

The infant is breathing without ventilatory support with some low flow oxygen to maintain his saturations. He has had his first dose of antibiotics and is currently on maintenance fluid.

vi) What do you do now?

A lumbar puncture is carried out and the result is below:

RBC	18,000/mm^3
WCC	12/mm^3
Protein	2.5 g/L
Glucose	1.4 mmol/L

CSF is moderately blood stained

vii) What does this result mean?

Six hours later the infant is more symptomatic having frequent apnoeas and desaturations. He is intubated and ventilated. Repeat bloods show the following results:

CRP	120 mg/L
Platelets	45×10^9/L
Neutrophils	0.8×10^9/L

viii) Which of the following treatments would you consider?
a. FFP
b. Immunoglobulin
c. Exchange transfusion
d. Platelet transfusion
e. Changing antibiotics
f. GCSF
g. Heliox
h. Pentoxifylline.

There is a phone call from the microbiology department the following day saying the blood cultures are growing Group B Streptococcus. The infant's CRP is now 40 mg/L, and his platelets have been stable above 100 after the platelet transfusion.

ix) **a.** How will you modify your treatment, if at all?

b. How long will you treat the baby?

c. What will you tell the parents?

QUESTION 7

A baby is born at term by normal vaginal delivery with good Apgars requiring no resuscitation. Membranes were ruptured just prior to delivery, and the mother was well throughout pregnancy and labour. The mother is a primigravida. You receive a phone call from the midwife looking after the mother, when the baby is 12 hours old to say group B Streptococcus is growing from a maternal high vaginal swab. The mother wishes to go home.

What do you do? Choose the best answer.

i) Admit the baby to the NICU for observation

ii) Admit the baby to the NICU for observation and routine surface swabs

iii) Admit the baby to the NICU for a septic screen (blood cultures, FBC and CRP) and await results before considering antibiotics

iv) Admit the baby to NICU, perform septic screen and start antibiotics

v) Reassure and discharge home

vi) Allow to go home with instructions if the baby becomes unwell to seek medical advice

vii) Discuss with the mother and say that she must stay in and the baby must be observed for a further 24 hours

viii) Observe the baby for another 12 hours; allow to go home with instructions if the baby becomes unwell to seek medical advice.

QUESTION 8

You are working on the Neonatal Unit when one of the mothers tells you that her other child has been sent home from nursery with suspected chickenpox. The mother is unsure whether she has had chickenpox. The baby is now 5 days old, corrected gestational age 35 weeks and is well. The mother is also well.

What do you do? Choose the correct answer.

i) Reassure the mother that no treatment is needed

ii) Reassure mother but isolate baby in side room

iii) Check the mother and baby's immune status and then give VZIG to both

iv) Check the mother's immune status and if negative give her VZIG

v) Check the baby's immune status and if negative give the baby VZIG

vi) Give the baby and mother VZIG

vii) Give the baby VZIG and aciclovir.

QUESTION 9

Which of the following organisms are known to commonly cause osteomyelitis? Choose four answers.

  i) *Bacillus fragilis*

 ii) *Bacillus cereus*

 iii) *Bacteroides fragilis*

 iv) *Campylobacter jejuni*

  v) *Haemophilus influenzae*

 vi) *Proteus mirabilis*

 vii) *Salmonella typhi*

viii) Group B streptococcus (GBS)

 ix) *Staphylococcus aureus*

  x) *Klebsiella*

 xi) *Serratia marcescens.*

QUESTION 10

Which of the following babies should receive hepatitis B immunoglobulin?

  i) Mother is HBsAg negative and HBeAg negative

 ii) Mother is HBsAg negative and HBeAg positive

 iii) Mother is HBsAg positive and HBeAg negative

 iv) Mother is HBsAg positive and HBeAg positive

  v) Mother had acute hepatitis during pregnancy

 vi) Mother where eAg and eAb status are unknown.

QUESTION 11

A baby presents with the following skin lesions.

  i) Describe the skin.

 ii) What is the diagnosis?

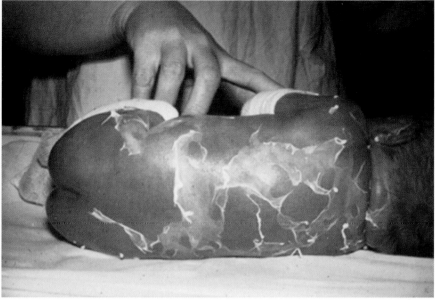

Figure 10.1 .

iii) What is the likely organism responsible?

iv) What is the treatment?

v) What is the prognosis?

QUESTION 12

Which of the following are true of congenital rubella syndrome?

i) It is a notifiable disease

ii) Causes hydrocephalus

iii) Causes thymic hypoplasia

iv) Causes corneal opacity

v) Causes bony abnormalities

vi) Causes IUGR

vii) Causes microphthalmia

viii) Causes conductive deafness

ix) Causes PDA

x) Causes aortic stenosis

xi) Infection during the first 12 weeks of pregnancy results in congenital infection and/or miscarriage in all cases

xii) Congenital infection can occur if mum is infected during the 2nd trimester

xiii) The infant is extremely infectious in the immediate postnatal period but this is no longer a risk after the first 4 weeks of life

xiv) Rubella is increasing in the immigrant population.

QUESTION 13

You are called to see a baby after delivery. The mother has had routine booking bloods and serology. The results are as follows:

> RPR reactive
> TPHA reactive
> Rubella immune
> Hepatitis negative

i) What do these test show?

ii) What test do you carry out to confirm this?

The confirmatory test is also reactive.

iii) What do you do now? Name two things.

iv) Which one test would confirm a diagnosis of congenital syphilis?

v) If the test is negative, what does this show?

vi) What information do you need from the mother?

vii) What other test might be helpful in assessing the risk to the baby?

On examination the baby looks normal, the non-treponemal serologic titre is less than four times the maternal titre, and the mother had treatment 2 weeks ago.

viii) What do you do?

QUESTION 14

On your neonatal unit, three babies are found to be growing an Enterobacter with identical antibiotic resistance. It is the opinion of the microbiologists that these must have been transmitted by staff contact. It is their recommendation that the three infants are isolated and barrier nursed and that there is a serious review of infection control procedures.

Which of the following statements are true?

i) Infected infants should remain in the cots they currently occupy; all staff involved in the care of the baby should adopt barrier nursing procedures

ii) Wearing of sterile gloves avoids the need for repeated hand washing

iii) Infected babies may be nursed by the same member of staff as uninfected infants

iv) Regular skin disinfection is of established benefit in most cases

v) Topical antibiotic ointment should always be used

vi) Use of separate gowns for each baby is an extremely important element of infection control

vii) Screening of all babies and all staff may be implicated

viii) Staffing levels are closely related to the incidence of nosocomial infection, as is the availability of hand washing facilities

ix) Units should be closed to all admissions as soon as the possibility of an outbreak is considered

x) Environmental screening is of no value

xi) Meticulous attention to hand hygiene is by far the most important element in reducing the spread of infection

xii) There is good evidence that standards of hand hygiene are normally very high in neonatal intensive care units

xiii) Soap and water hand wash is more effective than the use of alcohol-based hand rub

xiv) Topical cord care at birth has a major role in reducing the incidence of infection.

ANSWER 1

i) False – CMV is a DNA virus of the herpes virus group.

ii) True – it affects up to 2.5% of live born infants a year worldwide. In the UK the incidence is approximately 0.2%.

iii) False – fetal infection is more likely to occur and is more severe after primary maternal infection than after reactivation of latent infection. The earlier the infection occurs in pregnancy the worse the outcome.[1]

iv) False – the incidence is thought to be 1–4%.

v) True.[2]

vi) False – overall, only 10–15% of infected infants show clinical signs at birth but up to 90% of these will develop long-term sequelae.[3]

vii) True – reports state mortality ranges between 10% and 30% although much higher in premature infants.

viii) True – in the postpartum period, mother to infant transmission can occur as up to 88% of seropositive mothers shed the virus into their milk. Approximately 50% of these infants will become infected. CMV excretion is usually the result of reactivation in a seropositive mother; most infants will not develop clinical signs due to the presence of maternally derived transplacental antibodies. This is usually a benign and asymptomatic infection.

ANSWER 2

i) Echogenic bowel, intracranial calcification, cortical dysplasia.

ii) Answers **a**, **b**, **c**, **e**, **g** and **h** are correct. Hepatosplenomegaly and petechiae secondary to thrombocytopenia are relatively common manifestations of congenital CMV in the neonatal period. Jaundice is also common but this is usually a conjugated hyperbilirubinaemia as CMV hepatitis can cause both intrahepatic and extrahepatic bile duct destruction.[4] Intracranial manifestations of congenital CMV are microcephaly and periventricular calcification where the infection has caused brain necrosis. Lissencephaly and polymicrogyria can be present depending on the timing of the infection, lissencephaly occurring with an earlier infection. Defective enamelisation occurs in 40% of symptomatic infants at birth and 5% of asymptomatic infants. Inguinal hernias can occur with congenital CMV in male infants although the reason for this is unclear.

iii) Up to 80% of symptomatic newborns will develop sequelae such as mental retardation, cerebral palsy, visual defects and sensorineural hearing loss. Symptoms at birth are associated with a worse prognosis.[5]

iv) Up to 15% of infants who are asymptomatic at birth will have neurodevelopmental problems and sensorineural (SN) deafness. SN deafness is the most common abnormality seen in congenital CMV infection, occurring in 30–65% of symptomatic infants and up to 15% of asymptomatic infants. It usually develops after the newborn period and tends to be progressive. Cochlear implants have been used successfully.

v) Answer **c** is correct.

   a. Detection of the pp65 antigen has been used to detect active infection in immunocompromised people but due to the large quantity of blood required this test is less useful in neonates. However a recent paper showed that high levels of pp65 antigen in the blood were seen in newborns that developed sequelae.[5] This test is very rarely used in the UK as it has been superseded by PCR.
   b. High viral load in the urine is highly predictive of audiological impairment.[6]
   c. PCR is the gold standard for testing for congenital CMV.
   d. A positive IgG reflects passage of maternal antibodies and therefore does not diagnose infection in the baby. Maternal IgG can persist up to 12 months. A positive IgM test does suggest congenital infection but both false positive and false negative results can occur. The test has a sensitivity of approximately 75%. With the availability of PCR, viral serology should not be used to diagnose congenital infection.
   e. Skin biopsy – this is not used for CMV testing.

vi) PCR testing on a urine sample needs to be done within the first 3 weeks after birth. If the test is carried out after 3 weeks it is difficult to distinguish between a congenital, perinatal or postnatal infection. Infants infected at birth after exposure to infected secretions during delivery may start shedding virus by 3 weeks of age.

vii) There are currently a few antiviral chemotherapeutic agents, such as ganciclovir and foscarnet, that are available for treatment of serious, life-threatening or sight-threatening CMV in the immunocompromised patients. Cidofovir is also licensed for CMV retinitis. A randomised, controlled multicentre clinical trial investigated the use of ganciclovir for the treatment of infants with congenital CMV infection with evidence of CNS involvement.[7] Ganciclovir (or placebo) was given intravenously as an infusion every 12 hours for 6 weeks. The ganciclovir group were significantly more likely to have improved or normal hearing at 6 months of age compared to the placebo group. They also showed improvement in their liver function tests and head circumference. No change in mortality was demonstrated and currently there are no published data on long-term outcome. Ganciclovir is not thought to be beneficial for infants who show severe intracranial pathology antenatally. Several centres in the UK are using a six-week course of intravenous ganciclovir and then switching over to oral valganciclovir, with close monitoring of levels and viral load to assess response. The main side effects of ganciclovir are secondary to bone marrow suppression. Nigro[8] described a study using CMV specific hyperimmune globulin and found that pregnant women whose amniotic fluid was CMV positive, and who were given passive immunisation, had a lower rate of congenital CMV when compared to a control group. There are currently no randomised trials looking at this preventative treatment.

ANSWER 3

i) False.

ii) True – it was discovered in 1975 and is a small, singled stranded DNA virus consisting of about 5600 base pairs.

iii) True – it has a predilection for rapidly dividing cells, hence the affinity for erythrocyte precursor cells. A characteristic haemolytic anaemia can occur in the fetus.

iv) False – about 50% of adults show serological evidence of a previous infection with p antigen and are therefore immune.

v) False – there is an incubation period of about 10 days when flu-like symptoms and viraemia occur; 7–10 days after this, the second phase occurs with joint pain and the characteristic rash, but no viraemia. 30% of infections may be asymptomatic.

vi) False – there is no correlation between the severity of maternal infection and fetal infection.

vii) False – the incidence of parvovirus infection in pregnancy is 0.3–3.7%.[9] The overall risk of fetal infection is 30–50%. Most fetal infections are self-limited and do not result in adverse outcome. In 1–2% of fetuses with serological evidence of infection, parvovirus will cause abortion, stillbirth or hydrops. Between 10% and 25% of cases of non-immune hydrops are related to parvovirus.

viii) True – around 1 in 10 women infected before 20 weeks of gestation will suffer a fetal loss due to B19. The risk of an adverse outcome of pregnancy after this stage is remote. Infected women can be reassured that the maximum possible risk of a congenital abnormality due to B19 is under 1% and that long-term development will be normal.[10]

ANSWER 4

The combination of hydrocephalus, epilepsy, cerebral calcification and chorioretinitis is the classic presentation of congenital toxoplasmosis. Infection in the central nervous system causes extensive cortical and periventricular necrosis which then calcifies. The periventricular damage can cause obstruction to the aqueduct of the midbrain and cause hydrocephalus. Although the classic ophthalmological presentation is chorioretinitis, cataracts and microphthalmia can also occur.

ANSWER 5

i) False.

ii) True – the risk of congenital disease is lowest (10–25%) when maternal infection occurs during the first trimester and highest (60–90%) when maternal infection occurs during the third trimester. The overall risk of congenital infection from acute *T. gondii* infection during pregnancy is approximately 20–50%.[11,12]

iii) False – congenital disease is more severe when infection is acquired in the first trimester.

iv) False – about 30% of women are sero-positive in the UK.

v) False – congenital infection occurs in less than 1 in 1000 infants.[13]

vi) True – increasing gestational age at seroconversion is strongly associated with increased risk of mother-to-child transmission (OR 1.15, 95% CI 1.12–1.17) and decreased risk of intracranial lesions (0.91, 0.87–0.95), but not with eye lesions (0.97, 0.93–1.00).[14]

vii) True – the CSF will show raised protein, lymphocytosis and tachizoites (cysts of *T. gondii*). PCR on the CSF will confirm the diagnosis.

viii) False – infants with congenital toxoplasmosis should be treated for a year to avoid adverse outcomes. They should be given spiramycin for 4–6 weeks, alternating with 3 weeks of pyrimethamine and sulfadiazine, beginning shortly after birth and continuing for 12 months. The medications are synergistic against toxoplasma. A recent study[15] showed that in infants with moderate or severe neurological disease at birth, more than 72% had normal neurological and/or cognitive outcomes, if treated, and none had sensorineural hearing loss. 91% of children without substantial neurological disease and 64% of those with moderate or severe neurological disease at birth did not develop new eye lesions. All children without substantial neurological disease at birth who received treatment had normal cognitive, neurological and auditory outcomes.

ix) False – the mother can be treated antenatally if infection is diagnosed by PCR of the amniotic fluid. The treatment is with spiramycin as pyrimethamine and sulfadiazine are contraindicated in the first trimester as pyrimethamine is a folate antagonist. Spiramycin is a macrolide antibiotic.

x) False – in a recent study 24% of children developed retinal lesions over a six-year follow-up period. In only 11% was a diagnosis of retinochoroiditis made during the first month of life and half of the lesions were diagnosed after 1 year of age. The delay in onset of lesions is an important consideration when counselling families.[16]

ANSWER 6

i) The baby should be resuscitated using an ABC approach and taken to the neonatal unit for ongoing care and management.

ii) Ask about possible events that may make infection more likely. Was there prolonged rupture of membranes? Did the mother have any episodes of raised temperature? If there have been any previous pregnancies were any infants treated for infection? Ask about UTIs (these are important risk factors for neonatal sepsis) as well as increasing the risk of premature birth, pre-eclampsia and low birth weight infants.[17]

iii) Blood culture, urine culture, FBC, CRP and CXR. Blood culture is the definitive test. The majority of blood cultures taken will grow in 48 hours if they are going to be positive. The majority of neonatal infections are associated with a bacteraemia and thus a positive blood culture. Urine culture is an important investigation if sepsis is suspected. The drawback with urine analysis and culture is obtaining the specimen. If a baby is unwell and presumed septic, the easiest way to obtain a sample is by suprapubic aspiration of urine. This avoids the contamination which happens in the majority of bag urine specimens. If a bag urine specimen is thought to be positive, it must have at least 150 white cells/mm^3 and a pure growth of more than 10^5 organisms/mL urine. Be wary of any organisms other than *E. coli* or a mixed growth. If this is the case, an SPA will have to be obtained to confirm the infection.

A full blood count itself is not very useful. However a differential white count is of help. A low neutrophil count, <2.0–2.5×10^9/L in the first 2 days of life, suggests that there is a bacterial infection. After this time, either neutropenia or neutrophilia (>7.5–8.0×10^9/L) may occur. Other helpful markers of infection may be the ratio of immature to total number of neutrophils. The maximum acceptable ratio for excluding sepsis during the first 24 hours is 0.16. In most newborns, the ratio falls to 0.12 within 60 hours of life. An I/T ratio of >0.2 has been shown to be a good marker for infection. As well as being used in early onset sepsis, an I/T ratio >0.16 differentiated between Gram-positive, Gram-negative and fungal infections ($p = 0.007$) in late-onset infections. The sensitivity of the I/T ratio is in the range 60–90%, and elevations may be observed with other physiological events, limiting the positive predictive value of these ratios. An elevated I/T ratio should be used in combination with other signs when diagnosing sepsis.[18]

C-reactive protein is a good indicator of infection if serial measurements are made and the trend analysed. It is better than white blood cell indices as an infection marker. It takes a few hours to rise and therefore should not be used to decide when to start antibiotics. Culture-proven sepsis is unlikely if the CRP does not rise within 48 hours of the onset of the illness, and thus it is generally safe to stop antibiotics if the cultures are negative and the CRP is normal at 48 hours.[19]

All infants with suspected sepsis should have a chest X-ray.

iv) There has been much research and interest into procalcitonin. Procalcitonin (PCT) and C-reactive protein (CRP) concentrations in umbilical cord blood of 197 neonates were measured to evaluate their value as markers of infection. Sixteen of the neonates were infected. The sensitivity and specificity were 87.5% and 98.7% for PCT, and 50% and 97%, for CRP. It seems therefore that serum PCT in cord blood could be a useful and early marker of antenatal infection.[20] Other groups have made similar observations and suggest that a procalcitonin level >2.3 ng/mL or a CRP >30 mg/L indicates a high likelihood for neonatal sepsis, and antibiotic therapy should be continued even in the presence of sterile cultures.[21] Research has also shown that a raised interleukin-6 and TNF-alpha are good indicators of early sepsis.[22]

v) After resuscitation, stabilisation and investigations, antibiotics should be given immediately. Most units have policies for which antibiotic to use, but in general for early onset sepsis (which is most likely in this infant's case) the antibiotics need to cover group B Streptococcus, Listeria and Gram-negative organisms such as *E. coli*. A combination of a penicillin and gentamicin would be a good choice as there is synergistic action between the two against GBS. Cephalosporins alone will have no coverage for *E. coli* or Listeria.

vi) Most people in this situation with such a high CRP would carry out a lumbar puncture. If the platelet count was below 50, then a platelet transfusion should be given before the lumbar puncture.

vii) It is unlikely that this baby has meningitis. Generally in meningitis a polymorphonuclear count is >30/mm^3. When blood-stained CSF is obtained, the ratio of red to white cells should be calculated and if there is no infection, the ratio of red to white cells should be more than 500 to 1 (this can be most accurately calculated from the peripheral white cell to red cell ratio). The protein is difficult to interpret as the CSF is heavily blood stained. Without a blood glucose level, it is difficult to interpret the glucose of 1.4 mmol/L in the CSF. The CSF glucose should be at least 50% of the blood glucose level and a level <1.0 mmol/L suggests bacterial meningitis. Ideally a lumbar puncture should be performed prior to starting antibiotics. The one dose of antibiotics that has been given pre lumbar puncture may mean that cultures are less likely to be positive, but a lumbar puncture should still be performed in any baby who is sick with presumed sepsis as the cell count may be highly informative.

viii) a. Fresh frozen plasma is often given when infants are septic to try and boost their immune response. It has been shown in adults to improve neutrophil chemotaxis, but this is not the case in neonates. In fact, the only indications for FFP, as described in the document by the British Committee for Standards in Haematology, Haemostasis and Thrombosis task force, in 2002, are DIC, vitamin K dependent bleeding and inherited deficiencies of coagulation. It should therefore not be used in this situation.

b. Intravenous immunoglobulin infusions have been studied as a possible therapy for neonatal sepsis to provide type-specific antibodies to improve opsonisation and phagocytosis of bacterial organisms and to improve complement activation and chemotaxis of neonatal neutrophils. Cochrane Reviews in 2004 showed that prophylactic IVIG led to a 3% reduction in sepsis and a 4% reduction in any serious infection but is not associated with reductions in other important outcomes such as sepsis, NEC, IVH or length of hospital stay.[23] The use of IVIG in proven sepsis, as part of a treatment regime, has been less well researched. A meta-analysis showed a significant decrease in mortality in proven sepsis, however results were not as convincing in the suspected sepsis group. There are difficulties with IVIG therapy for neonatal sepsis – the effect can be transient, and problems associated with the infusion of any blood product can occur. Dose-related problems with this therapy decrease the usefulness in neonatal populations. At present, data do not support the routine use of IVIG in neonatal sepsis. Results from a large multicentre trial are awaited.

c. Exchange transfusions with fresh whole blood have been used in neonatal sepsis to remove toxins and cytokines. The available data show that exchange transfusion may improve survival, but there are only a small number of reports with small patient numbers. There are currently no randomised trials to confirm these findings.[24,25]

d. 50% of infants with sepsis will develop a platelet count of $<100 \times 10^9/L$ and it would be prudent to transfuse these infants with platelets. Thrombocytopenia occurs as a combination of increased platelet consumption, often without evidence of DIC, and reduced platelet production.

e. It would be sensible to continue with the first choice antibiotics for at least 24 hours or until you have identified the bacteria from blood culture. If, after 48 hours, the infant's condition is deteriorating with continuing rise in infective markers, consider other causes such as abscesses, fungal infection and osteomyelitis and treat appropriately with early discussion and involvement from microbiology colleagues.

f. Granulocyte-macrophage colony-stimulating factor (GM-CSF) and granulocyte colony-stimulating factor (G-CSF), naturally occurring cytokines, are used to induce granulocyte production, as their names suggest. There are many trials which show an increase in neutrophil counts and enhanced functional activity as seen by C3bi expression. Mortality rates have been shown to be decreased by up to a third with treatment with rhGM-CSF in critically ill septic neutropenic neonates. However, the Cochrane Review concludes that there is currently insufficient evidence to support the introduction of either G-CSF or GM-CSF into neonatal practice, either as treatment of established systemic infection to reduce resulting mortality or as prophylaxis to prevent systemic infection in high risk neonates.[26–28]

g. Heliox has no place in the treatment of neonatal sepsis. It can be used in bronchiolitis or other obstructive airway disease as it decreases respiratory resistance and enhances carbon dioxide removal.[29]

h. Pentoxifylline is a methylxanthine derivative with a broad spectrum of activity that modulates the inflammatory response, including the inhibition of TNF production. In animal models it has been shown to preserve micro-vascular blood flow, prevent circulatory failure and intestinal vaso-constriction, and improve survival. Two randomised controlled trials of pentoxifylline recruited 140 preterm infants with clinical sepsis. In the 107 with positive blood cultures, pentoxifylline was associated with 86% reduction in risk of mortality (RR 0.14, 95% CI 0.03–0.76). The recent Cochrane Review concludes that the use of pentoxifylline as an adjunct to antibiotics in neonatal sepsis reduces mortality without any adverse effects.[30–32]

ix) a. Therapy can be simplified to intravenous benzyl penicillin alone as GBS is very sensitive to this.

b. Without meningitis, GBS bacteraemia can be treated with antibiotics for a total of 10 days. If meningitis was also present, antibiotics should be continued for at least 21 days.

c. Up to 30% of pregnant women are colonised with GBS. The majority of neonatal infections present within the first 4–6 hours of life and about 90% of cases will present within the first 24 hours of life. His infection was picked up early and treatment commenced promptly. His infective markers are improving showing he is responding to treatment. The baby has no signs of meningitis and is on the correct antibiotics with maximum supportive treatment. Previously, mortality from early-onset GBS sepsis was approaching 50% with a mortality rate up to 100% for babies weighing less than 1.5 kg. Currently in the UK, the mortality rate is 10%. At this stage we would be cautiously optimistic with the parents.[33]

ANSWER 7

Answer **viii** would be the most appropriate plan of action. Most cases of GBS present within 4–6 hours after delivery and the majority of cases by 24 hours. This baby has no other risk factors for infection (e.g. prolonged rupture of membranes, prematurity, maternal infection, bacteriuria or previous sibling being affected) and therefore close observation without treatment for 24 hours is indicated. It is imperative the you inform the mother about the test result, and should the infant become unwell after discharge, for example becoming less interested in feeds or poor handling, that she seeks medical advice.

The incidence of early-onset GBS disease in term infants without antenatal risk factors in the UK is 0.2 cases/1000 births. This infant has none of the risk factors associated with GBS infection which are prematurity, rupture of the membranes more than 18 hours before delivery, rupture of the membranes before the onset of labour and intrapartum fever. If postnatal antibiotic treatment was completely effective and there were no adverse effects, 5000 infants would need to be treated to prevent a single case and at least 80,000 infants would have to be treated to prevent a single death from early-onset GBS disease. Most infants who develop early-onset GBS disease present with illness soon after birth and 90% have presented clinically by 12 hours of age, before culture results become available. This figure is the same for infants born to mothers who have received intrapartum antibiotics. Postnatal antibiotic treatment has not been shown to eradicate carriage of GBS or to influence the risk of late-onset GBS disease. It is therefore unnecessary to perform routine surface cultures or blood cultures on well infants, whether they received antibiotic prophylaxis or not.[34–36]

ANSWER 8

Answer **v** is correct.

Chickenpox is an extremely common infection, such that 90% of the antenatal population are seropositive for VZV IgG antibody. Contact with chickenpox is common, especially in mothers with other children, so primary VZV infection is rare – 3 in 1000 pregnancies.

If the mother is immune, there is no need to do anything as the baby will be protected by the antibodies. If the mother is susceptible and the baby is less than 7 days old, the newborn should be given VZIG. The mother does not require VZIG as she is no longer at risk of serious complications since she has delivered. Aciclovir is used with VZIG if the mother develops chickenpox between 7 days pre and 7 days post delivery as it appears to provide some protection and may reduce the chance of transmission to the newborn infant.

This baby should have his immune status checked using a varicella zoster enzyme-linked immunosorbent assay (ELISA). If it is negative and thus the baby has not acquired antibodies from the mother, he needs to be given a dose of zoster immune globulin, 100 mg. After significant nursery exposure to VZV, ZIG should be given to seronegative babies and to all babies born before 28 weeks gestation.[37–39]

ANSWER 9

Answers **i**, **v**, **viii** and **ix** are correct.

i) Yes – *Bacillus fragilis* is a Gram-positive bacillus that does cause osteomyelitis.

ii) No – *Bacillus cereus* is another Gram-positive bacilli that causes meningitis and pneumonia.

iii) No – *Bacteroides fragilis* is a Gram-negative bacillus that causes meningitis.

iv) No – *Campylobacter jejuni* is another Gram-negative bacillus that characteristically causes meningitis and gastroenteritis. It is, like other Gram-negative rods, part of the normal gut flora, but all can cause disease when they reach tissues outside the lumen of the gut.

v) Yes – *Haemophilus influenzae* is a Gram-negative rod that can cause not only osteomyelitis but pneumonia and meningitis.

vi) No – *Proteus mirabilis* is a Gram-negative bacillus that causes meningitis and abscesses.

vii) No – *Salmonella typhi* classically causes gastroenteritis and typhoid fever. This organism is much more common in the developing world.

viii) Yes – group B streptococcus is otherwise known as *Streptococcus agalactiae*. It is a Gram-positive coccus that can cause infection in most tissues – osteomyelitis, empyema, brain abscess, endocarditis, cellulitis and UTI. It is a commensal of the gut and the vagina and colonises up to a third of pregnant women in the UK. There are nine serotypes, but types I, II and III are responsible for most neonatal infections. The osteomyelitis seen with GBS can be a subtle presentation with only one site being affected. Commonly hip, knee, pelvis and humerus.

ix) Yes – *Staphylococcus aureus*, a Gram-positive coccus, is associated with a high mortality and morbidity. Some strains are more virulent than others, due to extracellular factors and toxins. It is the primary cause of infection in bones, joints and skin. Pustular skin lesions are classic and there is rapid seeding to bones, joints and lungs. It is a relatively rare cause of meningitis and very rarely a UTI. A clear association has been shown between the severity of bacteraemia and mortality.[40] The systemic infection leads to marked neutropenia and thrombocytopenia with a rapidly increasing CRP.

x) No – *Klebsiella* is a Gram-negative bacillus that causes urinary tract infections and meningitis. Gram-negative bacilli are thought to account for about 20% of cases of late-onset neonatal sepsis and even higher numbers in the developing world. The mortality from systemic infections is extremely high, especially in preterm infants. There is a link between Gram-negative bacilli and the severity of bronchopulmonary dysplasia.[41]

xi) No – *Serratia marcescens* is an opportunistic Gram-negative bacillus which is often seen in the developed world and typically infects compromised hosts. It commonly causes a septicaemia with associated meningitis, with a high mortality. It has been reported as a causative organism in infected ventriculo-peritoneal shunts. It occurs sporadically in the NICU, primarily in premature infants requiring support, and appears late in their hospital course. There are very occasional cases of neonatal osteomyelitis being caused by *Serratia marcescens* but affected infants had underlying immunodeficiency disorders.[42,43]

ANSWER 10

Answers **iv**, **v** and **vi** are correct.

HBsAg is a marker of the carrier state of hepatitis B and its incidence varies from 0.1% in parts of Europe to up to 20% in Africa and Asia. The presence of the e antigen greatly increases the risk of infection to the baby. Therefore the baby in part **iv** of the question is at greatest risk of infection and must receive both hepatitis B vaccination and immunoglobulin. The expression of the e antigen seems to be genetically determined with more Chinese women carriers being HBeAg positive than African carriers. It is recommended that babies born to mothers with acute hepatitis should also receive hepatitis B immunoglobulin as the risk of transmission is significantly increased. Where e antigen and e antibody status are unknown immunoglobulin should be considered.

ANSWER 11

i) The baby's skin shows desquamation which has been provoked by rubbing the skin's surface. This is called Nikolsky's sign. This occurs after an initial scarlatiniform rash, which is usually present on the face and in the flexures. If denudation occurs, this is followed by drying of the skin and a further desquamation phase that lasts for a few days. The mucosal surfaces are unaffected.

ii) The diagnosis is staphylococcal scalded skin syndrome, previously known as Ritter's disease.

iii) The responsible organism is *Staphylococcus aureus*. The commonest source of infection is an infected umbilical stump.

iv) The infant should be treated with intravenous flucloxacillin.

v) Infants respond extremely well to intravenous antibiotics and the skin heals with no sequelae.

ANSWER 12

i) Yes – rubella was made a notifiable disease in 1988, and is monitored through clinical and laboratory reports.[44]

ii) No – toxoplasmosis causes hydrocephalus. Rubella does not. It does cause microcephaly and delayed developmental milestones.

iii) Yes – although this is not present at birth, infants may develop this along with reduced cellular immunity and thyroid autoantibodies. Some infants with congenital rubella do not present in the neonatal period with the well described rubella syndrome including jaundice, thrombocytopenia and hepatosplenomegaly. They present in later life with neurological problems, heart disease, eye defects and deafness.

iv) Yes – corneal opacities are present in congenital rubella.

v) Yes – irregular lucencies in the bone and abnormal trabecular pattern in the long bones. The X-ray appearance is said to resemble a stick of celery.

vi) Yes – one-third of affected babies are growth restricted.

vii) Yes – micro-ophthalmia does occur as well as glaucoma. One study reported that up to 78% of affected infants developed ocular abnormalities and no significant association was found between gestational age at time of maternal infection and the incidence of individual ocular conditions.[45]

viii) No – conductive deafness does not occur in congenital rubella, it is usually sensorineural deafness and commonly bilateral. These deficits occur in up to 66% of affected infants.[46]

ix) Yes – cardiac abnormalities, especially PDA, occur in up to 58% of infants.

x) No – aortic stenosis does not occur. Peripheral pulmonary stenosis is a frequent finding and due to viral damage to endothelium of large blood vessels.

xi) No – although the risk of congenital infection is highest in the first trimester, not all infants are affected; approximately 10–20% are not.

xii) Yes – although the incidence decreases with increasing gestation. Congenital rubella is rare after 20 weeks' gestation.

xiii) No – the infants can continue to shed the virus up to months after delivery and therefore appropriate precautions should be taken with female nursing and medical personnel.

xiv) Yes – despite the incidence of congenital rubella dramatically falling with the introduction of the MMR immunisation programme, there are still cases occurring. The majority of the mothers are from the immigrant population and there is a drive by the World Health Organization to improve the global control of rubella and CRS.[45,47]

ANSWER 13[48,49]

i) RPR (rapid plasma reagin test) is a non-treponemal serological test and TPHA (*Treponema pallidum* haemagglutination assay) is a treponemal test. Both being reactive show that the mother may have syphilis.

ii) You must confirm with a treponemal test that is different from that used in screening such as the treponemal ELISA for IgG and IgM.

iii) You must:
   a. Examine the baby for any signs of congenital syphilis such as thrombocytopenia, jaundice, hepatosplenomegaly, rhinitis, periostitis (visible on long bone X-ray) and IUGR.
   b. Take blood for serology – from infant not from cord blood as the latter can become contaminated from maternal blood and give a false positive result.

iv) A positive anti-treponemal EIA IgM is consistent with a diagnosis of congenital infection. It should be repeated to confirm.

v) Serology can be negative in babies infected late in pregnancy. A negative IgM should be repeated at 1, 2 and 3 months of age as the IgM response may be suppressed.

vi) It is vitally important to see if the mother has been treated adequately for syphilis to assess the risk to the baby. The baby is at low risk if the mother has been treated fully in this pregnancy starting at least 30 days before the baby was born.

vii) Quantitative non-treponemal serological titres (VDRL/RPR) are useful to assess risk to the baby. If the titres are four-fold higher than the mother's titres, the infant is at high risk and needs treating. If the titres are the same or less than four-fold the maternal titre, treatment of the infant depends on the adequacy of maternal treatment.

viii) Due to inadequate maternal treatment, the infant needs treating with benzyl penicillin 30 mg/kg IV (50,000 units/kg) 12-hourly for 7 days and then 8-hourly for 10 days treatment in total. Follow-up at three and sixth months and one year with VDRL/RPR is required.

ANSWER 14

i) False – if several infants are affected by the same organisms, it is more sensible to cohort infants, separating them from uninfected infants. Although this is dependent on available space and staffing, it should always be attempted where highly resistant or highly infective organisms are spreading. Once cohorted, all staff involved in the care of the baby should adopt barrier nursing procedures.

ii) False – the use of gloves may have a role in the reduction of infection, but there is good evidence that scrupulous attention to hand hygiene is of paramount importance.

iii) False – nursing staff should care for segregated cohorts in this situation.

iv) False – there was a vogue for regular skin disinfection in the early years of neonatal care. This policy led to widespread damage of babies, including significant brain damage with the use of hexachlorophene.[50]

v) False – topical antibiotic therapy may be indicated but should always be targeted toward a specific organism (e.g. *Staphylococcal aureus* cord infection) and should never be routine and generalised.

vi) False – although the wearing of gowns may contribute to reducing the spread of infection, there is some evidence to suggest that the impact is minimal and other infection control measures are more important.[51]

vii) True – the source of infection often remains unclear but it is advisable to screen other babies to identify asymptomatic carriers. If the means of spread is uncertain, staff screening may sometimes be of value, but must be managed tactfully and diplomatically.

viii) True – staff numbers and the thoroughness of their hand washing have been shown to be very important elements in reducing infection rate.[52]

ix) False – although this may be indicated on rare occasions, such a decision should only be taken following advice from microbiology and infection control specialists. Proper barrier nursing and meticulous attention to hygiene should allow a unit to function without having to resort to closure.

x) False – there are documented cases where the source of the infection has been environmental and thus full screening including settle plates may be useful if all other actions fail to identify a source or means of spread.

xi) True.

xii) False – there are published data which suggest that effective hand washing of an appropriately high standard may be performed in little more than 20% of patient contacts. Even more worryingly, there are incidents where hands are not cleansed adequately (or at all) between patients – even when there has been contact with body fluids or excreta.[53]

xiii) False – there is now good evidence that the proper use of alcohol-based hand rub between patients is more effective in infection control than the use of soap and water.

xiv) False – there is no evidence that application of sprays, creams or powders is any better than keeping the baby's cord clean and dry at birth.[54]

REFERENCES

1. Yow MD, Williamson DW, Leeds LJ et al. Epidemiologic characteristics of cytomegalovirus infection in mothers and their infants. Am J Obstet Gynecol 1988;158:1189–95
2. Demmler GJ. Infectious Diseases Society of America and Centers for Disease Control. Summary of a workshop on surveillance for congenital cytomegalovirus disease. Rev Infect Dis 1991;13:315–29
3. Lipitz S, Achiron R, Zalel Y et al. Outcome of pregnancies with vertical transmission of primary cytomegalovirus infection. Obstet Gynecol 2002;100:428–33
4. Hart MH, Kaufman SS, Vanderhoof JA et al. Neonatal hepatitis and extrahepatic biliary atresia associated with cytomegalovirus infection in twins. Am J Dis Child 1991;145:302–305
5. Lanari M, Lazzarotto T, Venturi V et al. Neonatal cytomegalovirus blood load and risk of sequelae in symptomatic and asymptomatic congenitally infected newborns. Pediatrics 2006;117:76–83
6. Rivera LB, Boppana SB, Fowler KB et al. Predictors of hearing loss in children with symptomatic congenital cytomegalovirus infection. Pediatrics 2002;110:762–67
7. Kimberlin D, Lin C, Sanchez P et al. Effect of ganciclovir therapy on hearing in symptomatic congenital cytomegalovirus disease involving the central nervous system: a randomized, controlled trial. J Pediatr 2003;143:16–25
8. Nigro G, Adler SP, La Torre R et al. Congenital Cytomegalovirus Collaborating Group. Passive immunization during pregnancy for congenital cytomegalovirus infection. N Engl J Med 2005;353:1350–62
9. Gay NJ, Hesketh LM, Cohen BJ et al. Age specific antibody prevalence to parvovirus B19: how many women are infected in pregnancy? Commun Dis Rep 1994;4:104–107
10. Miller E, Fairley CK, Cohen BJ et al. Immediate and long term outcome of human parvovirus B19 infection in pregnancy. Br J Obstet Gynaecol 1998;105:175–78
11. Dunn D, Wallon M, Peyron F et al. Mother-to-child transmission of toxoplasmosis: risk estimates for clinical counseling. Lancet 1999;353:1829–33
12. Remington JS, Klein JO (eds). Infectious diseases of the fetus and newborn infant, 5th edn. Saunders, Philadelphia, 2001; 205–346
13. Hohlfeld P, Daffos F, Thulliez P et al. Fetal toxoplasmosis: outcome of pregnancy and infant follow-up after in utero treatment. J Pediatr 1989;115:765–69
14. Thiebaut R, Leproust S, Chene G et al. SYROCOT (Systematic Review on Congenital Toxoplasmosis) study group. Effectiveness of prenatal treatment for congenital toxoplasmosis: a meta-analysis of individual patients' data. Lancet 2007;369:115–22
15. Mcleod R, Boyer K, Karrison T et al. Outcome of treatment for congenital toxoplasmosis, 1981–2004: the National Collaborative Chicago-Based, Congenital Toxoplasmosis Study. Clin Infect Dis 2006;42:1383–97
16. Wallon M, Kodjikian L, Binquet C et al. Long-term ocular prognosis in 327 children with congenital toxoplasmosis. Pediatrics 2004;113:1567–72

17. Schieve LA, Handler A, Hershow R et al. Urinary tract infection during pregnancy: its association with maternal morbidity and perinatal outcome. Am J Public Health 1994;84(3):405–10

18. Gonzalez BE, Mercado CK, Johnson L et al. Early markers of late-onset sepsis in premature neonates: clinical, hematological and cytokine profile. J Perinat Med 2003; 31(1):60–68

19. Bomela HN, Ballot DE, Cory BJ et al. Use of C-reactive protein to guide duration of empiric antibiotic therapy in suspected early neonatal sepsis. Ped Inf Dis J 2000;19:531–35

20. Joram N, Boscher C, Denizot S et al. Umbilical cord blood procalcitonin and C reactive protein concentrations as markers for early diagnosis of very early onset neonatal infection. Arch Dis Child Fetal Neonatal Ed 2006;91(1):F65–F66

21. Turner D, Hammerman C, Rudensky B et al. The role of procalcitonin as a predictor of nosocomial sepsis in preterm infants. Acta Paediatr 2006;95(12):1571–76

22. Mishra UK, Jacobs SE, Doyle LW et al. Newer approaches to the diagnosis of early onset neonatal sepsis. Arch Dis Child Fetal Neonatal Ed 2006;91(3):F208–F212

23. Ohlsson A, Lacy JB. Intravenous immunoglobulin for preventing infection in preterm and/or low-birth-weight infants. Cochrane Database Syst Rev 2004;(1):CD000361

24. Mathur NB, Subramanium BKM, Sharma YK et al. Exchange transfusion in neutropenic septicemic neonates: effect on granulocyte functions. Acta Paediatr 1993;82:939–43

25. Vain NE, Mazlumian JR, Swarner OW et al. Role of exchange transfusion in the treatment of severe septicemia. Pediatrics 1980;66(5):693–97

26. Bilgin K, Yaramis A, Haspolat K et al. A randomized trial of granulocyte-macrophage colony-stimulating factor in neonates with sepsis and neutropenia. Pediatrics 2001;107(1):36–41

27. Miura E, Procianoy RS, Bittar C et al. A randomized, double-masked, placebo-controlled trial of recombinant granulocyte colony-stimulating factor administration to preterm infants with the clinical diagnosis of early-onset sepsis. Pediatrics 2001;107(1):30–35

28. Carr R, Modi N, Dore C. G-CSF and GM-CSF for treating or preventing neonatal infections. Cochrane Database Syst Rev 2003;(3):CD003066

29. Myers TR. Use of heliox in children. Respir Care 2006;51(6):619–31

30. Lauterbach R, Pawlik D, Tomaszczyk B et al. Pentoxifylline treatment of sepsis of premature infants: preliminary clinical observations. Eur J Pediatr 1994;153(9):672–74

31. Haque K, Mohan P. Pentoxifylline for neonatal sepsis. Cochrane Database Syst Rev 2003;(4): CD004205

32. Lauterbach R, Pawlik D, Kowalczyk D et al. Effect of the immunomodulating agent, pentoxifylline, in the treatment of sepsis in prematurely delivered infants: a placebo-controlled, double-blind trial. Crit Care Med 1999;27(4):807–14

33. Heath P, Nicoll A, Efstratiou A. Group B streptococcal disease in UK and Irish infants younger than 90 days. Lancet 2004;363(9405):292–94

34. Lin FY, Brenner RA, Johnson YR et al. The effectiveness of risk-based intrapartum chemoprophylaxis for the prevention of early-onset neonatal group B streptococcal disease. Am J Obstet Gynecol 2001;184:1204–10

35. Escobar GJ, Li DK, Armstrong MA et al. Neonatal sepsis workups in infants ≥2000 grams at birth: a population-based study. Pediatrics 2000;106:256–63

36. Bromberger P, Lawrence JM, Braun D et al. The influence of intrapartum antibiotics on the clinical spectrum of early-onset group B streptococcal infection in term infants. Pediatrics 2000;106:244–50

37. Heuchan AM, Isaacs D. The management of varicella-zoster virus exposure and infection in pregnancy and the newborn period. Australasian Subgroup in Paediatric Infectious Diseases of the Australasian Society for Infectious Diseases. Med J Aust 2001;174(6):288–92

38. Royal College of Obstetricians and Gynaecologists. Chickenpox in pregnancy. Clinical Green-top Guideline No. 13, 2nd edn. RCOG, London, 2001

39. Ng PC, Lyon DJ, Wong MY. Varicella exposure in a neonatal intensive care unit: emergency management and control measures. J Hosp Infect 1996;32(3):229–36

40. Schonheyder HC, Gottschau A, Friland A et al. Mortality rate and magnitude of *Staphylococcus aureus* bacteremia as assessed by a semiquantitative blood culture system. Scand J Inf Dis 1995;27:19–21

41. Cordero L, Ayers L, Davis K. Neonatal airway colonization with Gram-negative bacilli: association with severity of bronchopulmonary dysplasia. Ped Inf Dis 1997;16:18–23

42. Mayer CW, Bangash S, Bocchini JA et al. *Serratia marcescens* osteomyelitis in an infant. Allergy Asthma Proc 2006;27(6):544–48

43. Bizzarro MJ, Dembry LM, Baltimore RS. Case-control analysis of endemic *Serratia marcescens* bacteremia in a neonatal intensive care unit. Arch Dis Child Fetal Neonatal Ed 2007;92(2):F120–F126

44. Tookey P. Rubella in England, Scotland and Wales. Euro Surveill 2004;9(4):21–23

45. Best JM, Castillo-Solorzano C, Spika JS et al. Reducing the global burden of congenital rubella syndrome: report of the World Health Organization Steering Committee on Research Related to Measles and Rubella Vaccines and Vaccination, June 2004. J Infect Dis 2005;192(11):1890–97

46. Givens KT, Lee DA, Jones T et al. Congenital rubella syndrome: ophthalmic manifestations and associated systemic disorders. Br J Ophthalmol 1993;77(6):358–63

47. Robinson JL, Lee BE, Preiksaitis JK et al. Prevention of congenital rubella syndrome – what makes sense in 2006? Epidemiol Rev 2006;28:81–87

48. Screening Guidelines Steering Committee. Sexually transmitted infections: UK screening and testing guidelines. British Association for Sexual Health and HIV, London, 2006

49. British Association for Sexual Health and HIV. UK National Guidelines on the Management of Early Syphilis, Clinical Effectiveness Group (Association for Genitourinary Medicine and the Medical Society for the Study of Venereal Diseases), 2002, www.bashh.org/guidelines

50. Anderson JM, Cockburn F, Forfar JO et al. Neonatal spongioform myelinopathy after restricted application of hexachlorophane skin disinfectant. J Clin Pathol 1981;34(1):25–29

51. Pelke S, Ching D, Easa D et al. Gowning does not affect colonization or infection rates in a neonatal intensive care unit. Arch Pediatr Adolesc Med 1994;148(10):1016–20

52. Parry GJ, Tucker JS, Tarnow-Mordi WO. UK Neonatal Staffing Study Group. Relationship between probable nosocomial bacteraemia and organisational and structural factors in UK neonatal intensive care units. Qual Saf Health Care 2005;14(4):264–69

53. Cohen B, Saiman L, Cimiotti J et al. Factors associated with hand hygiene practices in two neonatal intensive care units. Pediatr Infect Dis J 2003;22(6):494–99

54. Zupan J, Garner P. Topical umbilical cord care at birth. Cochrane Database Syst Rev 2004;(3): CD001057

Index

References are mainly to the page on which the question appears. Where some items are mentioned only in the answer, then the answer page number has been referenced instead; such references are indicated with a bracketed A. Abbreviations used. FH, family history; PC, previous child/baby.

A

abdominal wall defect, 255–6A
acamprosate, 5
acetazolamide, 145–6
acidosis *see* metabolic acidosis; respiratory acidosis
activated partial thromboplastin time (APPT), 74, 75
acute lymphoblastic leukaemia, 9
acyl-CoA dehydrogenase deficiency, medium chain (MCAD), 13, 124
adrenal hyperplasia, congenital, 8
adrenaline, 143
African race, absent red reflex, 72
albinism (FH), 12
albumin administration, 113A
alcohol abuse, 4, 5
alkalosis *see* metabolic alkalosis; respiratory alkalosis
alpha-1-antitrypsin deficiency, 12
amino acids, parenteral, 262
aminophylline, preterms, 140
amitriptyline, 5
ammonia (blood), elevated, 124
anencephaly, 15
angiotensin II receptor antagonist, 126A
angiotensin-converting enzyme (ACE) inhibitors, 126A
preterms, 141
aniridia, 15
antenatal problems, 1–67
antiarrhythmics, 6

antibiotics, 181A, 276, 286A
Enterobacter outbreak, 281
preterms, 139, 140
anticoagulants, 6
anticonvulsants *see* antiepileptics
antidepressants, 5, 6, 7
antidiuretic hormone (ADH), syndrome of inappropriate secretion (SIADH), 121
antiepileptics
maternal, 5, 6, 7
vitamin K and, 99
neonatal, 91–2A
antihypertensives, 5, 6
antimalarial, 6
antithyroid drugs
maternal, 5, 7
neonatal, 109A
α-1-antitrypsin deficiency, 12
aortic coarctation (PC), 1–2
apnoea of prematurity, 142–3
arginine, hyperammonaemia, 134A
arrhythmias
fetal, 2
maternal, 2
see also antiarrhythmics; bradycardia
arterial line/catheter, umbilical, misplaced, 229A, 233A
arteriovenous malformation, intracranial, 226A, 248A, 257A
asphyxia, perinatal, 253A
aspirin, 117
atenolol, 5
azathioprine, 5

B

Bacillus cereus, 278
Bacillus fragilis, 278
Bacteroides fragilis, 278
barbiturates, neonatal, 92A, 113A
BCG vaccination, 12, 73, 99, 100
benzodiazepines, 6
    abuse, 4
beta-blocker (=atenolol), 5
betamethasone, 5
bile duct, cystic dilatation, 102
biliary atresia, 19, 112–13A
bilirubin, elevated *see* hyperbilirubinaemia
birth, problems at, 69–97
    asphyxia, 253A
birth mark and thrombocytopenia, 3–4
bladder
    exstrophy, 9
    thickened wall, 18
blood counts, 285A
blood culture, 285A
blood gases, 70–1, 163–93
blood transfusion and necrotising
        enterocolitis (NEC), 261
blue spot, Mongolian, 114A
bowel *see* intestine
brachial plexus injury, 74
bradycardia, fetal, 22A
brain
    congenital anomalies, 14–15, 19–20
    CT, 245, 246
    MRI, 236, 238–9, 241, 246, 247
    ultrasound, 237–8, 239–40, 241, 242–3,
        248
    see also central nervous system
breast (human) milk
    drugs in, 5–8
    nucleotides in, 261
    vitamin content, and maternal diet, 262
breathing, absent at delivery, 70
breech presentation, 109A
bronchiolitis, RSV-positive, 152A
bronchodilators, preterms, 140
bronchopulmonary dysplasia *see* lung,
        chronic disease
buprenorphine, 4
Buscopan, 260

C

C-reactive protein, 286A
caffeine, preterms, 142, 144

calcium
    blood, low, 122
    supplementation, 261
Campylobacter jejuni, 278
cancer (malignancy) risk
    undescended testes, 101
    vitamin K use, 99
cannabis, 4
captopril, 117
caput succedaneum, 74
carbamazepine, 5
carbimazole, 5
cardiac function/problems, etc., *see* heart
cardiofacial syndrome, 75
cardiomyopathy
    diabetic, 229A
    hypertrophic (FH), 2
cardiotocography (at delivery), profound
        decelerations, 70–1
cardiovascular collapse, 82–5A, 123
carnitine, hyperammonaemia, 134A
β-carotene supplementation, 261
case conference, prenatal, 19
cataracts, congenital, 16, 72
celecoxib, 117
central nervous system, congenital
        anomalies, 14–15, 19–20
    see also brain
central venous lines, 231A
    misplaced, 210, 233A
cephalhaematoma, 74
cerebral artery infarction, middle, 249A, 257A
cerebral function (analysis) monitoring
        (CFM/CFAM), 77
cerebral palsy (PC), 14
cerebrospinal fluid (CSF) analysis, 276
CHARGE syndrome, 75, 100
chest X-ray *see* X-ray
chickenpox, 11, 277–8
chiropractice, gastro-oesophageal reflux,
    260
chlamydia
    maternal, 11–12
    neonatal conjunctivitis, 100
chlordiazepoxide, 5
chloroquine, 6
choroid plexus cysts, 14
chromosome anomalies
    balanced translocation, 3
    encephaloceles with, 251A
    exomphalos with, 256A
    sex chromosome, 3

chylothorax, 226–7A
ciclosporin, 6
circulatory collapse, 82–5A, 123
cisapride, 260
clavicle fracture, 82A
cleft lip and/or palate
    fetal, 8
    paternal and PC, 8
cleidocranial dysostosis, 224A
clotting *see* coagulation
coagulation (clotting) disorders
    maternal, 9
    neonatal, 75–6
coagulation factor deficiencies, 9, 89A
cocaine, 4
codeine, 6
Coleif, 260
compressions, cardiac, 70
computed tomography, brain, 245, 246
congenital hypoparathyroidism, 100
congenital hypothyroidism, 8, 79
congenital infections *see* infection
congenital malformation/anomalies
    adrenal hyperplasia, 8
    bowel, 8–9
    CNS, 14–15, 19–20
    diaphragmatic hernia, 223A, 254–5A
    eye, 15–16, 72, 100
    GI tract, 228A
    heart *see* heart disease
    kidney, 17–18
    skeleton, 225A
congenital nephrotic disease, 17
conjunctivitis, 100–1
connatal cyst, 253–4A
continuous positive airway pressure
        (CPAP), preterms, 139, 182A
convulsions *see* seizures
corneal anomalies (FH), 16
corpus callosum, agenesis, 14, 252A, 254A
corticosteroids (glucocorticoids)
    systemic, 7, 34A
        BCG vaccination and, 99
        preterms, 140
    topical (=betamethasone), 5
cow milk protein intolerance (CMPI) and
        allergy (CPA), 11, 262
COX inhibitors *see* non-steroidal
        anti-inflammatory drugs
crack, 4
cranium (skull)
    fracture, 74–5

ultrasound, 237–8, 239–40, 241, 242–3,
        248
cromones (disodium cromoglycate),
        preterms, 140
cryptorchidism (undescended testes),
        9, 101
cultures, bacterial, 285A
cyclo-oxygenase inhibitors *see* non-steroidal
        anti-inflammatory drugs
cyst(s) (and cystic lesions)
    brain, 249A, 252–4A
    choroid plexus, 14
    kidney, 17, 253A
    lung, 18, 224A
    ovarian, fetal, 1
cystic adenomatoid malformation of lung,
        224A
cystic dilatation of bile duct, 102
cystic fibrosis (FH), 18
cystic hygroma, 8
cytomegalovirus (CMV), congenital, 232A,
        256A, 273–4

D

Dandy–Walker syndrome, 251A, 256A
deafness, maternal, 10–11
death
    mono-chorionic twin, 14
    sudden infant death syndrome, 14
decelerations (profound) at delivery,
        70–1
dehydration, hypernatraemic, 128–9A
dexamethasone, 34A
    BCG vaccination and, 99
    preterms, 140, 144
dextrocardia, 2
diabetes
    maternal, 8, 209, 212
    neonatal, 8
dialysis, hyperammonaemia, 134A
diaphragmatic hernia, congenital, 223A,
        254–5A
diazepam, 4, 6
diazoxide, 137A
digoxin, preterms, 141
disodium cromoglycate, preterms, 140
diuretics, 6
    preterms, 140, 141
dobutamine, 143
domperidone, 260
dopamine, 143

Down syndrome (trisomy 21)
  high risk, 3
  PC with, 3
doxapram, 143
drugs
  adverse effects
    neonatal renal failure, 117A
    osteopenia of prematurity, 156
  gastro-oesophageal reflux therapy, 260
  maternal intake affecting child, 4–8
ductus arteriosus, patent
  congenital heart disease dependent on,
    72
  preterms, closure, 141
Duffy antibodies, 9
duodenal atresia, 8, 228A
dysrhythmias see arrhythmias
dystrophic epidermolysis bullosa, 25A

E

echocardiogram, 83A
ectrodactyly (PC), 16
Edwards' syndrome, 75
electrolyte imbalance, 117–38
emphysema (pulmonary)
  interstitial, 230A
  lobar, 224A
encephalocele, occipital, 251A
endoscopy, gastro-oesophageal reflux,
    260
endotracheal tube, misplaced, 224A, 229A,
    233A
enoxaparin, 6
Enterobacter, 280–1
enterocolitis, necrotising (NEC), 223A,
    234A, 261
epidermolysis bullosa (FH), 3
epileptic fits see seizures
epinephrine (adrenaline), 143
Erb palsy, 74
erythromycin, 260
escitalopram, 6
exchange transfusion, 41A, 120, 122, 134A,
    142, 153A, 276
exomphalos, 255–6A
expiratory time (Te), decreasing, 71
extracorporeal membrane oxygenation
    (ECMO), 81A, 192A
eye conditions, 100–1
  congenital, 15–16, 72, 100
    rubella, 279

F

facial palsy, 75
facio-auriculo-vertebral (Goldenhaar)
    syndrome, 19
factor V Leiden, 9
factor VIII deficiency, 9, 89A
factor IX deficiency, 89A
factor XI deficiency, 89A
factor XII deficiency, 89A
fatty acids, long chain polyunsaturated,
    262
feeding, 259–72
  difficulties, 79
femoral head, ischaemic necrosis (Perthes'
    disease) (FH), 16
fetus
  ovarian cysts, 1
  renal disorders, 17–18
  ultrasound, 8–9, 240, 244–5
  see also congenital malformation/
    anomalies
fibrinogen values, 74, 75
fistula, tracheo-oesophageal, 225A
fits see seizures
flecainide, 6
floppy (hypotonic) baby, 70, 76–7, 79
fluid imbalance, 117–38
fluoroscopy in gastro-oesophageal reflux,
    260
folic acid supplementation, 261–2
foot deformities, talar see talipes
formula milks, 260
  hydrolysed, 260
  long chain polyunsaturated fatty
    acid-enriched, 262
fortified feeds and necrotising enterocolitis
    (NEC), 261
fracture
  arm/humerus, 225A, 231A
  clavicle, 82A
  skull, 74–5
fresh frozen plasma (FFP), 276
furosemide, 6
Fy^a antibodies, 9

G

galactosaemia, 13
gastrointestinal tract
  congenital anomalies, 228A
  perforation, 223A, 229–30A, 232A

gastro-oesophageal reflux (GOR), 259, 260
  apnoea of prematurity and, 142
  sliding hiatus hernia and, 223A
gastroschisis, 9
Gaviscon, 260
GCSF, 276
genetic diseases *see* inherited diseases
genital herpes, 12
gentamicin, 117
germinal matrix haemorrhage, 146,
      156–8A, 250A, 257A
gestational pemphigoid, 4
glaucoma, congenital, 72, 100
glucagon administration, 137A
glucocorticoids *see* corticosteroids
glucose, blood, low (hypoglycaemia), 120–1,
      137–8A
glucose-6-phosphate dehydrogenase
      deficiency (FH), 9, 99
glutamine supplementation, 263
Goldenhaar syndrome, 19, 75
gonococcal (*N. gonorrhoeae*) conjunctivitis,
      101
granulocyte-colony stimulating factor
      (GCSF), 276
Graves' disease, maternal, 7
gripe water, 260
growth, 259–72

H

H$_2$ receptor antagonists and necrotising
      enterocolitis (NEC), 261
haemangioendothelioma (birth mark) and
      thrombocytopenia, 3–4
haemangioma (birth mark) and
      thrombocytopenia, 3–4
haematological disorders, maternal, 9–10
haematoma
  subdural, 256A
  subgaleal/subaponeurotic, 74
haemodialysis, hyperammonaemia, 134A
haemofiltration, hyperammonaemia, 134A
haemophilia A (factor VIII deficiency), 9,
      89A
Haemophilus influenzae, 278
haemorrhage
  intracranial *see* intracranial haemorrhage
  retinal, 107A
haemorrhagic telangiectasia, hereditary, 12
Hallermann–Streiff syndrome, 100
hand hygiene, 280, 281

hearing difficulties, maternal, 10–11
heart
  compressions, 70
  dropped beats, 2
  enlarged, 225–6A, 248A
  failure, 248A
  rhythm abnormalities *see* arrhythmias
  see also entries under cardio-
heart disease, congenital, 2, 14, 228A
  duct-dependent, 72
  in PC, 1–2, 2–3
heat loss, preterms, 79
Heliox, 276
hemivertebrae, 19
Henoch–Schönlein purpura, 9–10
heparin, low-dose, 6
hepatitis B, 11
  immunoglobulin, 278
hepatitis C, 11
hereditary diseases *see* inherited diseases
hernia
  congenital diaphragmatic, 223A, 254–5A
  sliding para-oesophageal/hiatus, 223A
heroin, 4
herpes simplex
  conjunctivitis, 101
  genital, 12
hiatus hernia, sliding, 223A
high-frequency (oscillatory) ventilation
      (HFV; HFOV), 81A, 140, 175,
      189A
hip, developmental dysplasia
  maternal, 16
  neonatal, 101
Hirschsprung's disease, 9
histamine H$_2$ receptor antagonists and
      necrotising enterocolitis (NEC), 261
HIV (human immunodeficiency virus),
      11–12
  BCG vaccine and, 104
horseshoe kidney, 18
human immunodeficiency virus *see* HIV
humerus fracture, 225A, 231A
hydrocephalus
  PC, 14–15, 256A
  post-haemorrhagic, 252A
hydrolysed formula milk, 260
hydronephrosis, 255A
hydrops, 22A
hygroma, cystic, 8
hyoscine butylbromide, 260
hyperammonaemia, 124

hyperbilirubinaemia, 103
    conjugated, 100
    unconjugated, 111–12A
hyperglycinaemia, non-ketotic, 13–14
hyperinsulinaemic hypoglycaemia of
        infancy, persistent, 137–8A
hyperkalaemia, 133A
hypernatraemic dehydration, 128–9A
hyperoxia, 182A, 186A, 192A
    avoidance in preterms, 94–5A
hyperthyroidism, neonatal, 109A
hypertrophic cardiomyopathy (FH), 2
hypoalbuminaemia, 113A
hypocalcaemia, 122
hypoglycaemia, 120–1, 137–8A
hyponatraemia, 130A
hypoparathyroidism, congenital, 100
hypophosphataemic rickets, hereditary/
        familial, 13, 232A
hypotension, preterms, 143, 183A
    metabolic acidosis and, 183A
hypothyroidism, congenital, 8, 79
hypotonic (floppy) baby, 70, 76–7, 79
hypoxaemia, 191–2A
hypoxia, 179–80A, 181A, 186A, 188A

I

ibuprofen, 117
    preterms, 141
imaging, 195–258
    scans, 235–58
    see also specific modalities
immunisation, preterms, 143
    see also immunoglobulin and specific
        vaccines
immunoglobulin, intravenous, 276
    hepatitis B, 278
immunosuppressive drugs, 5, 6
incontinentia pigmenti (FH), 3
indomethacin
    necrotising enterocolitis (NEC) and, 261
    preterms, 140, 141
Infacol, 260
infections, 273–96
    maternal, 11–12
    neonatal/postnatal (incl. congenital),
        232A, 256A, 273–96
        eye, 100–1, 232A
        respiratory tract see respiratory tract
            infections
    see also sepsis

inherited diseases
    FH, 12–13
    metabolic, 136A
    renal see renal system disorders
    see also chromosome anomalies
injuries, birth, 73–5
    see also fracture
instrumental deliveries, 73–4, 74–5
insulin-dependent diabetes, maternal, 8,
        209, 212
    see also hyperinsulinaemic
        hypoglycaemia of infancy
intermittent mandatory ventilation,
        synchronised, 173–4
intermittent positive pressure ventilation,
        synchronised, 172–3
interstitial emphysema, pulmonary, 230A
intestine (bowel)
    fetal abnormalities, 8–9
    necrotising enterocolitis (NEC), 223A,
        234A, 261
    obstruction, 231A
    perforation, 223A, 229–30A
intracranial arteriovenous malformation,
        226A, 248A, 257A
intracranial haemorrhage, 146–7, 156–8A,
        248A, 249–50A, 251A, 254A,
        257A
    hydrocephalus following, 252A
iris, absence (aniridia), 15
iron deficiency and supplementation, 260–1

J

jaundice, 102, 119
junctional epidermolysis bullosa, 25A

K

Kasabach–Meritt syndrome, 26A
Kell antibodies, 10
keratoconus (FH), 16
kidney see entries under renal
Klebsiella, 278
Klumpke palsy, 74

L

La antibodies, 11
lactase (Coleif), 260
lactic acidaemia, 125
lamotrigine, 6

laser therapy, retinopathy of prematurity, 142
lens cataracts, congenital, 16, 72
leukaemia
  acute lymphoblastic, 9
  risk, vitakin K use, 104–5A
leukomalacia, periventricular, 159–60A
life support, neonatal, algorithm, 69
lobar emphysema, 224A
long chain polyunsaturated fatty acids, 262
losartan, 117
Lowe syndrome, 100
lumbar puncture, 276
lung
  chronic disease (CLD;
      bronchopulmonary dysplasia),
      191A, 192A, 262
    in nephrocalcinosis, 132A
    preterms, 151–2A
    X-ray, 205, 206, 227A, 228A, 230A,
      231A
  cystic lesions, 18, 224A
  emphysema see emphysema
  hypoplasia/aplasia, 229A, 231A, 253A
  surfactant see surfactant
lymphoblastic leukaemia, acute, 9

M

macrosomia, 109A, 125
magnetic resonance imaging (MRI), 235,
    236, 238–9, 241, 246, 247
malignancy see cancer
maple syrup disease, 125
Marfan's syndrome, 12
mastocytosis (FH), 4
maternal problems/disorders
  arrhythmias, 2
  diabetes, 8, 209, 212
  haematological disorders, 9–10
  infections, 11–12
  myasthenia gravis, 15
measles/mumps/rubella (MMR) vaccine,
    6–7
meconium
  aspiration syndrome, 226A
  failure to pass, 100
medium chain acyl-CoA dehydrogenase
    deficiency (MCAD), 13, 124
megacolon, congenital (Hirschsprung's
    disease), 9
membranes, premature rupture of, 166, 178

meningitis, 286A, 289A, 290A
metabolic acidosis, 180–1A, 183A,
    193A
  respiratory acidosis and, mixed, 70,
      180A, 181A, 183A, 184–5A,
      187A, 191–2A
  respiratory alkalosis and, mixed, 186–7A,
      190–1A
metabolic alkalosis, 186A
metabolism, inborn errors, 136A
metalloporphyrin therapy, 103
methadone, 4, 5
methylxanthines, preterms, 154A
  see also aminophylline; caffeine
metoclopramide, 260
microcephaly, 15
milk
  breast see breast milk
  cow, protein intolerance (CMPI) and
      allergy (CPA), 11, 262
  formula see formula milks
  soy, 262
MMR vaccine, 6–7
Moebius syndrome, 75
Mongolian blue spot, 114A
mono-chorionic twin pregnancy, 14
morphine, 7
mother see maternal problems/disorders
multicystic renal dysplasia, 17, 253A
multi-system/multi-organ failure,
    92–3A
mumps, 12
  see also MMR vaccine
muscular atrophy, spinal, 79
myasthenia gravis
  congenital, 79
  maternal, 15
myotonic dystrophy, 15, 79, 231A

N

naproxen, 7
nasogastric tube, misplaced, 231A
necrotising enterocolitis (NEC), 223A,
    234A, 261
Neisseria gonorrhoeae conjunctivitis, 101
nephroblastoma (Wilms tumour), 13
nephrocalcinosis, 122
nephronophthisis, familial juvenile, 12
nephrotic syndrome
  congenital, 17
  late-onset (FH), 17

nesidioblastosis (persistent hyperinsulinaemic hypoglycaemia of infancy), 137–8A
neural tube defect (PC), 14–15
neurofibromatosis, 12
neuroimaging see brain
neurological disorders, congenital, 14–15, 19–20
Nikolsky's sign, 291A
nitric oxide, 81A, 149A, 255A
non-ketotic hyperglycinaemia, 13–14
non-steroidal anti-inflammatory drugs (NSAIDs; prostaglandin synthase inhibitors; cyclo-oxygenase inhibitors)
    COX-2 specific (celecoxib), 117
    ibuprofen see ibuprofen
    indomethacin, preterms, 140
    naproxen, 7
nuchal fold, thickened, 3
nucleotide supplementation, 261
nutrition see feeding

O

occipital encephalocele, 251A
octreotide, 137A
oculomandibulodyscephaly with hypotrichosis (Hallermann–Streiff) syndrome, 100
oesophagus
    endotracheal tube in, 233A
    impedence in gastro-oesophageal reflux, 260
    manometry in gastro-oesophageal reflux, 260
    see also gastro-oesophageal reflux; para-oesophageal hernia; tracheo-oesophageal fistula
oligohydramnios, 109A
    pulmonary hypoplasia secondary to, 229A
omeprazole, 260
ophthalmological conditions see eye conditions
osteogenesis imperfecta, 225A
    paternal, 16
osteomyelitis, 278
osteopenia, 225A
    of prematurity, 156A
ovarian cysts, fetal, 1
oxygenation index, 71
oxytetracycline, 7

P

para-oesophageal hernia, sliding, 223A
parathyroid disorders, 100
parenteral nutrition, amino acids, 262
paroxetine, 7
parvovirus B19, 274–5
peak inspiratory pressure (PIP)
    increasing, 71
        preterms, 140, 183A, 185A
    reducing, preterms, 191A
pemphigoid, gestational, 4
Pena–Shokeir syndrome, 19
pentoxifylline, 276
periventricular leukomalacia, 159–60A
Perthes' disease (FH), 16
Peter's anomaly, 13
pH
    abnormalities see metabolic acidosis; metabolic alkalosis; respiratory acidosis; respiratory alkalosis
    measurements in gastro-oesophageal reflux, 260
phenobarbitone, neonatal, 92A, 113A
phenylketonuria, 124
phenytoin
    maternal, 7
    neonatal, 92A
phototherapy, 103
platelet
    counts, 74, 75
    transfusion, 276
pleural effusions, 226–7A, 233A
pneumopericardium, 224A
pneumothorax, 224A, 232A
    preterms, 143, 148A
    tension, 71, 134A, 183–4A, 224A, 234A
Poland sequence, 75
polycystic kidney disease
    autosomal dominant (FH), 17
    autosomal recessive, 253A
polycythaemia, 10
polymerase chain reaction (PCR), CMV, 274
polyunsaturated fatty acids, long chain, 262
porencephalic cyst, 249A
positive end expiratory pressure (PEEP), 71
    preterms, 140, 189A
positive pressure ventilation, 169, 175
postnatal problems, common, 99–115
potassium imbalance, 133A
Prader–Willi syndrome, 79

prednisolone, 7, 34A
premature baby (preterm), 139–61
  feeding, 262
    problems, 259
  fluid/electrolyte disorders, 117–19
  imaging, 237–8, 239–40, 241, 242
    X-rays, 143–4, 196–7, 198, 198–200,
      201–2, 203–4, 205–8, 208, 209,
      210–12, 213–15, 216–22
  preparing for delivery, 79
  respiratory distress syndrome, 143, 144,
    146, 147–8A, 149A, 152A, 164,
    167, 168, 172, 174, 175, 176, 177,
    217, 226A
  ventilation and blood gases, 163–4, 165,
    166–9, 170–4, 174–8, 178–9,
    230A
premature rupture of membranes, 166, 178
propionic acidaemia, 124
propylthiouracil, 7
prostacyclin, 81A
  preterms, 141
prostaglandin synthase inhibitor *see* non-
    steroidal anti-inflammatory drugs
protein, preterm intake, 262
protein C
  activated, resistance (=factor V Leiden),
    9
  deficiency, 10
Proteus mirabilis, 278
prothrombin time (PT), 74, 75
pseudohyperparathyroidism, 131A
pseudohypoparathyroidism, 131A
pseudomonal conjunctivitis, 101
pulmonary hypertension, persistent, 81A,
    191–2A
purpura
  Henoch-Schönlein, 9–10
  idiopathic thrombocytopenic, 10
pyloric stenosis, 102

R

radiology *see* imaging *and specific modalities*
ranitidine, 260
red reflexes, absent, 72, 100
renal failure, acute, 117, 119
renal pelvis, dilatation, 17–18, 255A
renal system disorders, 17–18, 122, 124
  inherited, 17
    family history, 17
    maternal, 12

ultrasound, 224A, 242, 244–5
  fetus, 9
Rendu–Osler–Weber syndrome (hereditary
    haemorrhagic telangiectasia), 12
respiratory acidosis, 183–4A, 184A, 185A,
    188–90A
  compensated, 191A, 192A
  metabolic acidosis and, mixed, 70, 180A,
    181A, 183A, 184–5A, 187A,
    191–2A
  respiratory alkalosis and, mixed, 192A
respiratory alkalosis, 182A, 184A, 187A
  metabolic acidosis and, mixed, 186–7A,
    190–1A
  respiratory acidosis and, mixed, 192–3A
respiratory distress syndrome (RDS),
    preterms, 143, 144, 146, 147–8A,
    149A, 152A, 164, 167, 168, 172,
    174, 175, 176, 177, 217, 226A
respiratory tract infections, 181A
  preterms, 151–2A
resuscitation, 69–97
retinal haemorrhages, 107A
retinitis pigmentosa (PC), 16
retinoblastoma, 72, 100
  PC, 16
retinopathy of prematurity, 141–2
rhesus antibodies, 10, 103
rheumatoid arthritis, 11
rickets, 232A, 261
  hereditary/familial hypophosphataemic,
    13, 232A
Ritter's disease, 291A
Ro antibodies, 11
RSV-positive bronchiolitis, 152A
rubella, congenital, 279–80
  see also MMR

S

sacral dimple, 100
Salmonella typhi, 278
scalded skin syndrome, staphylococcal,
    291A
scans, 235–58
schizencephaly, 19–20
seizures (fits/convulsions), 91–2A
  drug therapy *see* antiepileptics
sepsis, 72, 285A
septo-optic dysplasia, 15
Serratia marcescens, 278
sex chromosomes, numerical anomalies, 3

sickle haemoglobin trait, 10
situs inversus, 14
skeletal dysplasia, 225A
skin, staphylococcal scalded skin syndrome, 291A
skull *see* cranium
sodium imbalance *see* hypernatraemic dehydration; hyponatraemia
sodium valproate, 7
somatostatin analogue, 137A
soy milk, 262
special care baby unit, 277–8
spherocytosis, hereditary, 10
spina bifida (PC), 14–15
spinal dysraphism, 105A
spinal muscular atrophy, 79
Staphylococcus aureus, 278
    conjunctivitis, 100
    scalded skin syndrome, 291A
steroids *see* corticosteroids
stomach bubble, absent, 9
streptococcus group B, 166, 277, 278
subaponeurotic haematoma, 74
subdural haematoma, 256A
subependymal cyst, 252–3A, 253A
subependymal haemorrhage (germinal matrix haemorrhage), 146, 156–8A, 250A, 257A
subgleal haematoma, 74
substance abuse, 4–5
sudden infant death syndrome, 14
supplements, 261–2
supraventricular tachycardia
    fetal, 20A
    maternal, 2
surfactant, 81A, 94A, 182A, 230A, 254–5A
    deficiency, 128A, 254–5A
synchronised intermittent mandatory ventilation, 173–4
synchronised intermittent positive pressure ventilation, 172–3
syphilis, 292–3

T

tachycardia, 22A
    supraventricular *see* supraventricular tachycardia
tachypnoea, transient, 227A
talipes, 17
    equinovarus, 101
temazepam, 4

tension pneumothorax, 71, 134A, 183–4A, 224A, 234A
testes, undescended, 9, 101
thanatophoric dysplasia, 225A
thickeners and thickened feeds, 260
    and necrotising enterocolitis (NEC), 261
thrombocytopenia, birth mark and, 3–4
thrombocytopenic purpura, idiopathic, 10
thyroid disorders
    baby, 8, 79, 101
    maternal, 101
    see also antithyroid drugs
tolazoline, 81A, 149A
Tourette syndrome, 19
toxoplasmosis, congenital, 275
tracheal tube, misplaced, 224A, 229A, 233A
tracheo-oesophageal fistula, 225A
translocation (chromosomal), balanced, 3
transposition of great arteries, 84–5A, 228A
trauma *see* fracture; injuries
Treacher Collins syndrome, 19
Treponema pallidum infection, 292–3
trisomy 18 (Edwards' syndrome), 75
trisomy 21 *see* Down syndrome
tuberculosis
    maternal, 100
    postnatal vaccination (BCG), 12, 73, 99, 100
tubular acidosis, renal, 124
tunica vasculosa lentis, persistent, 100
Turner mosaicism, 3
twin pregnancy, mono-chorionic, 14

U

ultrasound
    antenatal/fetal, 8–9, 240, 244–5
    cranial, 237–8, 239–40, 241, 242–3, 248
    renal *see* renal system
umbilical arterial line/catheter, misplaced, 229A, 233A
umbilical venous lines, misplaced, 233A
urea cycle defects, 124
ureteric dilatation, 18
urinary tract disorders *see* renal system disorders
urine culture, 285A

V

vaccination *see* immunisation *and specific diseases vaccines*
VACTERL, 64A

vacuum (ventouse) delivery, 73–4
valproate, sodium, 7
varicella (chicken pox), 11, 277–8
VATERL, 64A
venous lines
    central *see* central venous lines
    umbilical, misplaced, 233A
ventilatory support, 70, 71, 163–93
    preterms, 79, 139–40, 163–4, 165,
        166–9, 170–4, 174–8, 178–9,
        230A
    weaning, 191A
    see also specific modes
ventouse delivery, 73–4
ventricles (brain)
    dilatation, 157A, 158A
    haemorrhage, 146–7, 156–8A, 249–50A,
        251A, 254A, 257A
ventricles (heart), septal defect (FH), 3
vertebral abnormalities, 19, 63A,
        230A
vesicoureteric reflux (FH), 18
villous atrophy, 125
vitamin A supplementation, 261
vitamin C supplementation, 262
vitamin D supplementation, 261
vitamin E supplementation, 261–2

vitamin K
    deficiency bleeding, 75, 104A
    parental concerns of administering, 99
von Willebrand disease, 10

W

Waardenburg's syndrome, 13
Walker–Warburg syndrome, 13
warfarin, 7
water intake, inadequate, 126A
    see also dehydration
West syndrome, 15
Wilms tumour, 13

X

X chromosome, numerical anomalies
    Klinefelter variant (47XXYY), 3
    Turner mosaicism (45X/46XX;
        45X/46XY), 3
X-rays (mainly chest and abdomen), 71–2,
        73, 236
    chronic lung disease, 205, 206, 230A, 231A
    preterms, 143–4, 196–7, 198, 198–200,
        201–2, 203–4, 205–8, 208, 209,
        210–12, 213–15, 216–22